Better Days Are Coming

Better Days Are Coming

Surviving Breast Cancer

by Marcy Browning

TIPS *Technical Publishing*

Carrboro, North Carolina • 2017

TIPS Technical Publishing, Inc.
108 E. Main Street, Suite 4
Carrboro, North Carolina 27510
1-919-933-TIPS
http://www.technicalpublishing.com

Library of Congress Cataloging-in-Publication Data
Names: Browning, Marcy, 1968- author.
Title: Better days are coming : surviving breast cancer / by Marcy Browning.
Description: Carrboro, North Carolina : TIPS Technical Publishing, 2017.
Identifiers: LCCN 2017038991 (print) | LCCN 2017039333 (ebook) | ISBN
    9781890586645 (ePub) | ISBN 9781890586652 (mobi) | ISBN 9781890586638
    (print : alk. paper)
Subjects: LCSH: Browning, Marcy, 1968—Health. |
    Breast—Cancer—Patients—United States—Biography. | Nurses—United
    States—Biography. | Self-care, Health.
Classification: LCC RC280.B8 (ebook) | LCC RC280.B8 B463 2017 (print) | DDC
    616.99/4490092 [B] —dc23
LC record available at https://lccn.loc.gov/2017038991

ISBN print: 978-1-890586-63-8
ISBN ePub: 978-1-890586-64-5
ISBN mobi: 978-1-890586-65-2

First published: October 2017

To my reasons: My children.
Quite simply, the three of you are why.
You always have been and always will be.

Contents

Foreword

I'm honored to introduce you, the reader, to this book. The topic of cancer is something that has touched most of our lives in significant ways. Chances are, either you or someone you love has been impacted directly. In this book you will be enwrapped in the story of a cancer survivor and the struggle of living when the monster of cancer engulfs your life.

I have had the privilege of walking alongside Marcy as her therapist as she has settled into her life as a survivor and what that looks like for her and her family. Part of her journey of healing emotionally has been writing her own story, which she has graciously and authentically shared with you in the following pages.

Each of us deals with hardship in life. It may not be cancer for you or your loved one but there has been and will be hardship nonetheless. In this book Marcy shares her experience of battling through that hardship. She wrestles with finding hope when things feel hopeless and living with a debilitating illness with nothing but questions about what the future may hold.

She shares pieces of what was most helpful in her darkest days and what brought light into her darkest nights. She honestly exposes her own self-doubt, times when courage was lacking, and the support she had that allowed her to cling to hope.

This book will increase your understanding of the journey of someone battling cancer and give you a front-row seat into their heart and mind. It will help you learn to better support a loved one going through a season of hardship, whether that is battling cancer or something else. It will redefine your idea of healing and hope following a life-changing diagnosis.

I invite you to enter her story, read her thoughts and experiences, and find hope in the pages of her life laid out before you.

—Cori Moschberger, MSW, LCSW, Clinical Therapist
Author of *Helping the Hurting*

Introduction
Entering Survival Mode

In March 2012, I dusted off my bike and took it to the Lucky Brakes bike shop for a tune-up, new tires, and chain. I had not ridden it since the divorce in 2010, when I moved to my rental home with my mom and two children. Having previously enjoyed long-distance riding, I was hoping that getting back on my bike would help me lose the weight I gained during the end of my marriage. During the next few weeks, the hopes of riding on the trails were shattered before I could even pick my bike up from the shop. I anticipated as I tucked my bike into the garage that this time it would only be a year and I'd be back on the saddle the following spring. In reality it would be three years before I was able to feel the exhilaration of being on the road or trails again.

As a high school nurse I had spring break off, and I had put together a long list of personal things to do. When a person works at a school, that list of things to do during weekdays grows quickly. I piled my appointments into spring break: activities with my kids, a job interview, and my annual physical and mammogram (routine for a forty-three-year-old woman). My planning and excitement were obviously weighed toward the first two. The second was the culmination of long thought and increasing excitement on my part. As much as I loved my job and felt my work as Hamilton High School's nurse had purpose, I couldn't afford to continue working there. School nursing is one of the lowest paid jobs in the nursing field. With summers off, I supplemented my income by working at a summer camp and doing home care visits part time.

I had worked as a home care nurse full time in the '90s and thought it would be something I would enjoy doing again with a better earning opportunity. Having a year-round job with a higher pay scale would lessen the financial burden I was feeling as a single mom again. My goal was to empower my patients and their families to care for themselves at home; I tried to teach them how to navigate the medical system so they could both stay out of the hospital and improve or maintain their health. Being invited into someone's home because they needed help inspired relationships with much meaning. If I could leave them in better physical shape, more comfortable, and happier than when I arrived, I knew my job was well done. Moonlighting reminded me how much I loved this area of nursing and I began looking for an opportunity to move from school nursing to home health nursing full time again. I was eager for the interview that had been scheduled for the end of March.

I started my busy schedule on Monday to get my routine physical out of the way early in the week. While doing the breast exam Dr. Bea asked if I had noticed "this skin thickening." Skin thickening? I'm a nurse but had never heard that phrase before. She didn't make a big deal of it but gave me the mammogram order and told me to schedule it soon. The hospital let me schedule it for Wednesday, after my job interview.

Interviewing with two of the clinical managers from a hospital-based home care company felt easy and comfortable. I have never been so relaxed in an interview. Both of them lived in the same town as I did. I connected with one of them almost instantly; Brooke's son and my son, Riley, attended eighth grade together, and our daughters were the same age too. Brooke said she would call me to set up a peer interview and I left their office fairly confident that I would be working with them, and happy doing so.

As the mammography technician prepared the machine so famous for turning a breast into a pancake, I told her what Dr. Bea had said during my exam. My thoughts shifted to past issues with my breast health: my breasts were fibrocystic, so they always felt lumpy and bumpy to me. I had gone to many visits at the gynecologist's office and had many mammograms and ultrasounds. The year before, in February, I had been called back to the hospital for additional views and an ultrasound for an area of concern. It turned out to be nothing. So this test felt like nothing as well. Looking back at it now, I see that I desensitized myself to my own abnormalities.

After taking the views of a routine mammogram, the tech asked me to wait for a moment while she asked the radiologist if she needed any more views. When she came back she said there were a few more the radiologist needed. I thought it was better to get it out of the way instead of having to come back later and agreed to more pictures. After, she asked me again to wait and said she'd be right back. When she returned this time her demeanor was pensive. She said the radiologist wanted me to stay and have an ultrasound of the right breast to further evaluate some abnormalities on the mammogram. Although I had not been trained to read a mammogram, I asked her if I could see the pictures, since sometimes medical professionals will make allowances for others in their profession out of courtesy. The area of "skin thickening" was easily identifiable even to my untrained eyes as a white outlining of a large area of my breast. I also saw a completely separate area of what looked like a white web of barbed wire deep in the breast. Pointing to it, I asked, "Is that the area of concern?" She softly said yes and didn't make eye contact.

She brought me to private room to wait. I had to get Riley out of the waiting area where I had left him because I'd dropped back home before the mammogram to pick him up. We were going clothes shopping afterward. I had told him the test was routine and would only take twenty to thirty minutes and he could play his game system while I was getting my test. When I gave him some money to go get snacks, he asked, "What's taking so long?" I apologized and told him it shouldn't be much longer, but I was going to do one more test while I was here. I promised to take him out to lunch wherever he wanted to go to make it up to him. I would never have brought him had I known it would take that long.

Although I saw what were clearly abnormalities on the mammogram, I still believed them to be my "normal abnormalities." As the ultrasound technician repeatedly rolled her wand over the same few areas of my breast and her facial expression changed to one of concern, I started to feel anxious. As a seasoned nurse, I was proficient at a poker face; this tech was not. After the anxiety built to the level where I could feel my breathing getting faster, I looked away and counted tiles on the ceiling to pass the time, a technique I'd taught myself in the dental chair. The "twenty-to-thirty-minute appointment" was now almost two and a half hours. She gave me a towel to wipe off the ultrasound gel and left the room.

Just when I thought she'd forgotten about me and was ready to walk out into the hallway, she returned with company: the radiologist. After introducing herself and sitting on the stool next to the exam table, the radiologist informed me that I would need to come back for biopsies. She said a few other things that I could not absorb after she said "biopsies." She did ask if I had any questions.

"Yeah, just one. Does it look suspicious?" In medical speak, suspicious is a term used when it appears unfavorable or cancerous but they can't confirm it until the biopsies are done.

Her response was, "Yes, I'm worried."

After I was dressed, Riley and I walked out of the hospital. I was still trying to process the comment the radiologist made. In my years of nursing I hadn't heard a physician tell someone they were worried. It seemed odd, even unprofessional, yet at the same time I appreciated her honesty.

As we were walking in the parking lot I got a call from Brooke at the home care company. It had only been hours since my interview. She asked to schedule the peer interview for Friday. "Yes, I will be there!" The rest of the day I focused on Riley and the promising new job opportunity. I was actually able to put the comment from the radiologist aside, thinking, "I won't know anything until after the biopsies anyway. I am sure they are just being super cautious."

The next day began as a relaxing spring break morning. I looked out over our little corner of the lake, which was a great fishing spot, and drank coffee on the deck. Then my relaxing morning was interrupted by a call from Dr. Bea. Hearing her voice immediately made me nervous; I had never talked to her on the phone, as it was usually her nurse who called with test results.

She jumped right in. "I spoke with the radiologist who read your mammogram and ultrasound. You have an invasive and aggressive form of breast cancer. We will know more about the treatment options after the biopsies." I did ask how she could say that I had cancer before the biopsies were done. She explained that the appearance made it obvious: it had the "spiculated borders" seen in cancer. Since I am a nurse I needed detail. She said the ultrasound showed a three-centimeter irregular mass. She also explained there was a seven-centimeter skin involvement and a lymph node of concern. The biopsies were scheduled for Monday, April 2. She gave me the name of a surgeon and suggested I make an appointment for the day after the biopsies, which meant I would have to call off work the first couple days after spring break.

I began calling a few family and friends to repeat the information and process what happened. After trying to process this news with a few people for support, I stopped telling others, mostly because the ones I did tell stated they wouldn't believe it until the biopsies were done. I understood that. Have hope, wait for confirmation. I wanted to have hope with them. I didn't want to think about the diagnosis, let alone the possibility of a terminal one. But I knew I had cancer. Not just from the mammogram, and the doctor's confirmation, but also from my own body. I had woken up and noticed things my friends could not. None of them were in my body. None of them could feel the swelling of my breast or the changes in me. It seemed like my breast started changing more drastically after the mammogram, or maybe I just paid more attention to it. I learned later that the orange-peel texture of the skin and the area that looked like a worm under my skin were actually where the lymphatic vessels were blocked. I don't know if it was from the compression from the mamogram or if it was bound to happen regardless. My right breast was larger and fuller and my bras didn't fit right. This knowledge was undeniable, and yet I did want to deny it and protect myself and loved ones from what we weren't prepared to handle yet.

After talking to my family and friends, I reached out by email to a physician I used to work with, now a friend outside of work. Of all the medical people I had come to know in my years of nursing, I reached out to him first. Alan was able to convince me that "better days are coming" when I was the most vulnerable to cancer and the complications of treatment.

This book, titled for the hope I held onto and the wisdom I gained that confirmed it, is a collection of emails (EM), Facebook statuses and comments (FB), my online medical journal on CaringBridge (CB), and posts from my blog, *Flight of a Phoenix*, that were written while I was struggling through cancer and the aftereffects. They are the raw truth with unfiltered emotions, woven together by my reflections written afterward.

It wasn't until I started getting serious about putting this book together that I realized the first week or two after the diagnosis had faded in my mind. I made appointment after appointment, but it was just one of those times where you bring your body and hope your mind catches up. The family and friends who came to all my early appointments and significant ones after that helped retain information while I couldn't. I have been in that type of a fog before; it's called survival mode. In survival mode, I do what I need to do, focus on what is in front of me, and process it later when I know I have survived.

As I wrote this, I looked through my calendars and called the people involved to clarify some of the things that were foggy. A big thank-you goes to Lola for suggesting I keep an online journal, which helped to document the medical details and emotions—not just mine, but also those of my friends and family, who made comments and offered hope and encouragement. Most names have been changed for this book, but it was invaluable to have that support. Although I would love to acknowledge every morsel of support I received from the more than one hundred people who routinely checked in on me and encouraged me in writing, I occasionally summarize the comments so that I can focus on the impact that collective support had on my emotions, thoughts, attitudes, and overall cancer journey. I maintained some of the original comments from people who had a thread that connected the stories together. I recommend online journaling or blogging as a form of communication for anyone struggling with difficult medical issues. One day, the fog will lift and you will be able to digest everything that's happened and all you've been through, as I now can. Reviewing this material years after it was written in order to put this book together has been significant to my cancer treatment recovery and survivorship.

— 1 —

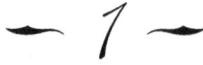

Chemotherapy

Walking for Breast Cancer

In April 2008 I considered joining the two-day-long Avon Walk for Breast Cancer. There were many neighbors who expressed interest in doing this to fundraise because they either had breast cancer themselves or someone in their family had. When it came time to commit and register, however, I was the only one who did. I went alone to a training event at a community college to find out more about fundraising, how the weekend would go, and how to train for it. The afternoon ended with an eight-mile walk where I met a new friend, Sasha, with whom I trained.

The Avon Walk was a two-day event in Chicago. The opening ceremony was held at Soldier Field, home of my beloved Chicago Bears. There were the usual speakers, motivational activities and stretching, along with announcements on where the money collected goes. The energy permeated through the thousands of walkers, supporters, and volunteers. Just before they released us to start walking, they made an announcement: approximately every three minutes a breast cancer diagnosis was made. They calculated how many people would be diagnosed during the weekend and showed us a white sash symbolizing a diagnosis. If you as a volunteer or walker found one in your belongings or were handed one, you were to wear it the rest of the weekend. It was supposed to provide a visual at the closing ceremony of just how many people were diagnosed over the weekend.

Saturday night we were exhausted, and after setting up our little tent Sasha and I both melted into our sleeping bags. I woke up in the middle of the night—not unusual for me—and went out to get water. As I stepped out of the tent I stepped on a rolled-up white sash.

I don't consider myself a superstitious person, but I had an eerie feeling that if I put that sash on, someday I would be diagnosed with breast cancer. I never put it on and I never told Sasha it was outside our tent. It got stuffed down into a side pocket of my backpack. The backpack then got stuffed in my closet and it wasn't until I was packing to move out of our home when I was getting divorced in 2010 that I found it, exactly where I had stuffed it down and ignored it a couple years before.

Coming to Terms

Email (EM): March 31, 2012

Subject: Little Did I Know

From: Marcy

To: Alan

Hi, I know it is weird sending this by email but I didn't want to call this late. It is coincidental, ironic, bad karma...call it what you will; I signed up for Relay for Life on February 18 and on March 29 my doctor called and told me I have an invasive and aggressive form of breast cancer. I guess now they can tell from the ultrasound by the way some cancers look, even before they do the biopsies. Biopsies are scheduled for Monday. I had to wait until then because I take daily aspirin [for heart health; they told me it could cause too much bleeding at the biopsy sites, especially as some of those sites are deep in the breast tissue]. I see the surgeon on Tuesday and I guess I will know the extent of it and the plan on Tuesday night. I didn't know a doctor would tell someone they have "a fast-growing cancer" based off a mammogram, ultrasound, and call from the radiologist. I thought they always waited for the biopsy. I wish I had asked more questions while I had her on the phone. I was stunned.

Thank you for donating to Relay for Life. I didn't know that the life I could be saving by participating in it or the Avon Walk years ago could end up being mine.

I hope life isn't throwing you any curves right now,

Take care,

Marcy

P.S. I don't know if Jack ever contacts you but I don't plan on telling him until I absolutely have to.

From: Alan

To: Marcy

Wow, sorry to hear that. I know it's hard but I would certainly wait for the biopsy and related work-up before jumping to conclusions. I will be praying for you.

I haven't talked to Jack since the night we all ate together. I emailed him a couple years ago but no response and nothing since.

Be strong and be positive. I promise you will be in my thoughts and prayers. I'll do my best to answer any questions. Keep me posted.

From: Marcy

To: Alan

Thanks, I will try to keep my head about it. Just sounded bad from what Dr. Bea told me on the phone. Do you know her? I started going to her a couple years ago when I moved because I remember Dr. Taft saying he knew her.

I know it would be hard for you to answer questions without all the data. I will try not to put you in that position.

Take care.

From: Alan

To: Marcy

Hi Marcy, I know who Dr. Bea is. I believe she trained at Memorial Hospital. I know her partner, Leslie Dunkin, well. She was a resident at Memorial when I was precepting. She's been my mother-in-law's doctor for twelve years. I talk to her a couple times a year.

I care about you. I'm happy to try to answer any questions.

Take care.

From: Marcy

To: Alan

My guess is I'll be getting to know Dr. Dunkin too.

TTFN (Ta Ta For Now)

Alan was a physician I worked with when I was a nurse at a family practice clinic. He and his wife Sophie, my former husband Jack, and I had
gone out together in the past. Alan and I maintained a friendship and occasionally after my divorce I would get together with Alan and Sophie. Alan
became a person I communicated with frequently via email and phone,
not only to clarify the things I was learning but to vent about my fears
and struggles, especially with the medical field. He was able to fill in the
gaps in my knowledge about my health and treatment from a physician's
perspective, and he always knew how to make me laugh. During some of
the busiest and most stressful times working together we used our humor
to lighten the burdens we were carrying.

My mom and my close friend Liza came with me when I returned to
the hospital for the biopsies. I expected that I wouldn't want to drive home,
especially if the biopsies were painful. I also thought it would be beneficial
to have someone in the waiting room with my mom. I was familiar with
the look of worry my mom had shown since I told her what Dr. Bea said
on the phone, as I had seen that look often in my teenage years and early
twenties. Liza took the day off work to drive us. We'd been friends from
the moment I walked into her business in 2003, and she had become like
a sister to me.

I had no idea that eight deep breast biopsies could be that excruciating.
Nor did I realize they had to take that many. With icepacks on my chest, I
spent the next couple days doing what everyone, especially a nurse, does
after diagnosis: researching. I was cautious and kept to reputable internet
sites. I was fairly reassured that breast cancer is not a death sentence. A
five-year survival rate was 90 percent or more likely. The only thing that
scared me was inflammatory breast cancer (IBC), which had a survival rate
of 25–40 percent (meaning that within five years of their diagnosis, 60–75
percent of women with IBC die). Thankfully that is a rare type of breast
cancer.

This time is a blur to my memory. I don't remember most of the conversations I had or whom I told about the cancer diagnosis. I do remember
two conversations with my children.

Dani, my eighteen-year-old, and I were in the car about to back out of
the driveway when I told her I was going for biopsies. I told her that, while
it would be confirmed with the biopsies, Dr. Bea had said I had breast
cancer. Without hesitation she demanded, "Well, just nip that in the bud
right now." I shared with her some of the research, telling her that cancer
is not a death sentence and is curable. As long as I didn't have IBC I would
be okay. She asked what that was. I told her it was the type of breast cancer

with the worst survival rates, but that it was very rare. I would come to regret saying those words to her.

Riley, my thirteen-year-old son, is always thinking and putting puzzle pieces together in his head. Not much gets past him. When I was icing my chest he saw the pamphlets I received after the biopsies. He asked if getting the biopsies meant that I had cancer. Although in my core I knew I had cancer, I told him people get biopsies all the time that identify other abnormalities, not just cancer. He seemed to accept that answer. As he walked away, I wondered if I sounded confident and convincing enough. He was younger than Dani, and a male, and I held more back from him. He often expressed discomfort when we started "girl talk" around him, and I couldn't blame him for that at the age of thirteen.

I know I also told my brother's wife, Patti, about the cancer suspicions shortly after the ultrasound, but I couldn't remember any details of the conversation. So recently, while I was trying to piece the early story together, we went for a long walk and she told me what she could recall.

She said that back in March of 2012, I walked the mile to her and my brother Steve's house and told her that they found something on my mammogram and did an ultrasound immediately. I told her I would be having biopsies the following Monday. She clearly remembers when I showed her my breast and the orange-peel appearance, which she could see and feel. To her it was "clearly abnormal." She continued to tell me that from her perspective things went at "warp speed." For me, the twelve days between Dr. Bea's call and starting chemotherapy were in slow motion, especially with the delay needed for the biopsy confirmation.

As I wrote this book, I talked to the key people in my life. These were some of my most ardent supporters who reached out and held me up in person or over the phone rather than online, making recording their efforts more challenging. Some of these people are described below.

My mom was one of those people. When she retired from being a Methodist minister in 2004 she moved from the central Illinois area and in with my husband, kids, and me. We lived in a developing area midway between Chicago and Rockford. I was working as a nurse in the endoscopy department of a nearby hospital and my then-husband traveled. She moved in to help me with the kids, especially with the requirement to be on call in my job. When I got divorced in 2010, she, the kids, and I moved into the rental home on a lake that was just a mile from my brother Steve.

As I wrote this book my mom and I talked about the difficulty I was having recalling some of the details of those early conversations, which are a little fuzzy to her as well. She could remember which appointments she went to with me, but not specifics of what I said. She does remember going with Dani and me to tell Grace and Harrison of the diagnosis.

Grace and Harrison are like second parents to me. We have been close since I was eighteen years old. I recovered from my wisdom teeth removal on their couch, cared for by their son, who was my boyfriend at the time, and their German shepherd. They have been grandparents to my children too; Grace was even in the delivery room with me when Riley was born.

It was just "us girls"—Grace, my mom, Dani, and I. Harrison recalls he was "just there and couldn't think of much to say that would be helpful." Grace was in denial; she says now of that time, "Denial is a very powerful tool when things are close to hurting us or the ones we love." As she listened, her mind rebelled—she thought she could save me with disbelief.

It was that conversation that made me realize I shouldn't tell any more people until it was confirmed. It was difficult for me for two reasons. One, I couldn't move forward in accepting what was happening and prepare myself for what was to come if I was trying to deny what my doctor and body told me. Two, I couldn't put anyone else through thinking I had cancer unless it was confirmed 100 percent true, even though I knew it was true. If Alan, who is a physician, and Grace wanted to wait for confirmation, then others would have a hard time believing it also. So I waited.

I didn't have to wait long in the perspective of society but to me, a newly diagnosed cancer patient, every delay felt like it could propel me toward the end of life.

EM: April 3, 2012

Subject: Confirmed

From: Marcy

To: Alan

Spoke with Leslie this morning. Biopsies show cancer. I hope Dr. Campbell can do the surgery ASAP.

From: Alan

To: Marcy

Hi Marcy, I hope it goes well. My thoughts are with you. Better days are coming.

Hang in there.

Meeting with the surgeon on April 3 for the first time is now a faded memory. My mom came, and would continue to come to all such visits. This first time I brought Patti as well. I was unprepared for Dr. Campbell to take more biopsies, this time of the thickened orange-peel skin. I asked her if that biopsy came back positive for cancer, would it mean I had IBC, that advanced and aggressive cancer I'd read about? She verified that it would. She also explained that she would only start with surgery if the biopsy was negative; otherwise, she would start with chemotherapy because if surgery was first, I would have to wait until I healed to have chemotherapy and the cancer could spread to other organs during that time. Wait, what? Not do surgery first? That sounded awful—I wanted this cancer out of me.

The surgeon then ordered an MRI of both of my breasts to verify that there wasn't cancer on the left side. Mammograms can't pick out small abnormalities in dense, fibrocystic breasts like mine, nor can they scan the deep lymph node, which had looked suspicious. This MRI would be important in deciding if I needed surgery on both breasts, either lumpectomies (removal of the tumor and a small amount of surrounding tissue) or mastectomies (removal of all or part of the breast and sometimes lymph nodes and muscles).

Dr. Campbell called just after I arrived home; she'd gone down to the MRI department but had just missed me. When she started the conversation with that introduction, it immediately put me on guard. I knew it had to be ominous news for her to walk down to another department during the middle of her morning rounds to find me. As much as she wanted to be able to share this type of news face to face, there was no time to see her in the office again. The skin biopsies showed cancer. Chemotherapy would be done before surgery. She'd called the oncologist and set up an afternoon appointment for that day. She suggested I bring someone with me. My mother immediately agreed, which lent me the clear thinking and support I needed, and thankfully Patti was off on Wednesdays and could bring the last ingredient, reliable hearing, in case we missed something important. Patti also had a calming effect on me. I often call her Saint Patricia for being the glue that held my family together for the last couple of decades.

Bringing my mom and sister-in-law to my first appointment with the oncologist was a wise idea. I don't remember much from that day. My brain shut down and my emotions detached. Those two things were the defense mechanisms I needed to get through that. I didn't cry and stayed as dispassionate in my interaction with the oncology staff as I could. I thought if I could maintain nurse mode instead of slipping into scared-cancer-patient mode, I could get through this without scaring my mom. The one specific question I asked was, "What stage is the cancer?" The oncologist answered that IBC was automatically staged as a three and since the cancer didn't appear to be in the chest wall it was B, not C. (C is the last substage before stage four, which is terminal.) The PET scan might bump that to a stage four, depending on the findings.

Before leaving the oncologist's office I had to schedule multiple appointments. I needed a baseline echocardiogram, as chemotherapy could cause heart damage. I needed an appointment with the chemotherapy nurse to learn about chemotherapy and what to expect. I also needed the aforementioned PET scan to further evaluate whether the cancer had spread to any other areas of my body.

We processed what we'd heard as Patti drove us home. After that oncology visit the phone companies must have been close to overload. I asked Patti and my mom to update the many family members I knew I would have a hard time sharing this with, not because I was worried about them being unsupportive but because I didn't want to start crying on the phone and didn't think I could handle the sound of worry in their voices. I did send out an email to family and close friends and provided a link to an information sheet on inflammatory breast cancer.

Looking back at this now, I regret sending that to my friends and family, as I know it made them worry more, just as it did me. Many told me they were glad I did so they "knew what we were up against" but I think it took the gray cloud over my head and turned it into a tornado that was about to suck them in as well.

Some of the friends I told of my diagnosis in person were Ron and Laurie. Friends are often found in unexpected places. I didn't expect a close friendship to develop with them when my husband and I started using their automotive repair shop years before. I joked with them that I fought for them in the divorce. To this day I stop by not only for automotive needs but for a quick hello and a long hug—Laurie calls me a "prolonged hugger"; I agree with her and have told her I prefer "holds not hugs." Ron has told me, "Most people see hugs as a motion but you hug with emotion." Laurie and I have had many conversations in their shop about life, love, and children. I asked her what she remembered from when I was diagnosed.

Laurie recalls that I told her about the cancer diagnosis in person at their shop. We cried and hugged a lot. Their shop was only a few miles from my oncologist's office, which made it easy to stop by often before or after chemotherapy, office visits, and labs to cry and hug. Ron and Laurie always allowed me to be me, whether it was the silly, playful me dancing and singing in their shop, or the sad, hurting me who cried on their shoulders.

EM: April 5, 2012

From: Marcy

To: Informed family and friends

Hi guys,

PET scan is schedule for Monday. That may or may not push me from a stage 3B to a stage 4. Chemo starts on Tuesday and will be every two weeks for four treatments (eight weeks) and then he will switch to another chemo. When he feels that chemo is sufficient to prevent recurrence and spreading he will recommend the surgery, then radiation, then oral chemo, something like that.

Here is the link.[1]

Love you,

Marcy

One of the first responses came from my friend Lola. She and her son Hawk have always been special to me; for one thing, she and I bonded over being single parents. I tried to do everything I could to support Lola as a single parent, as I knew what that was like from before I got married in 2003 and after I got divorced in 2010. Hawk reminded me a lot of my son Riley. They both needed much guidance and were very sensitive and empathetic. She still found time to encourage and support me in person, even with her busy life. She has always been the type of friend who doesn't need to be asked to do things, she always knew ways she could help. I saw this as our previous coworker slowly died from Lou Gehrig's disease (amyotrophic lateral sclerosis): as Curly slowly lost the ability to move her body, Lola routinely went to her home to give her massages. (Lola supplements her income as an in-home massage therapist.) Had I faced the same as Curly, I know she would have been there to the cruel end.

---

1.   The original site, at cancer.gov, has been taken down, but the same information is available here: https://www.cancer.org/cancer/breast-cancer/ understanding-a-breast-cancer-diagnosis/types-of-breast-cancer/ inflammatory-breast-cancer.html.

EM: April 5, 2012

From: Lola

To: Marcy

I don't like this!!!!!!

From: Marcy

To: Lola

I'll be okay, you know how stubborn I am, right?! I thought of you today when I was facedown in the MRI with my boobs hanging down and my face in the horseshoe. I was imagining I was on your massage table. LOL.

Talk to you soon, okay?

EM: April 5, 2012

From: Grace

To: Marcy

Hi Marcy, wish this could be a nice "chatty" email. I'm glad that you sent me all this info. It helps to know what's ahead and what we're facing. Just know that I love you and I will be there one step at a time, one day at a time. xoxoxoxo

P.S. The wisdom teeth were easier, I think!!!!!

From: Marcy

To: Grace

LOL, I could use Sandy right now (and Dylan) [their dog and son, my ex-boyfriend] but I guess I will have to settle for a peanut butter and chocolate shake from Baskin Robbins...

From: Grace

To: Marcy

I love you, just pure, plain and simple, I love you! xoxo

From: Marcy

To: Grace

Thanks. I have always known that but it is good to read every now and then. You do know I love you, right?

From: Grace

To: Marcy

There has never been a doubt in my mind. Can't get you off my mind today! Xoxoxo

Facebook status (FB): April 5, 2012

I honestly feel like I can get through this, thank you for your love and support. I have the best family and friends a person could ask for and I hope you knew that even before this week's events.

Messages of support poured in from others. One was my niece. Clara was born when I was sixteen years old. I spent a lot of time babysitting her at different periods of time during her childhood. Life seemed to make a full circle in our relationship because as a young adult she became a consistent babysitter for my children. She cheered me on through online messages, emails, snail mail, and various other ways. Although she lived in another state, we talked on the phone often.

Some of my other family and friends may not have provided written words of encouragement, but the phone calls and visits were consistent and abundant.

EM: April 6, 2012

From: Clara

To: Marcy

I know you're gonna get through this. And you are such an amazingly strong woman that I have respected and adored my entire life!!! You have helped mold me into the woman I have become and for that I thank you!

Roger, Dani's dad, had become very close to my entire family. Although we never married, we developed a friendship that is unwavering. He was devoted to both Dani and Riley. I told him about the cancer while he was in my home (he spent a lot of time with the kids and helping around the house). The following days he spent a lot of time reading about IBC. His mother had decided not to get treatment for her breast cancer and died from it in the summer of 2004. For this fight he was determined to learn what I would go through so he could help.

EM: April 7, 2012

From: Alan

To: Marcy

Hey Marcy, Do you still live in Round Rock? Can I get your address?

To: Alan

Why? Are you gonna send Shemar Moore to my house for a blind date?

From: Alan

I'm planning to send something. I was gonna send Shemar but it turns out the post office won't ship a person—go figure.

Happy Easter!

I sent him my address and heard from him again rather quickly.

EM: April 8, 2012

From: Alan

To: Marcy

Oops. I sent you something for good luck. I accidently hit "send" before I got to add the message. So when you get a small gift out of the blue it's from me, to let you know I'm thinking about you and praying/hoping for good health. And to let you know that I'm incompetent when ordering online.

Hope you had a good Easter

Although Shemar never came in the mail, a few days later I received a beautiful ceramic turtle. Her shell opened to hold trinkets and she played music. I kept that beautiful gift in sight when I was too weak to get up off the couch or out of bed. The turtle, named Hope, made me smile as it played "That's What Friends Are For," a song typical of Alan's response to praise for kindness that he showed.

One of my longest friendships is with Lucy. Lucy has been my "advocate" since I was a troubled fourteen-year-old enrolled at a family counseling center. An advocate was the Omni House version of a "Big Sister" from Big Brother Big Sisters of America. She volunteered for that role and remained in that role consistently throughout my life, even when I no longer qualified for that program after I moved. She went from a volunteer to a longtime friend. She was one of the first people I reached out to by phone. Although I would have loved to reach out to her in person, she lived eight hours away by car.

EM: April 6, 2012

From: Lucy

To: Marcy

Glad you got some information prior to the weekend. I look forward to hearing about the PET scan after you get the results. You have an oncologist now I'm guessing.

Thinking of you and praying for you.

From: Marcy

To: Lucy

Yep. He ordered the PET scan. I go for chemo teaching on Monday. My mom and sister-in-law, Patti, are going with me. Chemo starts on Tuesday. I can tell a visible difference in my breast in less than two weeks. I'll keep you posted.

Love you.

From: Lucy

To: Marcy

I wish I could be there with you! I took my brother to chemo so many times. It is crazy that so many people are getting cancer treatments daily—what is wrong with this picture??? I wish our monies were spent equally on prevention—back to getting foods healthy again and getting rid of so many preservatives, additives, etc. that have taken over our food industry.

Okay, I'll stop there before I go any further. It just makes me angry. The same thing for what we are putting on our skin with all the chemicals and our skin being our largest organ—just isn't right! I don't think God ever intended for us to do that. He provided all the foods, plants and herbs we needed, but we overlook that and complicate things so much. Wish we had more skilled herbalists around. We have a Chinese friend whose daughter has some type of cancer. They can't help her here in the US, so she goes back to China to get her the herbs and medicines she needs to keep the cancer away.

Take care dear friend and I love you too!

Lucy

From: Marcy

To: Lucy

So is this my fault for not preventing it by eating better and not using safer products on my skin?

From: Lucy

To: Marcy

No, silly, but I do think knowledge is power and we all need to know more about some of these additives, chemicals, and so forth that our foods and products are being made with, injected with, etc. I think our foods and products should be regulated more strictly. I read articles weekly about the grams of sugar in some of our foods that we are not aware of, chemicals that we are not aware of, etc. Why are these manufacturers doing this, or being allowed to do this? Between these things and the toxic environment we are in, our bodies are filled with toxins and yes, those toxins can compromise the body, setting it up for disease. It is very enlightening reading and I think slowly people are becoming more aware. But I feel more could be done to increase the awareness now. Toxins settle in fatty tissues of our body and unfortunately for women, breasts are made of fatty tissue. People can detox their bodies, but I don't think many people understand this process and feel the need for it—again a lack of knowledge.

It makes me angry, Marcy, that so many people are affected by cancer and yes, I do think a lot of it could be prevented by stricter regulations from the FDA and other agencies. I have heard so many stories from families affected by cancer. My brother wasn't aware that the chemicals he was around daily on his job and was inhaling, could lead to cancer, especially combined with other stressors he was dealing with at the time of his diagnosis.

I don't know if any of this makes sense to you, but I read a lot about it and hear many stories, have friends that own health food stores and do massage therapy and we all feel that given the food and product ingredients being used today (some that we have no idea about and I have been truly shocked about) it is no wonder that our bodies are being set up for disease and yes, with knowledge maybe some of that could be prevented. I have attended many health and wellness events over the last few years and their purpose is to educate about some of these issues.

Love you and I feel the fault lies in the manufacturers and regulators. If they aren't going to change anything, then I guess it is up to us.

Take care and Happy Easter.

From: Marcy

To: Lucy

I get what you are saying. There are definitely things people do to put them at higher risk, but like you said it is up to us. Yes, education and information is good but there is also a lot of misinformation out there from some companies that want to make their products appear better and they scare the public without any real data. Prohibition didn't work... We know cigarette smoking is terrible and they are still produced, are we going to stop driving cars or using lawn mowers because of the dangers of the exhaust? I think eating well and reducing exposure to things that we know to be dangerous is a good start but I don't think we can blame an entire industry or government. Bottom line is we make choices and sometimes we make the best choices we can and bad things still happen. I know you are passionate about what you do and the people you love and that is a good thing.

I love you, have a great Easter, Marcy

Throughout my cancer treatment and recovery, I painstakingly sifted through emails, facebook posts, articles, and verbal advice from well-meaning family and friends who I believe had my best interest at heart. There are many products out there touted to ease a person's suffering, to prevent or cure cancer. Wanting to validate their pure motives but not get caught up in unverified remedies had me researching medical journals or relying on Alan for accurate information. I could not blame the government or others for this merciless disease. I could not find one person or group to blame for the pain that was making a beeline toward me. Doing this required more energy than I had and there came a time when I had to believe in myself, the medical profession and my body for the cure. This proved to be exhausting to the point of having to squelch those topics for the sake of my sanity.

Strong for Me or Strong for Them?

I scheduled an outdoor portrait session. Looking back now I don't remember the thought process behind having the pictures taken. I had been growing my hair out for years, and I just wanted to have some professional photos before my cancer treatment, before I lost all my hair—and perhaps more than that. I think now that there may have also been some notion that if I didn't survive the cancer, I wanted my family to have recent professionally done photos to look at.

I knew Leeann from when she worked for Liza at a Fast Frame store. Leeann had come to my house and taught me how to scrapbook digitally. She and her husband had done Dani's high school senior photos at Chicago Botanic Gardens. I reached out to her.

I took Leeann's suggestion to take the photos at Independence Grove in Libertyville. It was a beautiful location. As she and her husband found interesting and beautiful areas for portraits, we talked and walked. We took time to play at the park and I had Leeann play on a teeter-totter with me. I stood on a rock and flexed my muscles, and posed near a tic-tac-toe game to show the hugs and kisses (Xs and Os) I had for my family and friends. I took some photos meant just for Liza, whom I'd met for lunch a couple days prior. She told me she wished she could duct tape me to hold me together. I brought a roll of duct tape and Leeann helped me tape across my chest as a message to Liza that I would be okay and hold myself together. I asked specifically to shoot some of my mother's ring, which I'd had custom made with a gold heart band and the birthstones of all three of my children nestled inside the heart.

After Leann and her husband left, I sat in a quiet area and called Dakota, one of Riley's previous teachers whom I had grown close to from volunteering as a room mom and art mom. Riley's fourth grade year was the only year we could afford to have me be a stay-at-home mom. Unlike the other moms in our neighborhood I worked every other year.

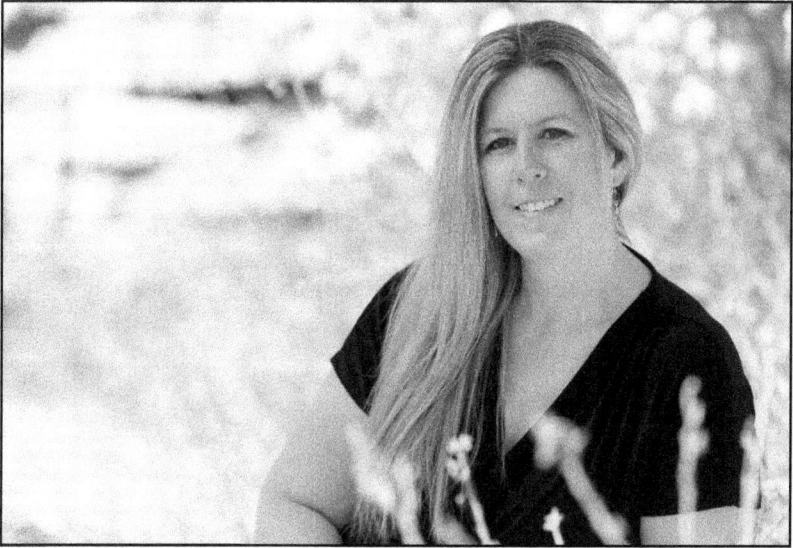

Figure 1-1. April 2012, just days before starting
chemotherapy (photo by Chang2 Studios)

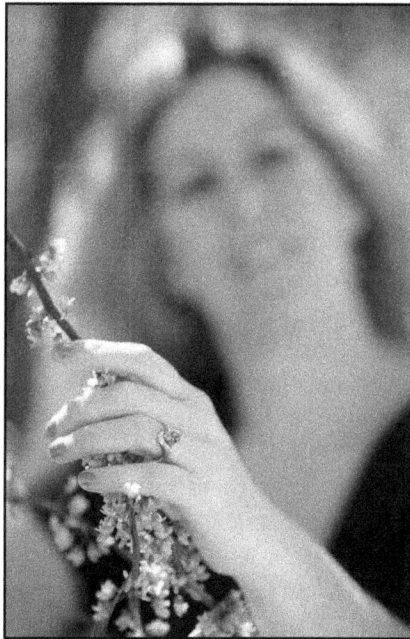

Figure 1-2. Showing my mother's ring (photo by Chang2 Studios)

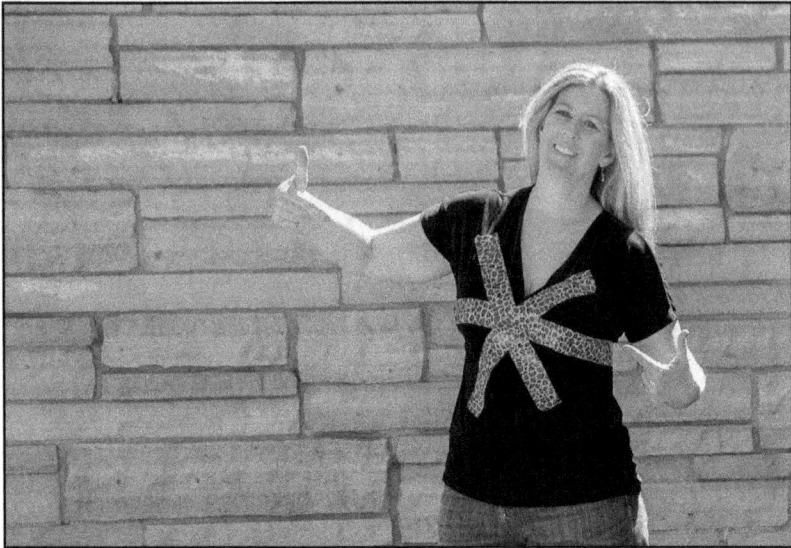

Figure 1-3. My picture for Liza using duct tape to hold
myself together (photo by Chang2 Studios)

Taking advantage of the many opportunities to volunteer, I grew close to
the teachers and staff. That year is still the only opportunity I have had to
actively participate in school activities during the day. Other than making
sure I kidnapped them for lunch once a year and chaperoned a field trip
once a year, I was not involved in their school days. I knew Dakota was
adopted and I sought her opinion on if I should contact Joey—the firstborn
child I placed for adoption.

I filled her in on the cancer diagnosis. Then I told her it was my belief
that it is the adopted child's choice to reunite and not the birth parent's. I
expressed to her that I didn't want to disrupt his life but at the same time
worried that if something happened to me and I died, my child wouldn't
be able to get the information he needed, if he did need it later. She recommended I wait, as it would be traumatic to him to hear of my illness. She
stated if the prognosis changed, I could consider contacting his adoptive
parents and letting it be their call whether or not contact with me would be
helpful. Although I really respected Dakota's opinions, it would take a few
more conversations with people who knew about adoption from different
perspectives before I could put the thoughts of contacting Joey on the back
burner.

Easter was the Sunday before I started chemotherapy and like most
holidays, we spent it at my brother Steve's house. Patti hosted her side

and our side of the family together on Easter every year. The diagnosis was still new and I had not started chemotherapy yet. I was grateful to be with family that day but also felt like the cancer diagnosis was the elephant in the room. Interestingly, the people who were the most open about discussing it and asking questions were the kids. Patti's niece in particular sat with me for most of the get-together and asked if I would lose my hair. I told her yes, but that it was okay because it would grow back. She asked if she could practice braiding on my hair. I said yes and felt relaxed as she braided my hair several different ways. It felt as if she was being extra gentle and made loose braids slowly, whereas when I braided Dani's hair I pulled securely as I weaved. I silently wondered what her innocent mind was thinking about my diagnosis. Did she think I was going to die? As she braided she asked more questions, which I encouraged. I wanted the younger ones to be comfortable asking questions and sharing concerns. She also wanted to know if I was planning on donating my hair since it was so long. I was disappointed to tell her that I'd wanted to but the bleach for highlights would cause some kind of interaction with the processing of the hair to make a wig, so I could not.

I tried to be as upbeat and positive as I could for my family, especially the kids. Before leaving their house, it was decided that I would come back the next day and get my long hair cut short so I could get used to the idea of it being short before I lost it all together. Riley asked if he could come with and cut the ponytail.

I was agreeable to Riley cutting my hair. I thought it would be less shocking for him and myself to have it shorter before I started losing it. I didn't realize at the time how impactful the hair loss would be for both of us. I knew it would grow back. I knew it might grow back a different texture—thin versus thick, straight versus curly. But what I didn't know was that the loss of my hair would affect not only others but also my mood. I wanted to believe I didn't care about my hair, but it was closely tied to how others perceived me and even how I recognized myself.

FB: April 9, 2012

I really like my shorter haircut, although I will only be able to keep it for a couple weeks. Riley thinks I look weird with short hair. Boy, is he gonna be the one who has difficulty with the hairstyle change. The positive side is when he wants to roll the car windows down, I will say sure because my hair won't get in my eyes.

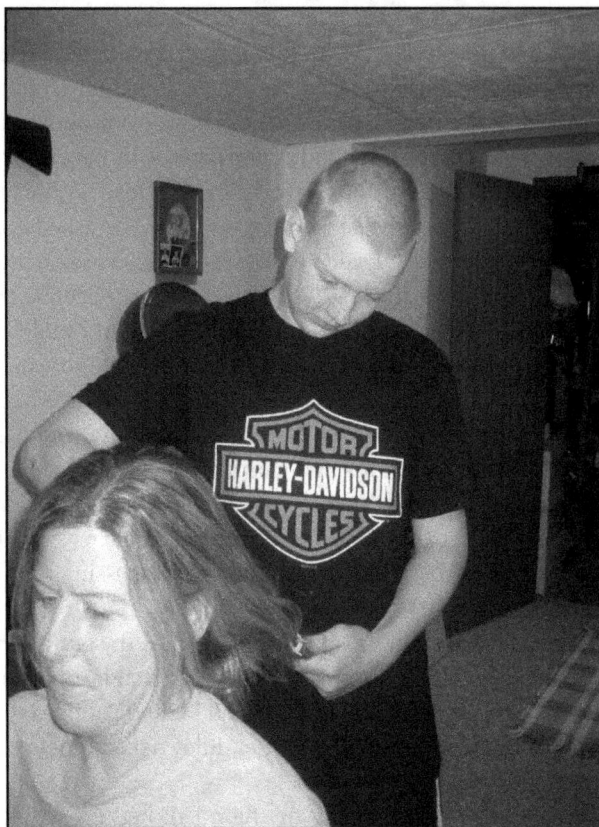

Figure 1-4. Riley cutting my hair

CaringBridge (CB): April 10, 2012

The Beginning

Little did I know on February 18, 2012, when I signed up for Relay for Life that today I would be sitting in an oncologist's office receiving my first chemo treatment for inflammatory breast cancer, stage 3B. It was diagnosed over spring break. The nurse commented that I was so calm and relaxed. I am calm and relaxed because I have an incredible support system. I am relaxed because just before chemo the doctor told me the PET scan was good and he didn't see any cancer in other organs. That meant I didn't have stage four cancer! I don't care if I lose my hair, I don't care if I lose my breasts, I just want life!

My biggest concern is my kids and always has been. My kids are the focus of my life.

I did the Avon Walk for breast cancer years ago. I just wanted to help. I didn't know the person I could be helping in the future might be me. I just ask two things: 1) Please keep up on your annual physical and screenings (this is for all types of cancers)! 2) If you are a woman, please keep up on your mammograms.

The cancer was discovered after I went for my yearly physical and the doctor noticed a "skin thickening." A mammogram showed an abnormality and more views were immediately taken, and an ultrasound was done immediately. Then I had biopsies five days later, more tests, and more time to diagnose a somewhat rare and aggressive form of breast cancer. At first I was disappointed that they didn't do surgery right away but then came to understand that since it is fast growing and aggressive that chemo would be needed to prevent the spread of the cancer before bilateral mastectomies can be done. So the plan is four months of chemo first, then surgery, then radiation, then hormone therapy. The goal is a cure. I plan to use this site to keep everyone informed of my progress through this journey. Feel free to write me a note or ask questions if you have them.

Thanks for coming here and reading this, stay healthy,

Love, Marcy

EM: April 10, 2012

From: Marcy

To: Alan

I got a call from Dr. Douglass, the neurologist I used to work for who said his friend is a radiation oncologist. He called the oncologist and told him about me. When I am ready for radiation it is good to know he is so highly recommended by a doctor I know well and trust.

From: Alan

To: Marcy

It's so much better when you get treated by people you're comfortable with. Stay positive! I'm sending good thoughts.

Post on my wall

Krystal: Hi Marcy, My sister Jasmine told me the news and I can't tell you how much I'm thinking of you! Just read a bunch of your posts and I can see how positive you are!! This is what will beat this!!!! Here for you. Miss you.

Marcy: Thanks Krystal, I really have thought about you and missed you a lot over the years. I looked up to you so much at the family practice office. You taught me a great deal about nursing and you are an incredible person. I am so glad you are on Facebook, I really love seeing the updates and pics. Keep them coming!

Martial Artist

I was six months from testing for my black belt in tae kwon do. I could have achieved that but my reward would have been a knee replacement earlier than expected, so I stopped. Besides yelling, one of my special skills was board breaking. Why? I knew if I didn't hit it hard and fast and aim through the board I wouldn't break it. Master Sun would make me do it until I succeeded. I did not want to try again with an already sore hand/foot, etc., so I broke my first board on the first try and it continued that way for a long time. That is what I am visualizing for this cancer. Hit it hard and fast and aim through it so I don't have to do it again in an already weakened state. When I have surgery, take them both! Let's hit it hard, fast and aim through it.

Maybe there is a little martial artist still in me, what do you think Melody [my martial arts teacher]? I am grateful for the many lessons learned in the dojo.

Kitt: I like the way you refer to it as this cancer. Don't claim it and go for it... Fight it like you've learned even if it takes you to a knee replacement...it will be worth it! You know what you want, so do it. Everything you've gone through has been part of the experience you needed to go through this... You can do it, girl!

Lola: Visualization and attitude to keep you focused on the positive end result!

Melody: Marcy, that is an excellent way to visualize it! I'm so proud to hear the lessons that you learned at the school are helping you now. Remember one of the Tenets is Indomitable Spirit and you my friend are truly exhibiting this. Love you and miss you! I forgot to say "hugs" to you!

Hannah: "Aye yah!"—picturing Marcy karate chopping the C cells.

FP: You have a warrior spirit.

The "Martial Artist" post received many compliments. It was received as strong and a great way to visualize fighting this disease head on. I was grateful to be able to use the martial arts training I was in with my son in such a profound way many years later. The value of martial arts for me was not just in the physical aspect for the fitness benefits, or the self-defense training; it proved significant to my mental strength and ability to visualize destroying my cancer cells and calm myself during my chemotherapy treatments. Melody was one of my martial arts instructors. It was heartwarming to read that she was proud of me.

I worried so much about how my illness would impact others, not only my family but also the teenagers at the high school. Some I was very close to as they came to my office daily or even twice a day for their medical needs.

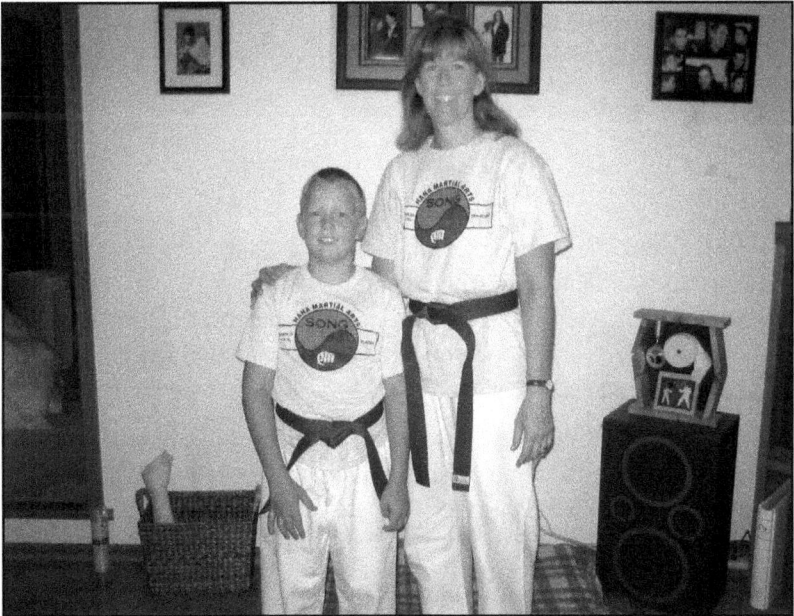

Figure 1-5. Riley and me in tae kwon do uniforms in July 2007

CB: April 11, 2012

Current Treatment Plan

Lots of questions on the plan: Chemo to start every two weeks. I get two types of chemo at the same time, for four treatments in two months then switch to another type for another two months. Three weeks off to get blood levels up and then surgery. Surgery will most likely be a bilateral mastectomy, meaning both would be removed. After that is healed, radiation and then after that a hormone therapy, most likely Tamoxifen. Which is not to be confused with hormone replacement therapy, which is estrogen replacement. The biopsies showed the cancer cells grow with estrogen. Tamoxifen reduces estrogen, whereas estrogen replacement would increase it. That is the plan so far. So far I am feeling good. I know it will eventually catch up with me but for now I am counting my blessings.

The outpouring of comments to this update had two things in common. First, overall support and encouragement. It was then that I first realized that I had my own personal cheerleading team. Second, the CaringBridge site would be valuable to keep friends and family updated. Many stated they didn't want to overwhelm me with questions but wanted to stay updated and aware of how I was and how they could support me.

EM: April 11, 2012

To: Willow

From: Marcy

Hi Willow,

I saw you went off Facebook a while ago. I have done that myself a couple of times and probably should have contacted you to see if you were okay. I think about you often and have been in your area a couple times recently and should have called. Can you forgive me for not being a great friend and let me try again?

I don't know if FP shared with you my recent diagnosis of breast cancer but it really makes a person think about who they felt good being with and who they felt bad being with. You are such a sweet person and I feel good when I talk, message, or have lunch with you. I hope you are okay.

I also have issues with the adoption now. It has always been my opinion that the adopted child should be the one to contact a birthparent when and if they are ever ready. I know I will beat this breast cancer but if things start looking bad, should I try to find him and contact him but then give him a choice if he wants to pursue a relationship or has any questions? I don't want to make issues if he has none. I don't know what to do. What do you think? Your opinion matters to me. Also, how would I even do that. Call and announce, "Hi, I'm your birth mom and I could die soon from cancer"? My gut is telling me that it is best to wait it out and not do anything, yet I wonder if something happened to me, would we regret not meeting again? Would he be mad if I died without giving him the opportunity to ask questions? Right now, I just need to believe that I will be okay and be ready when/if he reaches out to me. If I died before he sought me out, I would have to trust that my family and friends would give him the support and answers he needed, they would tell him how much I always have loved him.

If you want, you can email or call me but you don't have to if you aren't up for it.

Be well.

From: Willow

To: Marcy

I'm so sorry to hear about your diagnosis!! We do have a lot to catch up on. I should be the one apologizing!!! I went through a really tough year. I really hope to talk to you soon!!

Willow did call me back. We spent a long time talking about her experience getting to know her birth-mom. She was able to contact her and get to know her prior to her death. She spoke of the positive emotions and experience. She also shared that it had been her choice to search for her birth-mom. She understood the questions I wrote in the email to her. She also impressed upon me that those questions had no answers.

I had previously talked to Lucy about this as well because not only is she someone who knew me when I was a pregnant teenager, she had held the baby I placed for adoption when he was five months old. She also was an adoptive parent. She advised me not to seek him out. I spoke with multiple people with multiple different perspectives about this, as it weighed very heavily on my heart. I was able to come to the conclusion that as I did not want to disrupt his life, I would not try to locate him. If things changed with my prognosis and it looked like I would die from cancer, I could reevaluate my decision then.

CB: April 14, 2012

Wet Hair Mom

Please don't take this journal entry as not being positive anymore. If you will read anything here, you will read the truth. I do think I can survive this but as I was vomiting in the arcade bathroom the reality set in. I will not be able to continue to be the "Wet Hair" mom that I have always strived to be. What does that mean?

When we were at Disney World, we noticed that there were a lot of moms with perfect hair, makeup, nails, and diamond rings that would cause them to sink to the bottom if they fell in the pool. One mom was on a water ride trying not to get wet. My kids noticed that I was a "wet hair" mom. I want to be right there in it with my kids and swim with them instead of sitting on the sideline reading a book. I want to play in the rain and go on water rides with them. I want to participate in life and be a "wet hair mom."

When Riley's friend from California came in to see us on Friday I let Riley miss school (I know, the teachers are cringing right now). If I have learned anything in my life it is time with the people I love is the most important thing to me. I have not seen him or his mom in three years. So we took the day off to go to the arcade on Friday afternoon. I had been feeling okay but the bone pain from the shot to help keep white blood cells up was starting to kick in and my stomach was a little upset. We went out to eat. I then took them to the arcade. Immediately after I bought their game cards I went to the bathroom and got sick and spent the rest of the time in my car with my seat reclined back. I was hoping no one would see me in the parking lot. I told them later that I was not feeling well. I'm pretty sure I was able to hide it until after we got home. It saddens me that I probably shouldn't get season passes to the amusement park with Riley this summer and there will be times when I have to say, "No, I can't do something fun with you." I don't want my kids to start thinking of me as a dry hair mom from being sick. I will have to accept it is part of the journey to come out on the other side of the tunnel and be healthy again. I will have to get used to asking for help and asking other people to take Riley places so he doesn't have to see me sick. I hope other people will invite him to play and will enjoy life with him. I hope someone will enjoy his energy and sense of humor because I don't want that part of him to fade because I have cancer. I will probably be jealous, but I will also feel grateful that he has people in his life that will get their hair wet with him. Please enjoy your life and get your hair wet! Love you.

JH: I really appreciate what you wrote about being a wet hair mom. Going on water slides and playing in the rain with our kids is what they will remember most about us. Not how beautiful or perfect our hair was. You will get through this with strength and bravery, and your kids will remember that part of it. Not what you missed while fighting this. Stay strong!

CB: April 15, 2012

Encourage

I could tell when we hugged goodbye by the look in your eyes and the water building in them that you were trying not to cry. So was I. I could tell you were scared that we would not see each other again. Make no mistake about it, I will see you again! Yes, it had been too long but that is what happens sometimes. Feel what you feel and think what you think, I will never tell you that you are wrong for how you feel because that is the only way to keep it real, by living the truth. But know in your heart as I know in mine that we will see each other again.

I love you.

Alan: That is amazing. I honestly thought that was written by the Dalai Lama or a famous philosopher until I realized you were the author. Very cool. Don't forget to live in the present. Sending good thoughts.

Clara: Excellence is not a skill, it's an attitude. Auntie M, your attitude is not only inspiring but it makes me realize that no thing should ever defeat you. Sometimes in life we ask "Why me" and find ourselves living in a saddened confused state, but what you have taught me is why waste that time? We should always look at the problem, find the solution and move forward. Not stay stagnant because we can miss a whole lot of life experiences feeling sorry for ourselves. I only wish I lived closer so I can see you more. I miss you and love you so much!

CB: April 17, 2012

Planning Life

So today at work I am looking ahead to graduations, school registration, work schedule, and scrapbook retreats and I find my life is being planned around chemo weeks and non-chemo weeks... But hey, the key is *my life is being planned.* Which is better than planning for the alternative.

Today I went for my first post-chemo complete blood count. It is startling how much my blood counts can go down in one week, especially with a shot the day after chemo to keep the white blood cell count up. Here are boring numbers for those medical people or number people... The WBC (from 6.9 down to 2.6), hemoglobin (from 13.1 to 11.6—not too bad), platelets (291 down to 191—still normal range), and granulocytes (4.4 to 1.2). Several are low, but they are high enough to still get chemo next week. They will do a CBC just before chemo to check again and if the platelets are above 100 and granulocytes are above 1.0 the chemo will be given. If they aren't they would hold chemo and that would be one of the worst things for me to hear. I want to get this taken care of, I don't want to postpone chemo. So hope, pray, send good vibes, thoughts, or whatever you do that I can maintain my blood counts well enough to continue to get chemotherapy every two weeks with no interruptions.

CB: April 19, 2012

Good Information

A friend of mine who is a doctor I worked with helped me with my blood count concerns and I wanted to share what he said with all of you. I hope you don't mind, Alan. It is funny how when it is me I can't think rationally about this stuff sometimes but I knew the concept. I guess that is why it is important to share your concerns; how else will you get answers?

"One of the basic principles of chemo is that cancer cells are much more metabolically active than normal body cells/bone marrow activity. Hence, cancer cells are much more susceptible to chemo than regular cells. Choices of chemo regimens are usually based on cell type and several markers that are checked on the cancer cells to insure the greatest sensitivity. Just envision those cells getting their ass kicked."

Mom: Reassuring way to look at the CBC info. I think I knew the concept from when my mother had chemo but this was well put in "layman's language." Thanks, Alan. And this mama thanks you for the encouragement.

CB: April 20, 2012

Back at Work

Going back to work has been bittersweet. It was good to have a routine again, to be helping other people and to know I will get a paycheck soon, but it was exhausting. Physically and emotionally. Gradually I am telling people my story. Talking to staff, students, and parents, as they ask where I have been or why I cut my hair. I am concerned about how this may effect some of the kids that see me more often than others. Many seem genuinely concerned and I try to be as positive as I can. Some have stories of family members who have or had cancer and it brings up difficult times. I have received many hugs and well wishes. The parents who know have been very supportive, even ones I didn't really expect to be. One student went home and told his mom, who sent me a heartfelt email. Honestly, I didn't expect that from this particular person. My coworkers are awesome. It is such a blessing to have support from those around me. In about a week, the rest of the high school will know I have cancer because it will be obvious when my hair is gone. It isn't a secret, and I don't care who knows or who visits the online journal page, especially if my struggles/experience can help others in some way. If knowing my story helps others to not put off their physical or mammogram, then sharing my story is well worth it. I feel like I have the "fatigue ramble" going on here, so I will say good night to all and have a great weekend.

FB: April 20, 2012

My friend is going to Vegas this weekend; when he gets back I will either owe him a dollar for the slot machine or I will have money to pay my medical bills! (Hopefully my medical bills will not too bad as I do have insurance, at least for now.)

Lola: There's always fundraising events!!

Marcy: LOL, I know, that would be a last resort situation. There are so many people who need help and so many good causes out there for people who are able to help. I don't want to take away from those people unless I really am in dire need. I think I have a max out of pocket and although I am against credit cards it may be time to get one just in case, especially to cover the lost wages. It will all be okay, somehow the money comes when it is needed.

FB: April 21, 2012

Athena came to spend the weekend with us. I missed her and needed some canine therapy. Although in our rental house we could have dogs visit, we couldn't own one. Which is why she lives with friends now. Athena is old, fat, and limping. She doesn't want to get up on the couch. I'll eventually be on the floor with her. No more walks this weekend, stairs are enough exercise.

Kady: Aww. I didn't know you had a golden. How old is she? And OMG, you look so skinny!!

Marcy: She was nine last November. She seems happy but she is limping a lot. Riley was really trying to do something good for her but maybe he shouldn't have taken her for a walk. It was too much activity with the stairs too. We will keep her on one level now as much as possible. Riley is already saying he doesn't want her to leave. He says he "will suffer from separation anxiety."

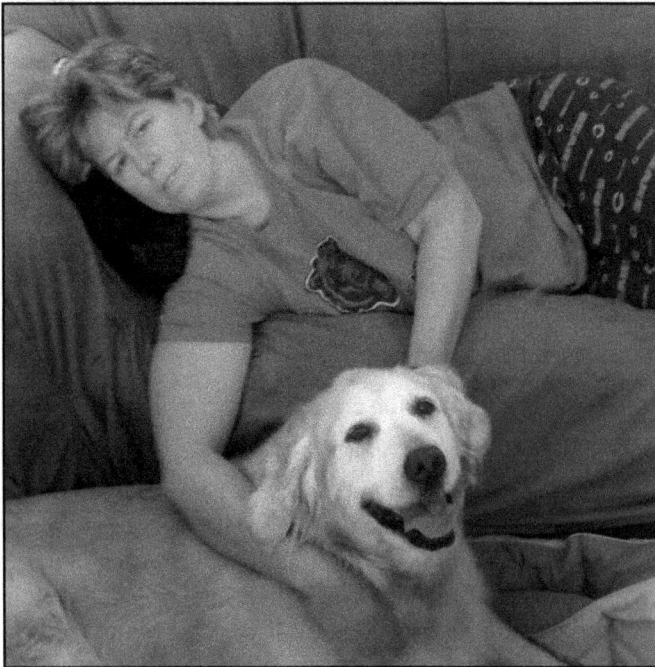

Figure 1-6. My last weekend with Athena before she died

CB: April 21, 2012

Fine Line

There is a fine line between being knowledgeable about your health and advocating for yourself and letting go, being the patient and trusting your medical team. Today I was getting organized and made the mistake of reading reports from tests. Maybe I shouldn't do that. I did learn things that my doctors never really verbalized. Maybe they thought they didn't need to. I am sure doctors need to get to know each patient and how much information they need to know and can process. I just want them to tell me everything and also the significance of what they know. Is that too much to ask? Then I will be less tempted to read my own reports, which can sometimes freak me out. I did tell my doctor to be up front with me. It is better to protect my life than my feelings.

Willow: I admire your strength and courage!! Definitely tell your doctors that you want to know everything. It's your health, you should be allowed to know all.

Alan: Hey Marcy, you should read any and all results/reports that you want to. A good doctor is happy to explain the findings and what the significance is. Radiology and pathology reports are written in a fashion that requires interpretation. Parts are to communicate with the doc, parts are trivial and parts are medico-legal. The true meaning is not always what's written. My advice, get your reports and get explanations. Be an advocate for yourself. I'm always happy to help. By the way you owe me a dollar. Be good.

I was always grateful when Laurie from the automotive shop commented, as she usually had a way to give me perspective, one of the many reasons I stopped by the shop to chat with her often.

FB: April 23, 2012

When people give their advice, I just let them talk and listen. I think it makes them feel better that they are helping. Even though it isn't always what I need, it is what they are capable of giving and I am grateful for the attempt.

Laurie: I think you either have the ones who completely avoid talking about it or don't know how to discuss it and then you have the ones who think they know all about it!

Marcy: True, and I have to remember either is fine. This is hard enough without placing unrealistic expectations on others or myself. It is good to know people care.

Because I was diagnosed with breast cancer at forty-three years old and Roger's mom also had breast cancer, I was concerned about the risk for Dani. Roger and I started looking into insurance coverage for genetic testing. I spoke with my oncologist about my concerns as well. We found out that insurance would not pay for her to have testing unless I were tested and carried the genes BRCA1 or BRCA2. The oncologist also thought it was important to have that testing to determine if I needed to have my ovaries out as well. After I made the appointment with the genetic counselor, the arduous mission of obtaining cancer history from both sides of my family was set in motion.

FB: April 23, 2012

Very frustrated trying to obtain genetic information from my family. It makes spending thousands of dollars on blood tests seem like a good idea! Overall, it has been a frustrating day in many ways, house/plumbing, technology/pictures, gathering genetic information/health. Time to go to bed.

Kitt: We're trying to help ya, hon. Mom passed away eight years ago and I don't remember things.

Marcy: I know, I have more than one person I have been talking to. You have been very helpful! The whole process is hard especially with information I don't need confusing information I do, it is a lot to sort through. Now, if you could only help with the plumbing.

Kitt: I can only imagine. Going through it with Mom isn't the same as going through it yourself and when you don't know the questions to ask, you don't get the info you need. All I really remember is how upset I was with the doctors because they gave her the chemo before they checked her lymph nodes and when they checked them they were clear but the cancer had already passed through them onto other sites and the chemo cleared the cancer from them so it looked good but it wasn't. We had trouble with Dad's doctors, too. His doctor told us when we were getting ready to take him home with hospice that he'd probably had the cancer for two years, Dad had been complaining of his stomach bothering him.

I'm getting started, I'd better stop before I get carried away. As far as your plumbing...not so much.

Marcy: So sorry you are reliving this because of me. Honestly your information has been extremely helpful and I really appreciate you for sharing it with me.

Kitt: I relive it every time I hear someone has received the cancer diagnosis, it's not your fault. It's mostly because I don't understand how doctors who are supposed to be taking care of us can be so careless and unthinking. Yes, they are human but they are paid big bucks to do the job, just wish they would. I've been told that it's my responsibility to ask the questions. That's true but if you don't know the questions to ask, someone needs to help you with it. Why shouldn't it be the doctor?!?!? Ok, there I go again, sorry!

My genetic questions were causing family to reexperience painful memories—just another thing to feel guilty about. Not only was I concerned for my immediate family and my children experiencing suffering for me, I was also concerned that my diagnosis was hurting my cousin Kitt, who followed my story closely. Both her parents died from cancer—her mom, who is my aunt on my dad's side, died from breast cancer and her dad died from colon cancer. She had passionate feelings from those losses that I am not sure she had ever been able to express before. I hope that somehow providing me with the information I needed allowed her to vent and move past the anger she still had.

FB: April 23, 2012

I don't know if I should feel honored or worried that many of Dani's friends want to see me. I'm *not* going to die. I'll see them this summer.

Lola: You should be honored that the young busy people are taking the time to let you know how significant you are and have been in their lives!

Marcy: I do feel that way but also worry they are thinking I won't make it. Maybe they just want a free lunch, LOL. I am close to a lot of her friends, others not so much, so am a bit surprised that some of them asked to see me.

KO: Dude, you're their second mom, it happens with cool moms.

Marcy: That made me smile. Nick, my daughter's best friend, wrote that in a letter to me. I would gladly have him as a son.

FB: April 24, 2012

Why can't I lose armpit hair and leg hair first? It is starting and I haven't even gotten the second chemo yet. I will probably shave my head tonight or tomorrow after work. So be it. I lose hair every time I touch my head but still have to pluck chin hair? That is just wrong!

PG: You will be beautiful!! BTW, my girlfriend (six-year survivor) highly recommends contacting the American Cancer Society for information on their Beauty and Pampering local events. Awesome!!

Looking forward to lunch with my big sister after chemo. Time to kick some big cancer butt!

CB: April 24, 2012

Better Blood Counts

Blood counts are awesome. Getting chemo now!

Feeling Better

Okay, so I try not to express my doubts to everyone but since I did share the concern over my CBC, I thought it would be good to give you an update. Wow! The Neulasta injection the day after chemo works! Knowing how effective it is will make it easier to deal with any bone pain I may have. My labs are actually *better* than before I started chemo in the first place. The second week they went on the up up up. Today, I actually made sure every little drop of chemo was out of the IV bag, my little Pac-Mans eating away at the cancer cells! I liked the nurse practitioner as well as I liked the oncologist and I think my oncology nurse that gives the chemo is great too (and being in the medical field I can be a little judgmental).

I'm finding out there is more family history of cancer. At least now I know. We have learned that when someone in the medical field asks, "Is there cancer in your family?" the response "Not that I know of" is not an acceptable answer. You have to ask the questions of your family or you won't know. I have found out that two paternal aunts had breast cancer and 1 cousin on the paternal side had breast cancer. My father comes from a family of six and at least three had skin cancer, including my dad but he didn't think it was "cancer" so he didn't tell me. Carcinoma is cancer, and now he knows. My grandma's colon cancer and stomach cancer, which I know all too well, was the only one I remembered at the start of all this!

All this information will be given to the genetic counselor in May, plus whatever I collect from my mom's side of the family. The genetics person can decide if it is significant. Many aren't genetically significant but that is not my call. If the family history and genetic counseling will change the screening recommendations for the younger generation, it is worth the time and money to do it.

Now, about the hair. It was starting to come out and it is gross to me when that happens. The flyaway hair when I touch my head and my clogged sinks are yucky. So after chemo today it was shaved. Looks funny because of the dark brown stubble, but when the stubbles come out it will be lighter and stubbles are easier to clean up than longer hair. Found cute little hats at....wait for it......K-Mart. I think they will do just fine! And by the way, not only does my hair dresser (sister-in-law) say I have awesome hair, she also said I have a "perfectly shaped head". My mom used to tell me that for being almost ten pounds when I was born I had a perfectly shaped head. So there! LOL.

It was a good day today. Thanks for keeping up with me. EVERYONE has been awesome! A big shout-out to my sister for keeping me company today.

Stay safe and be healthy, Marcy

P.S. Does my shadow scare you?

Marcy: For a couple days with the dark stubble, I look like GI Jane. Kickin' A

Clara: GI Jane kicked some major butt, looking hot doing it!!! As I know you do!

Miriam: GI Jane ain't got nothin' on you!

Hannah: If not for this, I never would have known how much your head is shaped the same as Riley's.

Marcy: You all are awesome and Hannah, you made me giggle-snort because I see it! Riley and I do have heads shaped the same!

CR: Who would have thought it would be handy for a woman to have a nicely shaped head? Truly, Marcy, it is not the shape of our heads or our bodies that matters, but the shape of our hearts and our souls, but, still, you do have a beautiful head.

Figure 1-7. Photo of my shadow after shaving my head for the first time

Being bald didn't worry me. I can't even say I was embarrassed or felt like I had to cover my head. I would have never imagined it would be handy to have a nicely shaped head! However, some of the little things about this process annoyed me. Every time I touched my head I got a handful of stubble, when I laid down I would leave black stubbles covering my pillow. More would come out when I changed my clothes. Overall I was thankful I had been gradually cutting my hair and didn't have to see large chunks of my long, thick hair coming out or clogging my drains. For the next weeks though, I spent much time trying to undo behaviors that I never even realized were so ingrained that I never had to think about them—the first time I held my bath towel and flipped my head down to wrap my wet long hair was a bit of a reality check. Those little changes in my routine and the inconveniences and worries of the cancer treatment started to add up into something more soul-chilling.

But I tried to deal with each new effect as it appeared. My scalp became sensitive for the first few weeks, similar to how it feels when you never walk barefoot and then step on concrete for the first time. I never wanted to wear wigs or expensive frilly scarfs. I did have some hair coverings and bandanas but I mostly wore hats. It was fun to shop for them.

The thing that brought me the most discomfort but took me awhile to identify was the look of pity and sometimes curiosity from people, often strangers, who weren't yet aware of my illness. The bald head was the first external physical sign that gave away that I was sick. It was a look that became very familiar to me and that affected me the most, which is why I often turned to humor to deal with the changes that I went through and covered my head most of the time.

FB: April 24, 2012

Here's to hoping the large dose of steroids don't keep me awake all night like it did last time I had chemo. I am hoping I can offset it with Xanax or Benadryl. Decisions, decisions. Alarm goes off at 5:15 a.m. tomorrow for work.

FB: April 25, 2012

PG posted on Marcy's wall: Marcy, I love seeing all the humor, support, friendship and love that you get from all your Facebook friends. But I think you would be shocked to know how many of my Facebook friends ask me how you are doing, and tell me they are praying for you. Some of them don't even know you. Anyway, you've got all kinds of good vibes being sent your way that you don't even know exist. You deserve each one of them!

FB: April 27, 2012

Although I will not walk at Relay for Life tonight as originally planned before I was diagnosed with cancer, I will drop off nourishment for the HHS [my workplace, a high school] team. Today I made an appointment to get a free wig, thanks to donations to American Cancer Society! Although I never saw myself wearing one, Riley asked me to wear one to his 8th grade promotion. If it makes him feel better, I will do it. If you haven't donated already and are able to, please donate. Best of luck to all those walking tonight and thank you for doing it!

FB: April 30, 2012

My goal on this Monday back to work is not to cry but instead be grateful that I have a job and health insurance. I am appreciative of the awesome people I work with.

I was so excited to be going to the second annual Chicago Cubs rooftop game with a group of faculty and staff from the high school. I was feeling pretty good since my last chemotherapy was April 25 and the game was on May 5. We all would meet at the rooftop since we were coming from different directions and most of us were on different train routes.

The excitement of being at baseball games was something that gave me energy. I got bored watching baseball on television but live games I enjoyed. When there wasn't action on the field there was usually action in the stands. I loved people-watching.

I felt normal being with my coworkers. I think I felt normal because they treated me normally. They all joked with me as they had prior to my diagnosis. They didn't coddle me or give me advice. When we were on the rooftop, we weren't teachers, nurses, secretaries, or administrators, we were just Cub fans. This game against the LA Dodgers ended in a loss, something we Cub fans are accustomed to.

A bunch of my coworkers were going to hang out in the sports bars in Wrigleyville but I was learning not to push myself and opted to head home. As we were making our way down the stairs, I saw an empty cup. Aware there was an elderly man coming down the stairs behind me, I picked up the cup to throw it away so no one tripped on it. The man behind me said, "Thank you sir."

I was taken aback for a moment. Does he think I am a man because I am wearing the doo-rag my brother Steve gave me? Certainly I don't look male. When I turned to look at him, the look of shock was clear on his face. He corrected himself by saying, "I'm sorry ma'am." I guess from the back maybe I looked like a man with that head covering.

Even with a Cubs loss and being misgendered, it was one of the good days I would hold onto. Even then I was pretty sure the good days would lessen as the treatments continued.

CB: May 9, 2012

Roller Coaster

So it has been a little more than two weeks since beginning chemotherapy. I know I have been quiet on here and I guess that is just me. When things get a little more roller-coastery I have a tendency to be quiet to try to work things out in my head. I have talked about some of it and appreciate all the support I get from family and friends. My biggest issue after the last chemo was going to the American Cancer Society for a wig. Sitting and looking at myself in the mirror with a wig on was harsh. It wasn't hard to cut my long hair or even to shave my head but getting a wig really affected me. I looked at myself, or at least I think it was me, and thought of Riley. The only reason I am getting a wig is for him and it made me cry a little (trying to keep it together in public or I would have bawled). I want to be there for him as he grows up. My sister-in-law, Patti, had no idea what I was doing just a half an hour earlier when she called to check on me. She knew something was wrong because when she asked how I was, I couldn't talk. I was driving in the car with my mom. I had to keep it together. We went right over to her house instead of going home. She assured me she could work with the wig. The thing that really touched me though was what my big brother Steve did. Sometimes I don't know how things in our family are affecting the men. They don't talk about feelings or show them much. When I got there he had a gift for me: A motorcycle-type doo-rag (do-rag, dude-rag, whatever you want to call it). At the Harley Davidson store the cashier asked if I ride when he said he was buying it for his sister. He said, "No, she has cancer." It just meant a lot to me that he was thinking of me and my bald head, and protecting it from the sun. I remembered when I was young, he was my protector from the outside world (he could "rough and tumble" me all he wanted but no one else could get to me…at least that's how I saw it). I wore the doo-rag to the Cubs rooftop game last Saturday. Awesome day with my coworkers!

I have the rest of the week off from work and won't see many of the senior students again. I felt so emotional and tearful. There is a particular senior student I have been working with and I felt compelled to tell him this: "My two hopes for your future are: 1) You take better care of yourself so you can live into your twenties, thirties, forties, and beyond, and 2) When you get to my age you don't have to look back at your choices with as much regret as I do. I hope that your theme song for your life doesn't become 'I Was Wrong' by Social Distortion." He gave me a hug and said he would come back and visit. So that is just some of the emotional/mental things I have experienced these past couple weeks. All these things have probably made my fatigue worse.

Physically, it is getting a little harder. I am more tired, bothered by reflux and indigestion, and it felt like there were sores in my esophagus. Unfortunately, it didn't keep me from gaining weight over the last two weeks. I don't eat well for a period of time and then make up for it by eating whatever, whenever. I need to stop doing that and eat healthier. Really, who gains weight on chemo? *Me!* I don't want to undo all the hard work I have done over the past year in Weight Watchers. The doctor gave me some more medicine to help with the indigestion and esophageal pain. He said to keep taking it until chemo is over.

Which brings me to the doctor's visit and chemo today. Since I have inflammatory breast cancer (IBC) the inflammation causes visible signs on my breast. The oncologist expected visual improvement with chemo. I can't tell a difference. He thinks that the dimpling, or orange peel appearance has improved and the skin thickening is less. That is great news. The nurses were as awesome as usual and I didn't have any issues with receiving the treatment. Hopefully, the headache and insomnia won't be too bad tonight.

Tomorrow I get the injection to stimulate the bone marrow to make blood cells.

I just want to feel good on Mother's Day to enjoy a late lunch at Beelow's Steakhouse with my children. I am looking forward to it. Since Dani works in the kitchen there, they told her she can come in later so she can eat with Riley and me before going back to the kitchen.

Maybe if I updated more often I wouldn't have such a huge entry.

TTFN

GC: I think the "doo rag" makes you look bad ass! I love it!

Alan: Glad to read the update. A roller coaster offers more thrills than the kiddie rides anyway. And a doo-rag is way cooler than a Cubs hat any day. Life throws you challenges and you keep rising to meet them. We keep praying for you. Happy Mother's Day!

LM: I only just read your news on Facebook this morning and spent some time reading your Facebook posts and your journal. I just want you to know you sound so incredibly strong and wise about your journey to recovery. You are a great mom! I will be keeping up with you via online journal and Facebook, and know that your support team goes all the way to Kuala Lumpur, Malaysia!

CB: May 16, 2012

Overtired = Overemotional

Today was an overemotional day. (Thank you to all the people at work for letting me cry on your shoulders.) I think I was overtired. Riley had an issue in school and I worry about him a lot, so when I was trying to sleep (going to bed at 8 p.m. now) he was on my mind and the doubts and fears creep in. I want to stay positive but I end up thinking what if I am not around to keep him on track, etc. Things got better by the end of today but while we were eating Riley said, "Mom, I know you are going to be okay but what if you and Grandma both died before I graduated high school, who would I live with?" Children should *never* have those thoughts or ask those questions. It was sad to me that he didn't even consider Jack as an option. I reiterated that I planned on being around but did tell him what the plans were and who would have decision-making power, etc. I think he was okay with that but add that to him telling me a couple of days ago that I am "the sickest person he knows." I just feel terrible. I am trying not to "act sick" and I try to spend as much time as I can with him, even if it is being the disciplinarian. Which is my way of trying to keep things as normal as possible. I try to make sure he knows I am planning on being around but also that I have a plan for him if I am not. He said he has heard that this is a "rare and aggressive cancer." I told him that is true but that does not mean it is not curable and the doctors are planning on a cure. Am I telling him the right things? Does he get it?

I have a busy weekend ahead with a scrapbooking retreat. I will be leaving that for a few hours for my nephew's HS grad party and Riley's eighth grade grad party. I am so grateful to my sister-in-law Patti for doing all the work and doing a combined celebration. I just feel unprepared and overwhelmed. I want to do my scrapbooking. I planned this weekend last January. It is very important to me that the kids have the photos and stories that go with them but I don't feel like I have the time and energy. This weekend may end up being more about the "get-away" than the productivity.

I hope I am not "acting too sick" in front of my kids because I think it worries them more and then they have less hope. So I try to push on at home and at work but then I'm overtired/overemotional. Any thoughts or suggestions?

Betty: One day at a time sweet Marcy. I think about you every day and am keeping you in my prayers. God's strength be with you, We know His love always is. Love you.

Nora: Darling, beautiful, strong Marcy. Don't add any more doubt or concern to your plate than you already have. Your children will be strong because you are strong. Your children will be OK. This, I promise you… without doubt or uncertainty. They will be OK. Say that, over and over again. You are honest with them, you are fighting, and they will be there with you, beside you, in your heart and you in theirs. *That is all that matters.* As mothers we forget ourselves too often, worrying so much for the children we bear, we forget that they are ours... They are of us... And you, my dear are one of the strongest women I know, and that is how I know your babies will be fine, no matter what. Keep the good fight... So many people are standing beside you...even people who you don't talk to regularly, you are an inspiration here at HHS... We love you...*Stay strong!!* And we will be here to pick you up on days when strength may leave you for a bit.

CP: I agree with Nora: Dani and Riley will be OK. They are strong children and love you very much. Sometimes I wish I had your strength. I know you'll be around for years to come. You'll look back and see how strong you really were. You're in my thoughts and prayers. If you ever need anything, just call me. I am there for you! Love you.

DA: I know you want to show your kids that you are strong and you *are*. But it's okay to rest when you are tired too! That will only make you stronger in the end. I will keep your whole family in my prayers. You can beat this! Blessings.

Sally: Hey, hey, hey!! I'm looking forward to our weekend getaway! I'm packed and ready to go! Tomorrow work is going to draaaaaaaag by because I'll be counting every minute 'til we can leave!

JH: Marcy, "I have heard there are troubles of more than one kind. Some come from ahead and some come from behind. But I've bought a big bat. I'm all ready you see. Now my troubles are going to have troubles with me!" By Dr. Seuss. Keep fighting!! I hope and pray for your health and strength everyday

I spent a lot of time on the phone talking to Miriam, who is my high school friend living in Florida, and Hannah, my grade school friend who lives in Arizona. Especially when I had days like that day and was worried about my kids. They may have lived in faraway states but they were always available to listen. This is one of the times I called and said hi and then there was a long silent pause as I began crying over the phone. I knew they would be comfortable with the silence as I tried to stifle the sobbing in order to tell them how I felt.

Liza especially was the person I could go to when I needed to verbalize my wishes. Most people were uncomfortable if I brought up plans for my family if I died. I would get responses like "Don't talk that way," "Have hope," and "Stay positive." Liza understood that it was important for me to plan for the worst while I hoped for the best. We spent a lot of time on my loveseat talking about the future of my kids if I wasn't around. I can't remember one instance when she told me not to feel a certain way.

CB: May 17, 2012

What a Difference a Day Makes

I feel better! What a difference supportive friends, family, and time makes. Thank you all for the guestbook comments, emails, and hugs both in person and virtual.

I was very productive at work today, which makes me feel better about the end of the school year and the preparations needed for the next school year. I am not as worried about not being there at the beginning of the year [fall] as I was before. Unfortunately, the timing for my surgery will probably be right as faculty and staff are expected back to work.

About this weekend; I took a lot of stress off myself by deciding not to focus on the pictures this weekend. I have a book called "Reflections from a Mother's Heart—Your Life Story in Your Own Words." I have had it for years and years and it is only partially done. My grandma filled out the one I gave her. When she was dying from stomach cancer she could no longer see well and write, she dictated to my mom and she wrote it in. It was important enough for her to finish though, partly because I asked her to do it and partly because I think she wanted to leave something behind that she knew would bring me comfort. It is something I cherish. Her stories, advice, and history remind me that I can be strong, it is in my blood. My mom has the same book, because I also bought her one. If we all do it, there will be three generations of "Reflections" for my children to read.

I will take the scrapbook I haven't finished journaling in and journaling supplies and my laptop so I can organize digital photos. I also have a book for each of my kids called "What I Love about You." It gives prompts to tell your kids things you love about them. Although they aren't little anymore, I hope they will like it someday and it will get the thoughts going for me to write to them. I bought one also for my oldest child. Although I only had him five months, I hope I can fill some of it in, maybe someday we will know each other again and I can fill more in later. I wish all three kids could be together. The decision of what I will be working on at the scrapbook retreat is an utter relief. I don't have to organize and pack as many supplies and carry as much to the car and into the hotel, etc. I am not pressuring myself to finish everything so if I want to walk around Lake Geneva, go to the pool or just take a nap, I *will*, guilt free.

Thanks again for all your love. I hope you know how much I love you back.

EM: May 17, 2012

From: Alan

To: Marcy

Hey Marcy,

Kids are more insightful than you know, and smarter too. Over the years when a parent brings in a sick child I've evolved to the point where I get my history from children as young as two or three if you can believe it. They're also better equipped to handle the roller coasters of life. That's why they're the ones on the roller coasters at the amusement park.

It's OK to have a bad day. It's best that the kids see the real you—good and bad. They'll be ok. You'd be surprised.

It's also wise to plan breaks and rests into your schedule. I live in chronic pain. For every event I plan on a weekend I plan a corresponding rest period, a "take care of myself" period if you will.

The weather has been magnificent. When I'm off on weekdays my dog and I go to the park, lay on a blanket and look up at the trees and the sky. It doesn't get any better.

Sometimes I wonder if the dinosaurs had the same experience on a day like this four hundred million years ago. I suggest you take the kids to the park, lay on a blanket and look up at the sky.

Be yourself and remember you genuinely love your kids. You can't do them wrong if you follow those principles.

Celebrate the good things and reach down deeper to overcome the bad. And know that a lot of people are rooting for you.

From: Marcy

To: Alan

Thank you so much, sounds like a plan. This makes me cry too.

I never wondered about the dinosaurs but sometimes when I am looking at fields, woods and the environment, I wonder what it looked like to the pioneers and how they got through it. I think I would have enjoyed the simplicity but hard work of the pioneer days. Thanks again.

From: Alan

To: Marcy

I was laying in the park with my dog today. A bird was chirping off to our left and then one would chirp back off to our right. It was kinda cool. Fortunately, no birds pooped on us, and we were not stomped on by a dinosaur.

I know your driving force is to be there for your kids. It's probably also your greatest source of worry. But you wouldn't have it any other way. I admire you for that. I wish and pray for the best. Take it easy.

From: Marcy

To: Alan

That is awesome!

Thanks for that. You are right about the biggest driving force and the greatest source of worry and you are also right, I wouldn't have it any other way. That is probably one reason my marriage failed, I couldn't put him before my kids and he couldn't live without being number one.

Quick medical question...is there any reason I can't go in a public pool? My WBCs seem to bounce back with the shot I get. I definitely would stay out of the hot tub, but I think the pool would feel nice.... No hair to get in my face, LOL.

I feel so much better today!

From: Alan

To: Marcy

A public pool is generally extremely safe. They are chlorinated so well that they're practically sterile. The only downside is dry skin. It's like swimming in bleach.

I'd avoid a hot tub though. They can grow pseudomonas at high temps which is not a concern in a pool. Use lots of sunscreen.

CB: May 20, 2012

Nice Weekend

Hi all, I hope you had a great weekend. My weekend is pretty much done, I'm tired and just glad to be home. I enjoyed the retreat. I took Christmas photo cards and put them in an album. It was nice to have them easy to look at and not in a shoe box somewhere. I did some writing and that was about it.

My sister-in-law Patti did an excellent job with the boys' graduation party and it was nice to visit with everyone. I love that my family has a sense of humor about all this. Many men in my family have a shiny head like mine. I teased them that I went bald to support male-patterned baldness, and bring awareness for them.

SS: Glad you had such a good weekend...sounds pretty busy to me. Happy you got to spend time with your family as well. Love you.

Abby: Hi Marcy, it was great to see you this weekend! I'll be thinking of you, especially as I look for those yummy Skinny Cow bars at the store! Stay strong, and I look forward to seeing you in January!

Alan: Hi Marcy, Glad you had a nice weekend. Looks like everybody had fun. That's what it's all about.

EM: May 22, 2012

From: Marcy

To: Alan

Hey you,

So it is my understanding that this type of cancer feeds off estrogen? I recently read a study that says stress levels can increase estrogen. More food for the cancer cells? I am not good at evaluating the accuracy or reliability of those type of studies and just wondering if you know anything about that.

I am sure my stress level will go down when work and school is over for the summer and when I get some financial stuff taken care of but just curious how much, if any, effect it has. Definitely need to go lie in a park somewhere.

From: Alan

To: Marcy

Hey Marcy,

The term "steroid" is a general category. There are basically three types—cortisones, male hormones (testosterones) and female hormones (estrogens and progestins).

Cortisones increase in times of stress with mostly beneficial effects. There is no significant conversion of cortisones to estrogens caused by stress and I sincerely doubt stress increases estrogen levels to a significant extent.

I believe in the mind-body relationship and the importance of being positive.

More specifically, I believe you need to enjoy yourself when you can and, at times, forget that you have cancer. Just live like you normally would as much as possible.

You had a great weekend with friends and family. Felt good, right?

I live in chronic pain but I get in bed at night and review the fun and accomplishments of the day, I smile and go to sleep. One more day of getting the most out of life with the limitations we're given.

I doubt stress has a direct biochemical effect on cancer via estrogens. I've never heard or read that.

Hang in there. Beautiful day to lie outside.

From: Marcy

To: Alan

Thanks, believe it or not, sometimes I do forget I have cancer, until I look in the mirror or something. I mostly have been living my life like I usually do with some changes of course.

Looking forward to the summer and getting scrapbooking done and spending time with family and friends.

Tonight I am looking forward to Riley's eighth-grade promotion and cake!

From: Alan

To: Marcy

Cake is always good!

When I look back at my calendar and the stories I posted on social media and the online journal, I never really talked about Riley's eighth-grade promotion. Maybe because it was one of the worst days of the year, at least to that point. Considering I put it "all out there," my life was and is an open book and yet for some reason I never wrote about this day. I wrote about the wig, the scrapbook retreat, and the graduation party, but I never wrote about the graduation day itself.

I didn't want to ask Riley about that day, what he remembered from it. I fear I made it a bad day for him, or maybe I'm afraid that it would turn what he remembered as a good day into a bad one. If he knew how awful I felt about that day would it change his memory of that milestone? I hope he remembers the fun family graduation party we had thanks to his Aunt Patti. When I talked to Roger as I started trying to fill in the gaps, he said he could remember that we were separated and I ended up alone. Even with "chemo brain," I seem to remember a bit more about this than Roger, my mom, or Dani.

The chemo brain plus the emotions combined to make it one of the worst days ever. I am hesitant to even write about it almost five years later as I don't want Riley to feel bad about that day. I was truly happy for him and proud of him, but I was in survival mode, trying to get through the day the best way I knew how. One foot in front of the other.

Since we'd already had a party for him, the night's events were just going to include the five of us—my mom, Roger, Dani, Riley, and me. Ceremony, then home for cake and ice cream. For some reason I thought it would be a good idea to drive in separate cars so I could get seats when I took Riley, and the other three could come a little later. The ceremony was at a church and combined the district's two middle schools in one ceremony.

After we were all dressed and ready, I reminded them that a few pictures were needed. I actually didn't want to be in the pictures, but since I have always been the one who forced them to do it I wasn't going to duck out of it. I knew that they would eventually come to appreciate the photos and scrapbooks. We took pictures in the front of the house.

From the moment the wig went on my bald, sensitive head, the day went downhill. The wig felt scratchy. I hated wearing it. Even though Patti trimmed it up to improve the style, when I looked in the mirror it wasn't me that I saw. I saw a sick person I didn't recognize. For some reason it was easier to be bald and recognize myself in the mirror than it was to wear that damn wig. However, since Riley specifically asked me to wear it, I did, and kept the irritation to myself, contrary to my usual openness.

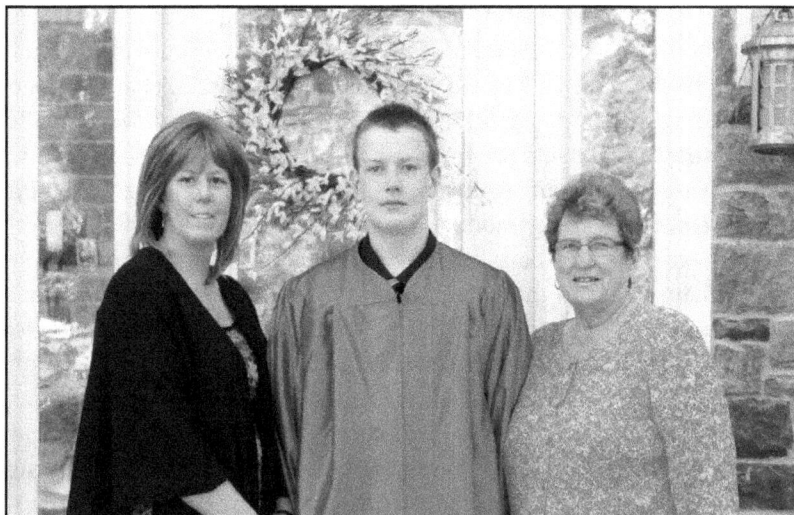

Figure 1-8. Me, Riley, and my mom before Riley's graduation ceremony

While driving there I realized that not only did I leave my cell phone at home but I left the tickets too. The traffic was horrendous. I advised Riley to call Roger and tell them to leave right away and also to look for the tickets on my desk, which is where I thought I had left them. After I dropped Riley off at the location he was to line up at, I was able to get in without a ticket and save seats. I was getting anxious about them not being able to find me as the start of the ceremony was drawing nearer. I left my belongings on the seat and started walking in the foyer back and forth trying to locate them. I felt really disconnected. When I saw some of the parents I knew I didn't stop to say hi as I would have normally done—they would have recognized me in a hat or bandana but not the wig.

Riley had taken his phone with him so I wasn't even able to call them to update them on where I was sitting. The announcement was made that the ceremony was beginning. I had to go back to my seat alone. I learned later that they were able to get seats elsewhere and were able to get in without tickets, and that they also had been walking around trying to find me until the announcement to sit was made. Most of the time I don't really care much about what people think of me as far as my looks go, but as I sat there I couldn't help but think that people had to know I was wearing a wig.

I spent the rest of the ceremony silently crying. Crying because Riley has been through so much with being bullied, health issues of his own, the divorce, and moving away from his friends. Crying because I thought I wouldn't be around for any more graduations. Crying because I was alone.

After the ceremony, the crowd was overwhelming. I didn't have a phone or a meeting point. I couldn't find anyone. It seemed like forever. I finally asked a stranger if I could use their cell phone, I called Riley and told him where I was so I could drive him home. I told him to call Roger and tell him to go ahead and take my mom and Dani home. By the time we were all together again, I was exhausted and so relieved to be home. Immediately the wig came off and the pajamas went on. When we discussed what happened with being separated and me forgetting the phone and tickets, I began to get tearful. Not much was said after that and I felt they were disheartened by the frustration and sadness they saw in me.

When I lay in bed that night, all I could do was think about the fear of leaving my kids. The embarrassment of not being able to handle my emotions. The despair and the anger. Anger at cancer and what the treatment was doing to me and my relationships.

Emotions were starting to become more difficult to manage as the chemotherapy continued. My friend Lola told me that I had "'roid rage." She asked to go out to brunch, I agreed only if she let me pay. I know what it is like being a single mom without support and Lola worked so hard, so I wanted to pay for brunch. When she gave the waitress her credit card behind my back, I got angry and raised my voice. It proved even more the 'roid rage. I felt terrible about my deplorable behavior. I didn't want to hurt her or anyone else but steroids magnified my emotions, and I wasn't sure how to let other people take care of me. Allowing others to care for me was something I would learn later, the hard way.

CB: May 25, 2012

Medical Update

Hi all, although there is a lot to say, my brain is a little tired. Just the update. Chemo number 4 is done. Next time, June 7, I switch to another drug. I will be in the oncologist's office about five hours including the doctor appointment. I actually think I can see and feel improvement, especially in the density of the affected breast. I saw the genetic counselor today and did proceed with some testing although she thinks the chances of this being genetic and being passed on to my children or that my siblings have it is about 10 percent. It is important to know because if I have the genes we are testing for it puts me at greater risk for ovarian cancer and I may opt to have them removed. To me that is worth the effort to test for.

I'm relieved to be done with work for a couple months. My focus this summer is going to be spending time with people. I have scheduled some dates already. I plan on resting, organizing, and scrapbooking. I hope you all have a great weekend, keep in touch.

Alan: Scrapbooking is a lot of fun. I'm not sure why but when I get home from an event or a trip I like to put on music and work on my scrapbooks. I started doing this when I was seven or eight before I knew it had a name. I'm up to volume thirteen or fourteen. There's just something about recording memories in that manner that's enjoyable.

But I'll tell you what's even more fun. Looking back through scrapbooks and smiling and remembering. Here's hoping for many more volumes.

You're in our thoughts and prayers,

Sophie and Alan

CB: May 26, 2012

Thank You

I just want you all to know I read all the guestbook comments, sometimes more than once. I wish this was set up more like Facebook so I could acknowledge the comments individually. Thank you all for keeping up with me and for your support.

FB: May 29, 2012

So you know how when things are not going well in your life you think, there are people who have it worse right now? My friend said when things get tough, she thinks of me, because I have it worse. I'm not really sure how I feel about that.

Hannah: It could be worse. You could still be married.

Marcy: I was just talking about that today. When I asked him to take a few minutes to call insurance, make sure Riley's school vaccine was covered, and order his generic allergy medication, he sent an email with the subject "Medical crap." Can you imagine if he had to deal with any of this cancer stuff? I would feel guilty that he had to spend time and money to help me fight my "medical crap." I never called his broken hip or giving him allergy injections every week "medical crap." I am so grateful I am going through this with friends and family as a single person vs. being married to Jack.

Thinking about making a new playlist, since the next four rounds of chemo will take four to five hours. So help me out. Is there a song that makes you think of me and why? Did it come out when we met, did we do an activity together while it was playing, do the lyrics make you think of me? Tell me what song it is and it will go on my playlist and be our song forever.

SV: Sorry but it's Sir Mix-a-Lot, "Baby Got Back." I like big butts and I cannot lie... *and* the reason is I remember that playing when we went to the FDN picnic.

Marcy: I will definitely add that. When I worked in endoscopy and had to have a colonoscopy, I made a CD they could play while I was under anesthesia, to crack them up, this was the first song. Well done!

SV: Thank you.

SB: The Judds, "Love Can Build a Bridge"...or anything by Alabama.

Marcy: Great song, I would have never guessed that made you think of me. Remember how many times we heard "La Bamba" and "Heart" on the way to Canada for our canoe trip. Sheeesh.

HC: Marcy, it will always be Shakira's "Hips Don't Lie." I have fond memories of being down in the "dungeon" [former medical clinic's basement] and singing that song and watching you dance. Now add it to your playlist and cut a rug.

Marcy: I thought you were going to say that... Good times!

SB: Rock of Ages.

Marcy: Love me some Def Leppard! There are so many awesome songs, trying to narrow it down to one or two. That was the first concert I took Dani to. Lots of high school memories too. I think one of the songs will have to be "Nine Lives"!

JG: Rush, "Closer to the Heart." Couldn't tell you why, just always has.

Marcy: JG, I love Rush, that's going on my list and I'll think of you. In my opinion Rush had one of the best drummers ever!

SW: I remember when we first connected on Facebook and I saw you were "friends" with Dio. I thought that was cool! So, if you have a favorite Dio song... My personal fave is "Holy Diver."

Marcy: "Holy Diver" it is!

Clara: Any Alanis Morrisette song pretty much makes me think of you.

Marcy: Yep, we listened to it a lot when Dani and I first moved back from Springfield. I'll pick one and think of you. Love ya.

Marcy: Will have to add "Closer to Fine" by Indigo Girls and think of CS. I remember my awful first studio apartment. She brought her guitar over and sang that song. So much talent, I was in awe.

Marcy: Clara, probably would have to be "Ironic." I remember driving in my car with you in the shotgun and Dani in her car seat in the back. I miss those days sometimes when you all were little.

Lola: I read your journal and am inspired by the strength and positive attitude you display. I know there are bad days and I wish more than ever that I had more time to spend with you, helping you and just, well, snoring on your couch! Know that you are *always* in my thoughts and prayers. My suggestions for music that will always bring us memories, let's face it, a little or a lot of Def Leppard. When you listen to it *please, please, please* don't forget the visual of the guitar player. And the rest of the good memories we have shared. To the moon and back with love.

Alan: Well I put a lot of thought into this. I reviewed four decades of songs in my head all day. I'm going back to 1980 with this one (when I was a Bison). What song does a tough girl need on her iPod? "Hit Me With Your Best Shot" by Pat Benatar. A good playlist makes time fly.

Good luck!

CB: May 29, 2012

Good News/Bad News

Grab a coffee or drink of your choice, this may be a long one.

I'll start with today and work my way back a few days, with good and bad news.

Today I saw my surgeon for the first time since she sent me to the oncologist. She is pleased with the appearance of the breast, as there has been physical improvement. She scheduled me for a double mastectomy with lymph node removal on the right side for August 13. I will not have reconstruction so she thinks I will only need to take three weeks (maybe two) off work. Then radiation will follow that. My last chemo is July 19 because she wants me to recover from chemo before surgery and that was the closest date she felt I will be in good enough shape that also coincided with her surgery schedule. The timing seems okay because I can work the week before to get Hamilton HS ready to go and also get Riley ready to start his freshman year.

This last round of chemo really seemed to get to me, maybe the heat didn't help, maybe it all caught up to me. I didn't do anything all weekend. I was supposed to go see Liza Sunday at 4 pm but cancelled because I just didn't want to sit up that long to drive and visit. I spent a lot of time on the couch. I now know that I can be very sick and tremendously tired but when my baby girl called at 4:20 p.m. and said she was in a car accident, I jumped up off the couch and beat the ambulance to the hospital. They did a CT of her head and abdomen and a chest x-ray because of the abrasions from the seat belt and the burns from the air bag. She was discharged to come home after about five hours. She is okay but totaled her car, no one else was hurt. I am very grateful she is alive with only minor bruises and abrasions.

The part that was really difficult for me and made me cry in the emergency department didn't even involve her accident. They brought a man in next door to us who had chemo on Friday. He got sick, the family was making end-of-life decisions and he was given about twenty-four to thirty-six hours to live. We couldn't help hearing all of these conversations outside of our room. At one point Dani asked, "Could that happen to you?" I told her "*No!* Different cancer (his was pancreatic), different situation." It was so hard to listen to, I felt heartbroken for them and for Dani to even have that as a concern. I don't ask "Why me?" but I often ask, "Why do my kids have to go through this, and will I ever see my firstborn child again?"

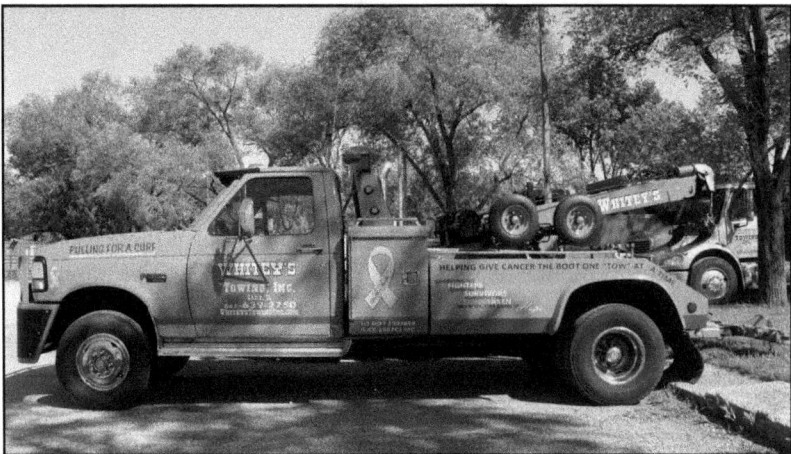

Figure 1-9. Whitey's Towing Breast Cancer tow truck

Today after I saw the surgeon I had a wonderful lunch with a coworker Monica, who has been by my side since I started working at school district D601. She helped me get involved with summer camp nursing, helped get me consistent work at D601, and she has always been supportive. I need more time with friends like that.

Lots of running around today, productive but exhausting. The last stop for the day was going to get the "junk" out of Dani's car. It was bittersweet when I saw the damage. I know if she didn't wear her seatbelt or have an airbag she could have been hurt much worse. When we pulled into Whitey's towing, I saw the pink tow truck. This truck made me cry. It had this painted on it; "In Memory of Debbie, 1970–2011" She was only 41, that is two (almost three) years younger than me. The truck said, "Helping give cancer the boot one 'tow' at a time. Supporting the fighters, Admiring the survivors, Honoring the taken, and never, ever giving up Hope."

Now, I am home and exhausted, physically and emotionally. I am with my mom and two of my babies (well, not babies, teenagers) and life is okay. We are here and safe.

Take care and be safe, Love you.

JH: I am glad Dani is okay and that everything is moving ahead with your treatment. Stay positive…it's inspiring.

Mia: Hi Marcy, I have been thinking about you and I stopped by now to read your last entry. I'm so glad your baby girl is ok. Hang in there my friend, keep strong, better days will be here before you know it. We send you lots of hugs and kisses…love you!!!

EM: May 30, 2012

Subject: Song Suggestion

From: Marcy

To: Alan

From a fellow Bison, thanks. I forgot you were a Bison but I know we talked about it before. I have ["Hit Me With Your Best Shot"] in my iTunes, will definitely put it on my playlist and think of you when it plays.

I have lots of fun activities planned this summer, it will be a great summer in spite of all of this. I actually played laser tag for the first time today.

Okay, I admit it, I sucked, but I couldn't be a "dry hair" mom and let Riley have all the fun, so I did try one round.

I made an appointment to go see the counselor Jack and I saw before the divorce. Mostly for keeping me on track, especially when things get hard with the kids.

I hope you are having a good week.

From: Alan

To: Marcy

My philosophy on life is... You take care of your family, You do right by others, you do what you need to do to live, and you squeeze in as many good times as possible. I saw a therapist for a while when I wasn't working. I found a tremendous therapeutic benefit just from talking out loud to an objective listener. A little counseling is good for the soul. Have a good evening.

FB: May 30, 2012

Okay peeps, I have ten songs, forty-nine minutes, that is going to be over quick. What else makes you think of me or me think of you? Did it come out when we met, did we do an activity together while it was playing, do the lyrics make you think of me or will it make me think of you? Tell me what it is and it will go on my playlist and be our song forever. I have to say I have such a variety in those ten songs, heavy metal, alternative, country, and rap.

Miriam: Wish I could get up there and we could headbang to our high school music!

Marcy: Someday, wait until the hair grows back so I "can let it down" LOL.

SS: Hi Marcy, I am a K-Love fan and the song that I have been listening to that reminds me of you is called "Live Like That" by Sidewalk Prophets. Will be thinking of you.

JH: I think this song is powerful and great to listen to, Alicia Keys "Superwoman." Sing along loudly!!

LM: We love you bunches and have you on all the prayer lists we know of! You were amazing with Megan and went out of your way to help her... You are such a giver. That being said, if you ever need something don't hesitate to ask! Meg is excited to be able to "walk" back into the school the first day back. So far she is on target for that. You are an inspiration to so many and when things get tough, just remember, we all know you can do this!!! Believe in yourself as much as we do!!! I can't think of a song for your playlist. The only thing in my head is the chant "Jamba-Juice" lol. Stay strong and never give up!!! Can't wait to see you back!!

It made me smile to be reminded of "the Jamba Juice Story." Meg, her mom, and I had worked together on the complicated aftercare needed following Meg's multiple leg surgeries, so Meg spent a lot of time in my school nurse's office with her mom. One time we were talking about putting full effort into what you want to accomplish and having the right motivation, I told them a personal story. When Riley and I were in tae kwon do we would often spar with each other. Sometimes he would barely lift his leg to kick or his arms to punch. Even his yelling was soft. I imitated his lackadaisical sparring for them, letting my arms flop like wet noodles. But when I told Riley we could go to Jamba Juice after tae kwon do if he really tried to fight me, he straightened up, the kicks were strong, and the punches were hard and in rapid fire. Every time he kicked me, he yelled, "JAMBA! JUICE!" I shouted that for them, and threw a roundhouse kick right there in my office.

I wanted to be a good role model for Meg. Even though she didn't have a song to recommend, I still thought of her and her mom during chemo when I was playing my music, smiling to myself as I replayed that day in my head.

EM: May 31, 2012

From: Marcy

To: Alan

Hey there, I don't think I have ever met Dr. Dunkin, although she told me my biopsy results on the phone when I called and asked for them. Gonna see her tomorrow for the first time, hopefully she can help me manage some of what might be chemo side effects related to dryness that the Replens (as suggested by the oncology NP) isn't helping with. Seems like I got a bit of itchy and dry areas, hopefully no infections.

So the note about scrapbooking, that was from Sophie, right? Any fun plans for the weekend or do you work?

From: Alan

To: Marcy

Hi Marcy, one of the products I like is RePhresh. It's mildly acidic to maintain the normal physiologic state which generally maintains the normal bacterial state.

I like Dr. Dunkin. I think she's a quality doc. Say hello if you think of it.

I'm actually the one who "scrapbooks," though mine are not traditional. My scrapbooks contain very few photos. Sometimes just one key photo from an event. It contains every ticket stub I've ever gotten, every boarding pass, every brochure from every tourist attraction I've been to, every hotel room assignment booklet, every card or matchbook from a restaurant/ meal of significance including the receipt from the meal, every table assignment from weddings and Bar Mitzvahs, every nametag from every conference, etc. If I go to something and there's something with a logo or company name on it then it goes in my scrapbook—sometimes it's just a napkin. I like looking back. I've been to more than I realize.

I just picked up my dog from the vet. He had knee surgery. We're gonna spend the weekend nursing him.

Hope yours is more fun!

Be good.

From: Marcy

To: Alan

That is so cool. The scrapbooks I had when I was younger were mostly memorabilia. I put some memorabilia in with my books/pictures, especially in the kids' school scrapbooks. But I really like telling the stories about the pictures. It is fun to look back. They act like they don't like pictures or sometimes make fun of me for the scrapbooking but they have been known to sit down and go through them page by page, Riley too. For their school albums I even got all their teachers to write to the kids. I put their little notes in the book. I think I realized how important journaling names and stories along with the pictures was when I worked for Dr. Douglass the neurologist. We took care of so many dementia patients.

I hope your doggie heals fast. How old is it?

Really? "Be good"? All I can say is, I will try to be good and if I can't I will be sure not to get caught. Now...where did I hear that advice from?

From: Alan

To: Marcy

Tommy is ten. He had his knee rebuilt yesterday including moving bone and metal plates. He's on Dilaudid but he won't share. We don't have pet insurance so we won't be getting new carpeting this summer. We lost our other dog in February—he was seventeen.

The only thing better than good memories is making new ones to add to the scrapbook.

Be good, or don't get caught!

From: Marcy

To: Alan

I got the book today that you sent to me. *You're Only Old Once!: A Book For Obsolete Children* by Dr. Seuss. Thank you so much, I heard of this book but never read it. I am going to read it to my mom in a few minutes. (Kind of backwards, instead of reading to my kids.)

FB: May 31, 2012

Ugggh, don't want to listen to these strangers tell horror stories about cancer while waiting for Riley at the dentist office. It's everywhere I go. I just want to forget for a while.

Sally: Pretend like you're deaf, maybe they'll leave you alone. Or you could just lean over and lick their face. That pretty much guarantees that they'll stop talking to you.

KB: Omg! Sally...almost laughed out loud in the quiet library!!! Marcy, I think pretending you're deaf leads to less germs!!

Sally: You gotta admit, if someone licked you in the face you'd leave them alone. Am I right or am I right?

Marcy: I can't even tell you how creeped out I get when I see people lick other people. I agree with KB, and would not risk the nasty germs. I did ignore them but my hearing is just too good and it was a small lobby. Just like having to listen to the family making end-of-life decisions on a cancer patient in the ER. I am much more aware and sensitive to those conversations.

Duh, wasn't even thinking that they wouldn't clean my teeth while I'm getting chemo due to infection risk. I should've known better.

Kitt: You can't think of everything all the time. You are human, ya know.

FB: June 1, 2012

Got two more prescriptions today. Since starting chemo two months ago, I have been given eight additional prescriptions, and recommended to take/use five over-the-counter medications plus what I was on before. I am glad those things are available to help me get through this but still it is very frustrating.

FB: June 5, 2012

Ahhh, which head covering should I wear today, doo-rag, baseball cap, wide brim straw hat... The options are endless.

Lola: The wide brim hat in a convertible while we run away sounds spectacular!

CB: June 6, 2012

I Don't Want To Go!

Ugggh, I don't want to go to chemo tomorrow. New stuff, a little nervous because it has been going fairly good so far and I'm a little afraid it will get worse. Whatever it takes though, it is only temporary.

Another great day today, spent the first part with Riley and my nephew Parker. The second half with Dani. I think it helps that I got to spend some fun times with them. I feel less guilty about the stuff I miss (so far it hasn't been a lot). I wonder if I will ever not feel guilty about all the times I wasn't there for Joey after placing him for adoption. I think about him so much. Being sick really makes a person do a life review.

I am hoping I feel up to going to a family birthday party in Wisconsin on Sunday. That is the plan.

DA: Hi Marcy, Glad to hear that chemo has been going well! Hopefully the new treatment will go just as well. Nice to take the time to do fun things!! Do what you can and enjoy it—let the rest go!

Alan: I think the scary part is not knowing how you'll feel afterwards. But you know in your heart whatever happens you can and will make the best of it. It must be hard to keep fighting but find strength in knowing that you're in a lot of people's thoughts and prayers, including mine. Feed off the energy of those cheering you on. I hope it goes smoothly.

FB: June 7, 2012

Kicking some big fat cancer ass right now! Listening to my playlist thinking specifically about each person who suggested them and the good times. It's making my "allergies" kick up bit.

CB: June 8, 2012

Roses and Thorns

Hi all,

When Riley was in Boy Scouts, after an activity or camp out we would often ask the scouts for Roses and Thorns. They had the opportunity to say what they didn't like or what could be done better (thorns) and what they enjoyed (roses). The catch was they couldn't do a thorn unless they had a rose, as they do go together. So this is my approach to this update. At the moment I think I have more roses, even some of the things that started as thorns became roses. So here it goes:

Rose: The biggest, most beautiful fragrant rose is the call I got from the genetic counselor today. I don't have the breast cancer gene mutation they tested for. There are other less likely genes but not at all worried enough to have them tested with less than a 1 percent chance it would be positive. She made some recommendations for Dani and myself and I will touch base with her if anything new comes up or every couple years to see what is new in the world of genetics.

Thorn that became a rose: Steroids give me insomnia and when I don't get enough rest I don't feel well and I am overemotional... Yeah, I know, nothing new. With the new chemo I have to take steroids the day before, day of and day after a treatment and Wednesday night I got less than two hours of interrupted sleep = *thorn*. Discussed this with my doctor and he gave me Ambien = *ROSE*. Last night I got about 9 hours sleep and when I did wake up, was able to go back to sleep quickly.

Rose: Saw my surgeon last week, she is pleased with the progress. I guess the advantage to this type of breast cancer is its effects are visible. When the cancer blocks the lymphatic vessels it causes inflammation and the orange peel appearance of the skin and a skin thickening you can feel as well as a fullness in the breast. All that has improved and the cancer is shrinking and not blocking those vessels as much. Can I get an "OH YEAH!"

Thorn: Immunosuppression has made the yeast in and on my body flourish; those opportunistic little bastards. The medication is helping but I know it is going to be a struggle to keep this under control.

Rose: The new chemo went well and didn't take as long as I was told. The playlist from my friends is growing and I think of my family and friends as I listen to my variety of music. It really makes time go faster and I feel so grateful for all the great memories you have all given me, whether I have known you for decades or months, don't underestimate how much you really do mean to me.

Thorn: The hot flashes and sweating as well as some of the emotions are in part because... the chemo did kick-start me into menopause. The steroids seem to cause "roid rage." I guess this just caused me to slam into it instead of a gradual thing. The way I look at it is, why not get it over with during this time period? Hopefully it won't outlast the breast cancer treatment.

Rose: I have spent some wonderful times with my kids and nephew, Parker. I have many visits with awesome people to look forward to. Activities upcoming include: horseback riding, camping, parties, hanging out with my niece Clara and my sister Becky, lunch with friends like PH, and Dani's graduation from Le Cordon Bleu and the ceremony in Chicago. *And* since I will get chemo two days before this and won't want to drive, take public transportation or stay in a hotel in Chicago, my mom is treating us to a limo. After the ceremony I will treat us to lunch at The Signature Room in the Hancock building. I will also get to see all of Dani's friends at a small get-together at my house. Dani has an awesome group of friends and I can't wait to see them all together again.

Thorn/Rose: To be determined: So far I feel good after the new chemo but the doctor did warn me some things that could occur are significant muscle pain that may start in a few days, worsening decrease in blood counts (will get it checked next Thursday) and my fingernails/toenails could discolor and separate from the nail bed causing some to fall off, ewwww. May not happen but at least I can be prepared and not freak out.

So those are the roses and thorns. I think the roses certainly are worth the few thorns.

Here is to hoping your roses are worth the thorns in your life. Stay safe and healthy,

Love, Marcy

FB: June 10, 2012

Okay, yeah, so this is the pain my oncologist warned me about. I just hope it doesn't last too long. I'm missing a birthday bash today for my great niece and great nephew. It makes me sad.

Lola: Anything you need??

Marcy: Someone to hit me on the head and knock me out for a couple of days? No, I'll be fine, it is good the family is going out, so I don't have to look pathetic in front of them. Thank you.

Lola: Maybe a piece of Portillo's chocolate cake can make it better?

Marcy: You bring cake and ice cream. I'll order pizza. What time?

Marcy: Riley's been wanting pizza and I'd love to see Hawk.

Lola: I will call you. I have Hawk. I can bring pizza.

Marcy: Yay, sometimes the spur of the moment stuff works out the best.

CB: June 14, 2012

The Truth Is... (Long Story)

Hey. The truth is I haven't updated in a week because I have had a rough time and don't want the truth of what I am experiencing to make anyone think I am not being positive or strong.

Honestly, I have moments where I feel weak and frustrated, emotional and beat down. At the same time, I know I could have it worse. The chemo caught up to me and I will tell you about that. Before I do, keep in mind, I know that as hard as it has been, I have not had to go to the hospital for transfusions, fluids or IV antibiotics. I feel awkward and embarrassed sharing my struggles and frustrations because I know there are young kids and elderly, getting the same, similar, or worse treatments.

So here is the physical update. I was feeling pretty decent after the new chemo. Docetaxel was started last Thursday. It took less time than I expected and I didn't have any immediate adverse reactions. The doctor gave me a sleeping pill to use around the days I have to take steroids prior to treatment (the steroids are to prevent fluid buildup). The previous yeast infection had improved and my throat felt a little better. Friday and Saturday were good, Saturday afternoon I started to get achy. Sunday I was really getting bone and muscle pain. Struggling to get comfortable, it hurt to move and it hurt to stay still. I alternated between acetaminophen and ibuprofen. I tried to decide which parts of my body hurt the worst and gave those parts the attention with the ice packs. I still had a nice visit with my friend Lola and her son Hawk. But the pain kept getting worse. Sunday night I took a Norco that Dani had from her car accident (I know, not supposed to do that...arrest me).

Monday morning the throat and chest pain were terrible and my body hurt so bad it was debilitating. I almost passed out but I made it up the stairs and called the doctor. They called in my own Norco for the muscle and bone pain. There was also a "swish and swallow" medicine with the assumption that this was a yeast infection in my esophagus. Yeast! Those opportunistic little bastards at it again. Turns out that medicine is specially mixed and only certain pharmacies make it. I couldn't even get it for twenty-four hours and my poor mother had to run all around for me to get it. I was on the couch and my sister-in-law, Patti, called to check on me. Of course, as usual, I couldn't talk at first, I could only cry. As I was crying suddenly my teenage son who usually acts like he isn't affected by anything, showed up with ice packs to try to make me feel better. Patti came over and eventually I calmed down. Taking the Norco helped but I still didn't have the swish and swallow medication.

Tuesday I had a very nice visit with my niece, Clara, and her husband, Todd, from Texas. It was so enjoyable to see them. I wasn't going to go to the pizza party that night but was asked/invited a couple times and so I did. The fantastic part about going was seeing one of my nephews, Kurt, who I had not seen in a while. When I got home I had a temp of 100.2. The threshold for calling the doctor is 100.5 so I didn't. In the meantime, the yeast rash was now in a lot of personal places, under my breasts and under my arms, etc. It was raw and starting to weep. I also noticed a small cut on my hand and on my foot that was getting a red circle around it. No streaks or drainage so thought I would see what things were like in the morning.

Wednesday morning, I called the oncologist and asked if I could come that day. I was scheduled for the next day for the CBC. I wanted to have them look at these skin things also. I told them about the minor temp the night before. Can I just say I very much appreciate and love everyone at the oncology office? The receptionist said, "Come in today, we will take care of you." Boy, did they ever. Such compassionate, patient, understanding and competent staff. Blood levels are out of whack but not terrible. Saw the nurse practitioner and got two more medications. I am now taking Diflucan orally for ten days for the yeast, which seems like it is everywhere and Cefadroxil to treat the bacteria areas that are raw and draining and the skin wounds that should have healed but have red circles around them.

So that brings me to today. Although those medicines will take time to work, I feel better knowing it is being treated. My throat and chest still hurt, especially when I swallow. I don't even enjoy my morning coffee anymore. Hopefully that will get better soon (probably in time for the next round of chemo). Again, this was a lot of complaining but now you know what it is really like. I have to say again...I'm grateful I am not in the hospital with complications that require fluids, blood, or IV antibiotics.

[....]

Today was a little better and I expect things will continue to improve over the next week until the next chemo. I am now concerned that I will not tolerate the next three chemo sessions since things got so much worse with this last one.

Thank you to those who helped me through this week in many different ways. I hope after reading this you still think I am "positive and strong." I am trying to be that for you...

Love ya, Marcy

P.S. Please forgive spelling and grammar on this long post. Too lazy to go proofread right now.

I wrote more to the CaringBridge journal entry, but was struggling between expressing my emotions and remaining private and tactful about family matters. Personal and medical issues were mixing more than I had ever expected.

When I brought my kids to a family get-together, feeling tired but happy to be there, I wasn't thinking it could be a potentially explosive situation. The short notice get-together at Steve and Patti's was planned because Clara was in town from Texas. I love that my family gets together to see the younger generation when they are available, and not just for holidays. My dad was a high school football and wrestling coach when he was a teacher and my five siblings played in a physical and competitive way. Over the years, the piles of Brownings wrestling on the floor grew, sometimes holding a few generations. But I had gotten more sensitive, so when my son and his cousins were roughhousing and running around in and out of the house I boiled over. All eyes turned to me when they heard me scream at them. I think they must have been in shock at my explosiveness. My reaction was more intense than usual in dealing with this and because I felt guilty about it, we left shortly after. I was upset that I couldn't keep my emotions in check.

On my post, my niece wrote to assure me she was still there for me.

Clara: Auntie M, it was amazing seeing you, and I feel so bad that maybe I pushed you to be out and perhaps that caused your high temp! I'm so sorry...I just wanted to spend as much time as I could with you. You are more than positive and every now and then it's OK to share your pains and frustrations, it's not good to keep them inside anyway. Without sharing you wouldn't be able to have as much support (hope this makes sense, it does in my head anyway). I can't help but to feel a little responsible for the situation. I love you so much and hopefully will be back once more before Christmas to see you! In the meantime remember always I think of you every day, most days all day and that I can't even begin to express the gratitude I have for all you have done for me and helped shape me into the woman I have become. As always, Your inspired niece

Message response to Clara: Being at the pizza party didn't cause my temperature, you didn't push me to overdo it. My temperature wasn't even very high. As we discussed on the phone Clara, no matter where I was, my body was going to do that due to an infection I developed myself. It was not from being tired or other people having germs. I probably had a low grade temp all day and didn't know it.

I have realized that over the years I became more uncomfortable with this type of play the more people got hurt and the more Riley got bullied. So yes, I was very sensitive to that, and during the chemotherapy that made me so emotional I stayed away from large family events. I loved visiting with my family but had to take visits in small groups. Being able to be with them was so important in my cancer journey. I needed to maintain my role and place in the family environment. I didn't want to be lost or excluded because people were afraid of getting me sick. I needed to be present with and for them. Sadly, that day I realized the cancer treatment would in fact affect my interactions: it wasn't going to be family business as usual.

EM: June 14, 2012

From: PH

To: Marcy

Your job is not to be strong for everyone else. You can be strong and positive for yourself and your kids. That's what is important...and if you cannot...so be it. I am sure that Riley and Dani will understand! Give yourself some slack...with all that you have been and are going through you are entitled to some down time! See you tomorrow. I hope that it is not going to be too much for you! If you have a hard time talking, it will be like when you had your braces on with the rubber bands! Love you.

From: Marcy

To: PH

I get what you are saying but sometimes I can't be strong for me. If it was just for me, I might not be as motivated to fight through this. Riley and Dani have really been great; I am so proud of them. I also want to be around for Joey (my firstborn that I placed for adoption), if he ever needs me.

I am doing better today.

EM: June 15, 2012

From: Alan

To: Marcy

Hi Marcy,

These things you've been going through sound pretty awful. It sucks to feel bad all the time. The thing is, don't make it worse by being hard on yourself. You don't have to be the perfect patient, mom, relative, friend.

You've been doing a hell of a job so far. Give yourself some credit. You're a strong woman but none of us are flawless. It's OK to lose it once in a while—everybody does—usually for a lot more trivial things than what you're going through.

Hoping and praying these things get better.

Your friend Alan

From: Marcy

To: Alan

Thanks, I am actually surprised I haven't lost it more than I have. My kids are so impressive (not trying to brag) but I cannot believe how well Dani and Riley have done with this. I am going to be glad when Riley goes to camp at the end of the month and is gone (but only ten miles away) for two weeks. He has been looking forward to it and I will feel good knowing he is active and having fun. I have begun to realize it is important for them to see the times that I need help. It is good for them to be able to help when they can. It gives them some power over the situation. Dani and I were talking yesterday how only strong people can admit and accept help. I'm working on that.

You have been a consistent cheerleader for me and you look really good in the skirt and pom-poms I imagine you in. Just kidding. I don't *really* imagine you in a cheerleader outfit.

The pain in the muscles and bone is very manageable now, mostly gone. I'm not using the Norco or the sleeping pills. Now I know what to expect and the timing and will have them for the next round. It is the skin stuff that will take more time to get better. I'm so glad I went to the doctor and didn't wait.

Have a great weekend.

From: Alan

To: Marcy

There's a song I listen to a lot, "Superman" by Five for Fighting. It's basically how we're all human and that's ok. Check out the lyrics if you get a chance. Don't watch the video though—it kinda sucks. It might make you cry, but the good kind of cathartic crying.

I don't look good in a cheerleader uniform, but I still like to wear one when Sophie's not home.

Let's Go Marcy!

Hope you have a good weekend as well.

CB: June 15, 2012

Thank You

Thank you to all the people who reminded me that I don't have to feel bad about feeling bad. When I do that to myself, I feel twice as bad.

EM: June 17, 2012

From: Sasha

To: Marcy

Marcy, please don't reply to this message. I have been thinking about your posts all weekend. I am sorry that I am so old-fashioned but I am not comfortable posting this note on the online journal guestbook. I wanted to say it to you privately but not for you to reply.

I was very, very sorry to read of your suffering but I have no clue what to say or to do to help. Over the weekend I have thought a lot about our training walks and the conversations that we had, particularly on the longer ones that took hours. I heard something of your life up to then and I wanted to let you know the lasting impression that those conversations have left, particularly because your posts talk about staying positive and strong.

You came through as a remarkable mother, devoted to her children, always on the lookout for opportunities for them. You were "with it" enough to keep their attention but still the grown-up and at times the disciplinarian. You hadn't had an easy life and yet you had met the challenges in your past and emerged from them with a better life than before. From that time on I have known that you are a strong person, a survivor. Dealing with physical illness does not diminish that character. Honestly acknowledging pain is not weakness or negativity. You do not deserve all the challenges that you've been given but now you have yet another one to face. As you have in the past I believe that you will conquer this one too and find a better life on the other side of it. You have a great deal to offer, not only to your children but to the rest of us also. It has been and continues to be a privilege to know you. You have my respect and admiration. I am not a religious person but I will keep you in my thoughts and hope that the remaining chemo that you need will go better than this first round.

Hang in there. I'll follow your online journal when you feel up to posting. Take care and do whatever you need to do to get through this fight. Your friend always no matter what.

CB: June 20, 2012

Your Support

Your support has meant so much to me. I know some don't feel comfortable signing a guestbook and others are, some call or send cards or email or just give me a hug when they see me, but I know you are reading, praying, cheering, learning, and sending good vibes. Thank you.

American Cancer Society Gift

Feeling pretty good now, just in time for chemo tomorrow.... Ugggh. American Cancer Society called me today and invited me to attend a make-up/beauty class at the cancer center tonight. I am not a big make-up person but I have Dani's culinary certificate ceremony in Chicago on Saturday and lunch at the Signature Room in the John Hancock. Dani doesn't care if I wear the wig, which I got (also provided by ACS). I hated every second of wearing it and will never wear it again. I can at least wear make-up to her ceremony. Wearing new makeup may be a good pick me up and they give me almost $300 worth of stuff. A lesson wouldn't hurt, my eyebrows are almost gone and with the steroids and sensitivity, I can get red in the face and blotchy. Although I almost said no, I did decide to go. This night made possible by all those who have donated to American Cancer Society/Relay for Life.

Thank you.

Even though chemotherapy was becoming more brutal I rarely brought anyone with me after the first couple when my mom or sister sat with me. I didn't want to burden anyone with watching me get chemo and I looked forward to some quiet time. The after-chemo activity usually included treating myself to lunch—truth be told, most of the time only dessert—and a visit with Ron and Laurie. Sometimes we would talk about the cancer treatment and plan, sometimes the kids, and sometimes we talked about things not related to me at all. The distraction was helpful. Even if I didn't have time to stay, it did my soul good to stop by and get some warm hugs. I was really looking forward to escaping at their RV campsite in a couple weeks. I knew I could rest or play. I could just do nothing and it would be okay.

CB: June 22, 2012

Milestones and Daily Moments

Hi all,

I hope you all have a great weekend. My oncology visit and chemo went well yesterday. I am becoming difficult to start an IV on for the first time in my life but I have skilled and creative nurses. Thankfully I only have two more treatments left. I am hoping that since this is my second time on this particular chemo, there will be fewer surprises and I will have a better handle on the timing of the side effects. I already have the proper medications to minimize them and head them off before they get bad.

Emotionally: Feeling kind of fragile. We are going downtown tomorrow for Dani's Culinary Certificate ceremony. So proud of her and all she has done, especially with all the challenges we/she have/has faced these past two years. I hope I can keep it together better than I did for Riley's 8th-grade promotion. Sometimes on big events like this my mind trails off and sneaks to the "what if" I am not there for the next major milestone. I am going to try not to let those thoughts sneak in. I want to enjoy the moments I have. I hope you savor every moment with your loved

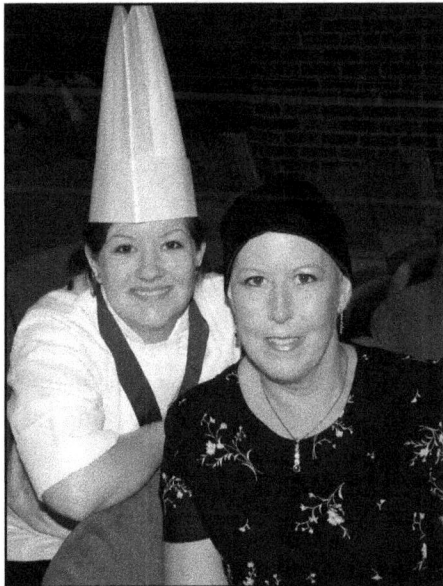

Figure 1-10. Dani and Me at Dani's Culinary School Graduation Ceremony

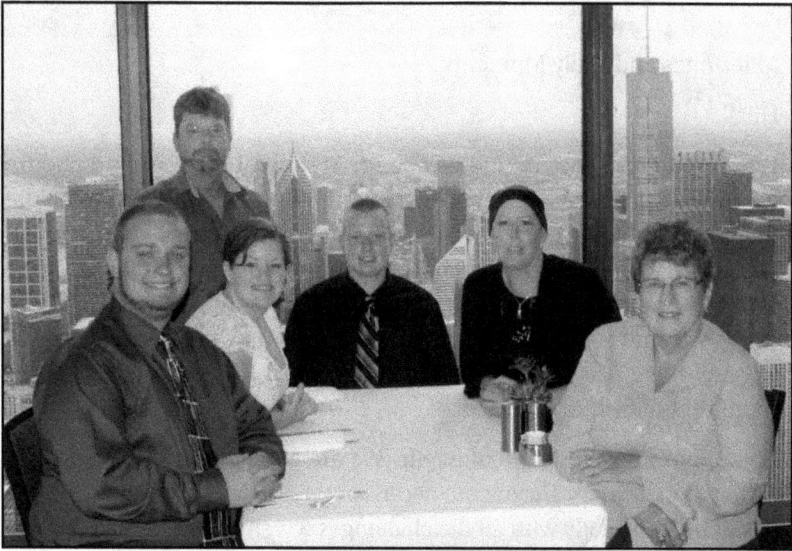

Figure 1-11. Eating at the Signature Room of the John Hancock Building in Chicago; sitting from left to right are Nick, Dani, Riley, me, and my mom; Roger is standing

ones, big events or the daily moments. Tonight we played Uno and it was nice to just be together playing cards. I love my friends and family; I want to stay with them a long long time.

Have a safe and happy weekend,

Love, Marcy

Sally: Hey, Marcy! As tough as I try to be, I still find myself getting emotional at events like graduations and birthdays. Sometimes I have to mentally check out and think of other, more mundane, things for a few minutes so I can pull my emotions in. For example, I will make a mental list of things I need at the grocery store or a list of things I need to do at home in order of importance. Once I feel like I'm in control of my sniffles I pay attention again to whatever may be happening. I particularly use this diversion at high school graduation ceremonies of the kids I have worked with. You may miss a few minutes of the ceremony, but you are able to keep control of yourself. I hope you have a great day with Dani!

CB: June 26, 2012

Moving Along

Okay, well I am sick of this. Two more chemo treatments to go. Today I saw the surgeon and at least my appointments are scheduled. Surgery August 13. I have my pre-op physical with my primary care doctor scheduled and my consult with the radiation oncologist scheduled.

Yeast came back, pain came back, slight temp came back but I am doing what I can to keep it under control. The most painful days are Sunday and Monday after chemo, which I get every other Thursday. Today I am really tired and achy but not in as much pain. Riley is at camp for two weeks so I feel less guilty about being a bum. I am looking forward to feeling better and enjoying the upcoming weekend away with my friends Ron and Laurie.

Stay safe and healthy, Marcy

It All Matters

The priceless gifts of support that I have received are, well, priceless. Those gifts have come in many forms: prayers, gifts, cards, words of encouragement, hugs, suggestions to help me manage my comfort level, donations in my honor, luminaries lit, and even the silent support knowing I am being thought about. I can feel it all and I will not forget what I have received. Thank you. I must go to bed now before I get myself too worked up. Good night friends.

LM: Marcy, the kids at school are rooting for you! Meg can't wait for you to see her walking. The two of you amaze me with your strength. They say you never know how strong tea is...until you put it in hot water. Same goes for you. You have shown your strength and you are a survivor!!!

EM: June 26, 2012

From: Alan

To: Marcy

Hi Marcy,

Let me preface this by saying I'm not nearly going through what you're going through. I thought sharing my story might make you feel better and help me draw some strength from you.

I have chronic neck and back pain. It's sucks being in pain every waking moment. Every day I tell myself, "You can make it through another day." But thoughts creep into your head and you begin to wonder when you just can't do it anymore. That's when I (you) need to find inspiration somewhere—family, friends, a song, nature, something good on the news, and remember, you're important to others.

Now for my story:

Yesterday I had more cortisone shots in my back. (I've had at least twenty-five over the past ten years for my neck, back and foot.) I always get sick for several days afterwards—severe muscle aches, flushing, heart racing, and my sugars top 300. The doctors don't really believe this can happen from local injection, but it happens every time.

I'm at work. I'm so achy and hot and tired. I don't know how I'll make it until 10 p.m., but I will. I always do. Again, I won't pretend this is nearly as bad as what you're going through but I know how you feel. Basically, you just get tired of feeling like crap and you wonder how much more you can take. There is light at the end of the tunnel. Better days are coming.

You've made it this far. You always make it through one more day. You can and you will.

I've been following your journal. It gives me strength. And I think you have a future in journalism too.

Hang in there and never give up.

From: Marcy

To: Alan

Hey there,

I cannot tell you how grateful I am for your emails and support. You seem to really understand me and have the ability to "read between the lines" and know exactly what to say. It really helps to hear other people's stories. Monday morning, I called my friend, Hannah, in Arizona and spent forty minutes on the phone with her because I was in pain and I knew if I was on the phone with her, getting caught up, listening to her stories and struggles and verbally supporting her that I would be distracted from my own pain and it would help both of us. For some reason she thinks I am very "wise."

I have often wondered what "your story" was. I knew you had chronic neck/back/foot pain. What is it from? Pain is pain, it is a challenge to get through, but I know there is a difference between acute and chronic pain and it sounds like what you are dealing with is worse than what I have ever experienced. I respect and admire that you not only work but that you are so supportive of others. Before any of this cancer stuff I was dealing with pain from "unspecified spondyloarthropathy". The pain started after Riley was born when I was working at the family practice office. My S-I [sacroiliac or hip] joint MRI does show early ankylosing spondylitis (although that MRI is old, probably shows more damage now) and I have the HLA-B27 gene. I know, many people do have that gene and never develop the autoimmune arthritis of ankylosing spondylitis. I was not in daily pain but had flare-ups to the point I could not walk or bend over and had to have my kids untie and take my shoes off. Medrol Dose Pak helped for flare-ups but I couldn't find preventives. Mobic seems to be working okay now. The chronic arthritis with flare ups have affected my daily functioning at times in my life.

This pain is different; in a way it feels worse but I am better able to deal with it knowing that it will get better in a few days. It just seems to get a little more intense with each treatment. It hurts to move, it hurts to stay still. I hurt from the inside out. The esophageal pain isn't pleasant either, but again, I know that will heal. You are right, I just need to make it through and you are also right that I always do make it through. Sometimes I wish though that I could just "be put out" for a few days until the bad days are gone.

How frustrating that you feel such severe systemic symptoms after the injections. I wish some physicians would listen to their patients more. You have received enough injections to know the way you feel after; why wouldn't the doctors believe it can happen with local injection? I have run into several times when physicians didn't take my evaluation/opinion seriously, and because of that my kids have suffered until I could get someone to listen. The first time was when I was seventeen, with an infant. They wouldn't believe a teenager, but I knew something was very wrong. He had pyloric stenosis and needed surgery. If they had listened and investigated based off my report, he would have been healthier going into the surgery. I try to always listen to my patients and their families. I think that is why I do well in home care.

The emotional stuff is hard right now. I am seeing the counselor I saw when I was trying to save my marriage and after the divorce. When you buy a new car you suddenly notice how many of them are on the road. Now everywhere I look it seems like there is cancer or people dying. Yesterday morning a nurse I worked side by side with and who was also my rheumatologist's nurse died suddenly. I got a text from another former coworker about it. We worked closely for a couple years but I only saw her when I went to the rheumatologist over the last couple years, it hit me so hard. It literally felt hard to breathe. Her family, her daughter and husband, what they must be going through.

At Dani's ceremony there was a short segment to honor a woman who passed away last year. She earned her Culinary Certificate but died before she could attend the ceremony to receive it. Her son spoke about her. As touching as it was, I never want my kids to have to speak about me like that.

I am so raw. I try to be positive but honestly I will confess to you, sometimes I wonder. What do the doctors really think? Are they holding back anything? Do they really believe it will be okay? When I first had my ultrasound and was waiting to go back for the biopsy I was looking up types of breast cancer and I thought...as long as I don't have "inflammatory breast cancer" it will be okay. It just scares me. I know they say I am responding and things look improved but I am scared that it could spread, especially with the concern over the lymph nodes.

Another confession? There have been times after the divorce that I felt suicidal and if not for my children, the two that I have with me and the one I only got to be with for five months, if not for them, I would not even be here. Now I have to fight this, honestly, if I didn't have kids I wouldn't be fighting. I know that sounds terrible and I need to look for other purpose but really all I have are my kids.

As far as journalism, I think not. I used to want to write my story. I have been through a lot during my life and thought I would want others to be able to benefit from it in some way, if at all possible, but I do not feel like that is something I can do. Little snippets of stories are one thing but journalism or a book is well beyond what I think I could do.

Hang in there my friend and thank you ever so much for understanding and reaching out to me.

From: Alan

To: Marcy

I have degenerative discs in my neck and back from living life—playing football with friends, shoveling snow, etc. My spine is much older than me for no really good reason. I also had a botched foot surgery a few years ago with left me with nerve damage. My foot alone has been injected with cortisone and alcohol—no exaggeration—at least twenty times. Probably a lot more.

If it weren't for Sophie, I don't know where I'd be—maybe not here anymore. But I keep going so I can be here for my family and friends, have some good times and hope that better days are coming.

Sometimes I'd just like to feel great for five minutes. It seems like everyone else plays golf and tennis and runs races and I do all I can just to go to work and keep some self-esteem. I know how you feel when your mind has all these great ideas, things you want to do, things you need to do, but your body can't get off the couch.

It's wonderful that your kids keep you going and keep you fighting. Do it for yourself too.

I've followed your treatment, which has certainly been aggressive. My honest opinion is you will come through this. I truly believe you can beat this. You won't always be feeling this bad.

I hope tomorrow is a good day.

(And if I may go all doctor on you: If the yeast/fungal infections are external—skin or genitals—I've found that lathering with Selsun Blue (selenium sulfide) can really diminish the load of fungus on the body.)

You won't always feel like this. Better days are coming.

From: Marcy

To: Alan

Before my Tarsal Tunnel surgery, I had a shot in my foot. When I think of the 0–10 pain scale I use that as a benchmark for a 10. I actually said bad words to that doctor and I am not like that normally. I can't imagine what that is like for you to do those repeatedly.

Thank you for what you said about my treatment. I was worried it wouldn't be aggressive enough and although I don't like feeling this way, knowing it is temporary and will do the job helps. I would hate to think they made the decision to spare me the hard times and then not have it be successful when they could have been more aggressive. I would rather go through a hard treatment once than a slightly less hard treatment and have to do it twice. That is part of the reason I am not doing any reconstruction. I don't care, I will get prosthetics. I don't want more surgeries, more complications, etc., etc. Thank you for keeping up with the medical side of things and for your opinions.

As far as going "all doctor on me," let me have it, as far as I am concerned I cannot have a big enough medical team right now. No one has suggested that before for the yeast/fungus. I actually had nizoral here (expensive stuff) that I bought for one of the kid's dandruff. That would work too right? The yeast/fungus is external (under breasts, arms, and groin at times) but also internal (vaginal and throat).

I hope you have relief from your pain soon.

From: Alan

To: Marcy

Hi Marcy, I'm feeling somewhat less ill this morning. I really appreciate your concern.

I completely agree with your choices. In my limited experience reconstruction just makes for a longer surgery/more surgery and a harder recovery. Personally, I think the prosthetics appear more natural—they are contoured naturally unlike a bag of saline. They have a natural texture. They are easily managed. You will be pleased and glad you went that route.

Terbinafine, available as Lamisil (you gotta read the label because Lamisil makes many different versions) is the best topical antifungal for the skin. Clotrimazole (i.e., gyne lotrimin) is probably the best vaginal product. Daily washing with Selsun really helps. There is a prescription strength Selsun for lathering on in the shower. I'd ask your doc about it. And of course there's always oral Diflucan.

I hope you feel better today and are able to do what you want to do today. I'm really really praying/hoping/cheering for you.

Be good.

Being Remembered

So this is what has been rattling around in my brain lately. It would be foolish for me not to prepare for the worst even though I have more hope for the future than I did even two days ago.

The reason I have more hope is thanks to Alan, a friend of mine who is also a doctor. He has been keeping track of things, like my treatment plan. He is intelligent, supportive, and funny. If he says, the treatment I have been receiving "has certainly been aggressive. My honest opinion is you will come through this. I truly believe you can beat this. You won't always feel this bad," I believe him and so should you. I know that he understands how much value I place on honesty. I can handle the truth, just never lie to me.

At the same time, we are all human and the "what ifs" always are there, even in the most positive, hopeful people. My nephew, Parker, was honest enough with me to say that we all sometimes think "What if?"

So about the subject of this entry… "Being Remembered." I think it is human nature to want to be remembered. That is why we have memorials and tombstones, pictures and poems…children. We want to know that our lives made a difference, that we mattered somehow. Yes, I want to know that too but more importantly, remember my kids.

What do I mean? In hoping for the best but preparing for the worst, I don't worry as much about you remembering me but please remember my kids. Today I am thinking about the memorial for my former coworker Liz. I can't go. I am so sorry I can't go but really I just can't. Right now it isn't a physical "can't," it is an emotional "can't." I think of her though, and her family…her daughter and I hope that the people who are closest to Liz remember her by remembering her family. Not just now but six months, and six years from now. I worry that my kids won't be remembered over time and they will feel alone. Will they always get the support they need when I am not here? Sure in the beginning they will but who will take a long-term interest? Especially Riley, I know he is going to be a handful, who will deal with that and see past the exterior to what he can become? Who will keep him on the straight and narrow? I have so many wonderful people in my life who love us, and I know intentions are good. It is just something I worry about because I know life gets busy and things get hard and when that happens, checking in and guiding someone else's children may become less of a priority. God bless my mom, but she won't be around forever either and parenting and grandparenting are so very different. I also think about Dani: If I am not here, who will help her through career stuff, relational stuff, parenting stuff? When Dani is in labor, who will dress in a cheerleader outfit and cheer, "Push em out, shove 'em out, waaay out"? I promised I would do that, after we watched *Bill Cosby, Himself.* Who will wear the handmade bead necklace Riley made for me to his wedding, like I told him I would?

So the bottom line is, I think it would be nice to be remembered if I die but more importantly, please remember my children.

With that said, on to better days, with a stubborn will, and a great weekend with friends planned. Stay safe and healthy, hug your family and smile.

JH: Marcy, I can't imagine how you must be feeling, physically and mentally. It sounds like you are doing a fantastic job of staying positive, but if you feel like being emo...then be emo!! Please know that I think of you all the time and wish I had that magic wand to make it all better.

CB: July 3, 2012

Business and Pleasure

Hello All,

Business: I met with the radiation oncologist yesterday. He was kind, as was his entire staff. He comes highly recommended by the neurologist I used to work for and the ophthalmologist who did my vision correction laser surgery. She said they would roll out the red carpet for me and I felt like they did. I will see him two weeks after surgery and, depending on the pathology from the surgery, will most likely be doing radiation Monday through Friday for thirty treatments. They will be able to see me after work so I should be able to start work as planned three weeks after surgery.

Pleasure: I had an amazing, relaxing, stress-free weekend at Ron and Laurie's RV campground. Next time I am invited back I promise not to end the weekend in tears from bonking my head. It was weird but quite awesome not to be responsible for anything. Thank you for taking such good care of me, Ron and Laurie. Also got some good canine therapy, thanks to the big guy Jagger.

When I got home Sunday night I had a birthday present waiting for me, a gold chain from my mom to put my mother's ring on. Just what I wanted. I am afraid my ring will slip off and don't want to have it resized yet. We had cake and ice cream too.

On my actual birthday (Monday), I did a ton of errands and when I got home in the afternoon, Dani and I were just hanging out and decided to go to Key Lime Cove hotel and water park. Such a nice night. She bought me dinner, we did some rides, but mostly round and round in the lazy river. When we were leaving the house to go there she said she was glad that I was the type of mom that did stuff like this. She meant the spontaneous stuff. We talked about how surprises and spontaneous stuff were fun but also how planning things is exciting and gives you something to look forward too. I have had such a great balance of that lately. I have made a lot of parenting mistakes but it is nice when my kids express something that I'm doing right. Spending time with them both together and individually. Now I am sitting here waiting for her to wake up. We will swim some more and go home. Unfortunately, I am already thinking about the next treatment because I start the steroids again tomorrow. Inside I feel like a four-year-old stomping her feet and saying, "I don't want to do it," but I will because I have to and that is that.

Have a safe Fourth of July, Love Marcy

Laurie: We almost made it tear free! You are an awesome, easy to please guest! Thank you!

DA: Hi Marcy, I always stop what I am doing to read your latest posting. I'm glad you are taking the time to do some fun things! We can all learn something about life's balance from you. Wish I was there too! You and your family, as always, continue to be in my prayers. I know you will be just fine! God has a plan for a hope and a future (Jeremiah 29:11). Hang in there. Soon this will all be in the rearview mirror.

Alan: Happy Birthday! Always good to read what's going on in your life. It's always nice to hear about the good times, but also important to keep posted on the not-so-good things. I count myself among your many fans and followers. It's hard to feel OK for a few days knowing you're scheduled to get beat up some more. Hang in there. There is light at the end of the tunnel. Smile when you think about the good times you had over the weekend and at the waterpark. It sounded like a lot of fun. Be good!

CB: July 3, 2012

Mastectomy Preparation?

I am a little creeped out as I investigate online fake breasts that I can take on and off and mastectomy bras. I will have to work my way up to it. Not quite ready yet, I guess. I know someone will visit me in the hospital to teach me about that. I am sure it will be fine, and still would rather do that instead of the reconstruction surgeries and permanent replacements.

FB: July 3, 2012

The insurance authorized 7 days in the hospital for my surgery. I was thinking surgery Monday, be home by Wednesday.

FP: Don't rush it. Take your time to recover.

Laurie: Yeah, don't rush it, they allow seven... Take seven!

Marcy: I really honestly don't think I will need 7 and think I would be absolutely sleep deprived and crabby if I had to stay that long. As soon as my pain is under control and there are no complications, I am leaving. I know I can handle the drains at home.

CB: July 4, 2012

Tears

I'm sorry I am not as strong as everyone thinks I am because right now I am in tears thinking about how much I don't want to go to chemo tomorrow. The actual administration of it is fine, Friday and most of Saturday will be okay. I just don't want to feel bad again but from Saturday night to about Tuesday I know I will feel beat up, will feel fair after that for about four days, then when I start to feel good again I will have a few days before I have my last one. I am more afraid of what will happen to me if I don't go than I am of dealing with the pain and the other side effects. I guess venting helped turn my thoughts around, a little.

Lola: Big hug!!! You can do this you have made it this far and you only have two more treatments left!!!!

Marcy: I know, they just seem to be worse now every time. You are right, only two more. Riley will be home again. I hate when he is around and sees me not doing well. I need to figure out something to do with him to get him out on Sunday. Monday he gets a filling and will probably want to rest too.

Lola: I don't think we have much on Sunday if you want me to come get him. Don't know if he will be bored here.

Marcy: Lola, thank you so much for offering to take Riley. I called Roger and he is going to take him on Sunday, maybe even Saturday night. It is so cool that he spends time with Riley.

PO: You are woman and we all hear your roar. The roar of a mother fighting for her life and that of her children. Take a deep breath, you got this Marcy!

Clara: It does suck but you're right, Auntie M, you do it because you have to and in the long run it's worth it!!! And it's always OK to vent and share your frustrations, you're one of the strongest women I know and that doesn't make you any less strong!

Miriam: I love you! You are the bravest person I know.

Marcy: Wow, coming from a woman who is a police officer and knowing all the people you know. That means a lot! Thanks Miriam

LM: Marcy...tears and fear do not make you weak...you are VERY strong and it is OK to be tired of being strong...that is why you are surrounded with people who care about you so much. When you feel weak, let us be strong for you! You have been there for so many of us...let us be there for you!!! And know that you are NEVER alone! We are all sending thoughts and prayers daily for you. You inspire so many... You can beat this!!!

EM: July 4, 2012

From: Alan

To: Marcy

Hi Marcy,

You're right. It just plain sucks to be feeling OK for a few days knowing that you're gonna get a treatment that will make you feel like crap (understatement) for several days. I don't think people understand what it's like to continuously feel awful and not have relief for even a few minutes no matter what you try. Each time is a little different and you don't know what to expect but you hope that this time it's not so bad and it will get better quickly.

I feel for you Marcy. It's hard to keep the big picture in mind when you just want to stop feeling ill. But please try. You're stronger than you think. It's OK to cry but don't give up. I promise, you're stronger than you think.

I'm sorry you have to go through this. Take care of yourself as best you can. Do something enjoyable tonight to take your mind off of it for a while. Other stuff can wait. I'm praying and hoping for you. I hope it helps.

From: Marcy

To: Alan

It does help because I know you understand, especially sharing your story knowing you will feel bad after the steroid injections but being in pain and having to make the choice to feel bad to relieve pain... What kind of choice is that? I pray for you too.

I think of my grandma, she quit chemo one round early. Not for the same reason but because she believes the nurse gave her the wrong one (it looked different). I don't know if that is true or not. Thankfully, she had already had her radiation, surgery and most of chemo for the colon cancer and was cancer free. I won't quit but that doesn't mean I didn't think about it. I would not tell many people that.

I finally got my scrapbook stuff organized and can work on that tonight. Guess what, I am dog-sitting a little gal that looks like Tommy Friday and Saturday. Heard she was a real lapdog and likes to snuggle. Canine therapy, yay!

EM: July 5, 2012

From: Sasha

To: Marcy

You are incredibly strong and please do not reply.

Hi. Once again I wasn't comfortable posting in the guestbook but please do not reply. Marcy, because you share with us the realities of the illness and the treatment that choice does not make you weak it makes you honest. If any of the rest of us ever have to face a health crisis we won't have some sanitized deceptive notion of serious illness.

Let me know if you are up for a visit perhaps after your last treatment and before your surgery in the beginning of August. Keeping good thoughts for you always.

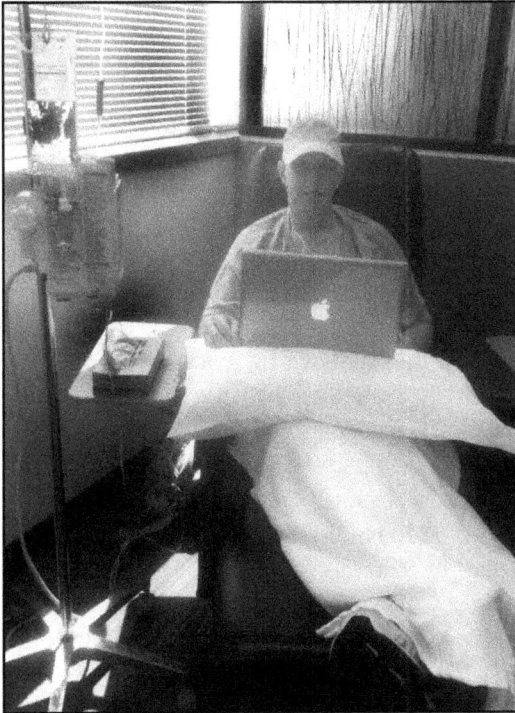

Figure 1-12. Receiving chemotherapy

FB: July 5, 2012

One chemo appointment left after today, keeping busy editing photos and listening to my "chemotherapy playlist" that are either songs suggested by you, make me think of you or I found to be motivational. Have a good day.

My chemotherapy playlist grew over time. It had suggestions from others for inspiration, songs that made others think of me or suggested by others, and songs that made me think of someone close to me. I usually played it on shuffle, in no particular order to keep myself from becoming used to it. I would visualize the memories and people the song made me think about.

The Chemotherapy Playlist

"The Climb" by Miley Cyrus
"The River" by Garth Brooks
"Stronger" by Kelly Clarkson
"Baby Got Back" by Sir Mix-a-Lot
"A Thousand Miles" by Vanessa Carlton
"Holy Diver" by Dio
"Hit Me with Your Best Shot" by Pat Benatar
"Ironic" by Alanis Morissette
"Somewhere over the Rainbow" by Jewel
"Hips Don't Lie" by Shakira
"Rock of Ages" by Def Leppard
"Nine Lives" by Def Leppard featuring Tim McGraw
"Closer to the Heart" by Rush
"Closer to Fine" by The Indigo Girls
"Live Like That" by Sidewalk Prophets
"Superwoman" by Alicia Keys
"I'm Gonna Love You Through It" by Martina McBride
"3 a.m." by Matchbox Twenty
"Superman" by Five for Fighting
"I Won't Give Up" by Jason Mraz

CB: July 5, 2012

Medical Update

Hey there, gonna get right into the medical nitty/gritty. Went to chemo today. The doctor told me to go on the oral antifungal (Diflucan) on Saturday to prevent the massive yeast attacks I get. I didn't know if I could do ten-day courses that frequently but he said to this time and the next. He also refilled and upped the quantity of Norco. He told me I don't have to be tough, if it helps...take it. I was a little teary-eyed when I was talking about sending Riley out of the house to do something on my more painful days and he wanted to give me something for depression... temporarily, but I don't feel depressed all the time, really just sad and frustrated sometimes, isn't that kind of normal? I did agree to go to their "wellness center" in a couple weeks, they have counselors and yoga and I don't know what else. I will go but I am also seeing the counselor I went to during/after divorce and that has been good because he knows me.

I mentioned to the nurse that lately I have had a runny nose but have not been sick or anything...duh, the chemo is killing the hair in my nose (cilia) too and that is what she says the runny nose is from. Hmmmm go figure. So now there is a tissue box in every room in the house.

I can blame my laziness (fatigue) on anemia. Normal range for hemoglobin in women is 12–18 and mine is 9.6, not low enough to hold chemo or for a blood transfusion, that would happen at a level of 8 or if symptomatic. I already am a little short of breath with activity. I have had bleeding hemorrhoids for a while and use a prescription cream, they are against suppositories due to risk of infection but I really think that the hemorrhoids are higher up internally where the cream won't help. I know the chemo is the cause of the anemia, not the hemorrhoids, but it could be a contributor and if the bleeding gets worse I will call. I will recheck the CBC next week.

I am getting worse on the IV stick. She only needed two sticks but when I have my surgery they will take lymph nodes from the right side and my "good stick" arm will no longer be an option. I guess I will have to deal with that for the rest of my life, may have to get one of those medical bracelets [alerting first responders of the condition].

Speaking of lymph nodes: I know there was cancer in one, not sure if more. I know she is going to take many out, don't know how many. I confirmed that with the chemo there shouldn't be any cancer in them by the time treatment is over, but asked if there were would I do more chemo? He said no, they have done all the chemo they can do now. The radiation oncologist would take it from there. Let's just hope, pray, cross our fingers that all the lymph nodes are clear.

All you wanted to know and maybe some stuff you didn't, huh? Well that is just the way I am, I guess. It may help someone, sometime if I share what my experience is, even the yucky stuff.

After chemo, I treated myself to Chili's and made myself eat some protein, veggies too, if you count the spinach and artichoke in the dip. Then I had an awesome dessert, which was all I really wanted anyway. Then went to Sam's Club and with a heat index of 113 degrees, and with everything else going on, I am inside and done for the day.

Can't wait to see Riley tomorrow, but I will have to play it cool when I pick him up. He will be tired too, so we will just hang out most likely.

Love you all.

EM: July 5, 2012

From: Alan

To: Marcy

Hi Marcy,

Hope you don't feel too bad over the next few days. As far as I know you can take Diflucan daily for a long time. It's a pretty good, safe med. Also, as you know, internal hemorrhoids tend to bleed and not hurt too much. Sitting in a hot bath ten to fifteen minutes daily can still help if you're permitted to do that.

Your posts are very well written. I still think you have a future in journalism. I think you're doing a hell of a job keeping people informed on your life and course of treatment.

As for yoga, I tried that once. It was the only time in my life I was the worst student in the class. Oh well. The instructor really tried to help me but I kinda sucked at yoga. I still recommend it to people though. I watched old ladies do things I could never have imagined.

Don't get overwhelmed by the future's uncertainty. In yoga they tell you to live in the present. Not bad advice. You're always in my thoughts.

Be good.

From: Marcy

To: Alan

Thanks. I liked pilates and did what I could. I would like the stretching part of yoga, it is good for the arthritis and not stiffening up.

If Diflucan is that safe, I will take it, especially because it isn't all external. Yeast in the mouth and throat and the vaginal yeast flourish too. I do think the Selsun Blue helps and have been using it daily. Thanks for that.

I am glad to have people who care enough about me to read the online journal, it definitely cuts down on telling people and the telephone game and getting things wrong in translation, this way people can get it straight from me.

Take care.

FB: July 7, 2012

I guess the day or two after chemo I can be pretty productive with all the steroids in my system but I know the crash is coming probably late afternoon or early evening and that sucks. Just hoping I will be good for work next Tuesday, Wednesday, and Thursday. Got to get those high school kids registered, a paycheck (even a partial one) might improve my mood too.

CB: July 9, 2012

Energy Battle

"An internal battle ensues when there is a deep realization that there is not a moment to lose, yet there is not a joule of energy to use in that moment." By me

DA: Sometimes words just won't come. It does say in scripture that Holy Spirit can take our groans before the throne and make sense of it all. There have been times when that was all I was able to do. Know that it's okay to feel that way sometimes. We don't have to have all of the answers just know that God is in control. I pray for you daily—sometimes many times in a day.

EM: July 9, 2012

From: Alan

To: Marcy

Hi Marcy,

You hit the nail on the head [with your last CB post]. It's extraordinarily maddening. I think that's what people don't get until you live it.

Since the shot two weeks ago I've been in serious pain. I have a follow-up in the morning. There's so many things I have to do and want to do and I just can't. What I've tried to do over the past few years is budget time and set small goals. I save most of my energy for getting through a work day. On days off I budget one or two errands and then a few hours on the couch. Sometimes it's even hard for me to make lunch.

I know it's really hard for you. My guess is there are days you can't do much at all. It's frustrating because the brain never stops but the body is hurting.

Set small goals and do what you can. Sometimes getting just one thing accomplished feels good. I hope things get better soon. You're always in my thoughts.

EM: July 10, 2012

From: Sasha

To: Marcy

Hi. I worked the weekend and yesterday and just read your latest post this morning. When this crisis has passed you should think about writing; you're good at it. Take care.

FB: July 11, 2012

I may have worked full 8-hour days in the beginning of chemotherapy but I can't do it now. I worked two days and left an hour early today. Thank you AV for covering for me. I don't know how those who get chemo and work full-time do it. I am so exhausted and have such a bad headache and body aches right now. I will be interested to see what my blood counts are tomorrow and if the anemia is better or worse.

AV: Don't even mention it, what are friends for? Just take good care of yourself.

Post on my wall

Miriam: I just wanted to tell you how much I admire you—your strength and your courage—and I love you as much as a friend can love another friend. You are a beautiful woman, inside and out. I wish I lived closer so that I could help you during this difficult time. I know you are going to be "okay," because you are an amazing person and I know you won't accept anything less than amazing. Okay, that's the end of my serious thoughts.

Marcy: Your post was perfectly timed as I was just beating myself up for not being able to work until eight tonight and telling them I couldn't work tomorrow. I am exhausted and don't know how people work full-time while getting chemo. I did it in the beginning but just can't anymore.

Miriam: You need to do what's best for you. It doesn't matter what other people did. You are not other people! Rest and heal. I'd like to have you around for a long time, and something tells me I'm far from the only one.

Marcy: You're right. I wouldn't be as upset about having to rest if resting actually made me feel better. I didn't even get dressed Sunday and Monday, rested a lot but still feel very tired and weak. I am sure I will feel better when the hemoglobin goes back up.

FB: July 13, 2012

Who can say "no" to an offer to be picked up and taken to Dairy Queen? I guess I will have to get dressed today. I love Peanut Buster Parfaits.

Marcy: Back home and in bed again already. Parfait didn't taste as good as usual, taste buds are off when it comes to dairy but the lemon lime Arctic Rush is hitting the spot.

With only one chemotherapy treatment left to go, the side effects of the chemotherapy compounded exponentially. By this time the fatigue was overwhelming. I had been spending a lot of time in bed. Riley appeared to be doing well, although I did notice that the more I was in bed the less active he was. We were able to enjoy a pajama day together. We had a *Big Bang Theory* marathon, so then we decided to play the *Big Bang Theory* board game. Riley pulled up a chair to my bed and put the board game on it. He then sat on the floor on the other side. It was nice to be able to play with him and laugh with him, even if I was too tired and weak to sit up for long periods of time. I was exceedingly gratified that he came up with a way to have fun with me while allowing me to stay in bed. I was tremendously dispirited that he had to.

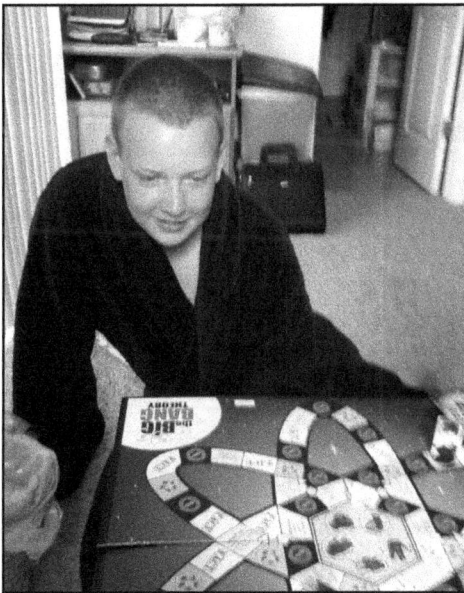

Figure 1-13. Riley playing *Big Bang Theory* board game on a chair pulled up to my bed

CB: July 14, 2012

My Journey

Hi all, did you miss me while I was gone?

I have just returned from my journey to a moonlit, healing mud bath, followed by a therapeutic massaging waterfall.

Okay....by "journey," I mean "walk to the bathroom."

By "moonlit", I mean "bathroom lights were dim."

By "healing mud bath," I mean "medicated dandruff shampoo as body wash."

By "therapeutic massaging waterfall," I mean, "sitting in an empty bathtub with the shower pointed at my back."

Nothing wrong with a little fantasy, is there?

Have a great rest of the weekend, Marcy

P.S. Now I am "on a beach in a seaweed wrap, feeling the ocean breeze"; by that I mean, "lying on my bed in a green towel with the fan blowing on me." Yes, it works for a second or two. No pictures posted with this journal entry, for obvious reasons.

FB and CB: July 15, 2012

Got Mammograms?

What is on my mind? In less than a month I will be having surgery to remove both of my breasts and some of my lymph nodes. If this cancer wasn't found during a routine yearly physical and mammogram, it surely would have spread to the other organs (fast-moving type) and I would not have the fighting chance I have now. So my question is to my women friends...are you current on your physical and mammogram. If not, why? Call me so I can talk you into going. If your excuse is no medical insurance, please call me and we will find some resources.

PO: Tuesday 3:30 mammo.

CC: Did it right after your diagnosis. Yes, you were my inspiration. Forty-seven years old and never had a mammogram. Shame on me.

Marcy: No shame, you are all good now. I know you did it right away and was very happy about that. I know there are some out there who haven't and I just am trying to go from the gentle nudge from a few months ago to a little heavier push. I think there are one or two people in particular who know I am thinking of them.

BC: I need to go, thanks for the push. I'm overdue. Calling for an appointment tomorrow!!!!!

Marcy: Glad you are calling for an appointment BC. We need to keep all of us women here and healthy.

EM: July 16, 2012

From: Alan

To: Marcy

Hi Marcy,

Hope you're feeling alright. I had physical therapy today and now I can't move. I guess that's the point—no pain, no gain right? Lots of Aleve and Tylenol will get me through tomorrow.

I've been thinking about your upcoming surgery. Talk about mixed emotions. I can't imagine the thoughts that go through your mind.

I think if it were me I'd want to rid myself of cancer any way I could and that is how I would be looking at it. Get a good night's sleep. You're in my prayers.

From: Marcy

To: Alan

Hi,

Sorry about the pain. Physical therapy always hurt me too. It did seem like they made things way worse before they started getting better.

I have felt good the past few days and have had some great visits with friends and family. Start the steroids again Wednesday and last chemo on Thursday.

Yes, as far as the surgery, I would be very upset if she didn't take as much as she needed to or could to make sure it is all gone and reduce the chances of it coming back. She did tell me on the side of the cancer it would be malpractice for her to try to do any "tissue-sparing" surgery. I don't have a problem with that. Take them both, take it all, don't save nipples or skin or anything that could cause me problems later, take whatever lymph nodes were suspicious, test the others. Whatever it takes. I've had many different surgeries, they have all had their little challenges and I am sure this one will. Maybe emotions will sneak up on me just before or after...who knows. But I think surgery is easier than the last couple months of chemo has been.

Starting the Diflucan on Saturday and using the Selsun Blue did the trick, no skin or vaginal yeast to speak of...the throat symptoms were the same and I had the nasty tastes and white fluffy tongue. I don't think my taste buds will recover for a while...the reflux and heartburn sometimes gets worse. I have Carafate for that.

About ready to go to bed. I hope you are able to get comfortable enough to sleep well.

Take care, Marcy

EM: July 17, 2012

From: Alan

To: Marcy

Glad you are doing relatively well and you're comfortable with the surgery. One day after they're all done beating you up we have to get together. It would be nice to see you.

I'm so sore from therapy. I'm probably burning a hole in my stomach with Aleve. A big Russian lady named Magdelena gave me a "massage" yesterday—more like torture. I'm at work. I hope it's quiet tonight.

My dog and I sat outside this morning but it's so freaking hot we couldn't take it. Someone needs to do something about this weather. Be good.

Alan

CB: July 18, 2012

Untitled

Going to try to focus on my friend and a day at the movies, and try not to think that I have chemo tomorrow. It is like scheduling to go in the boxing ring with Ali, you know you're going to be beat up, okay more like (pardon the language) get the shit beat out of you. At least this is the last round...get it? Do you like what I did with that boxing round and round of chemo? I crack myself up.

Alan: Just don't punch out any of the nurses or techs. That's generally considered wrong. Have fun today and good luck tomorrow.

Sally: Nice play on words there, Marcy!

SS: Thanks for the giggle!!! You are amazing Marcy... Love you.

I Am Rich

So the meaning of the title may not be clear until the end of my little steroid-induced, emotional rant, but I hope it will be worth it to read to the end.

The last five days or so I have been feeling pretty good. I have seen people I love and care about every day since Saturday night. Many of them I haven't seen lately and who I don't see enough.

It has been wonderful to feel well enough to catch up.

Today I had a wonderful day with a friend, laughed at the movies, shared good food and great conversation. We were talking about money, kids, and how we would not trade the time we have had with our kids for wealth because we know we are so rich.

But then there was the drive home and I was thinking about my diagnosis and how since the diagnosis of cancer my brain has worked overtime. I am not lying when I tell you that I have spent countless hours and days thinking about people.

I have thought about every house I have lived in, my family, my extended family, those not blood related that I call my family. I think about every classmate I can. Pictures have helped where childhood memories faded. I have looked at a lot of pictures. Some, I remember situations but not names. Many I have been reunited with, some have died way too soon. I have thought about neighbors, each job I have had and every coworker I could think of including Creative Memories scrapbooking consultants and customers. I have thought of patients I have had, all the kids at Parkside Youth Center that I lived with or worked with when I was a substance abuse technician there. I have thought of people that have become friends because of a business transaction. We are so close now because we shared personal things about ourselves and discovered our connections. There are those that I went to school with all the way from kindergarten to college. Those I studied with who helped me succeed and those who...well, if it was not for hanging out with them, I may never have been arrested (you know who you are...and I wouldn't trade our time together for anything). People I have been in church with, single parents' groups, people I've volunteered with, my students, their parents, and my coworkers at D601. I think of the people who have made an impact in the lives of my children...their friends and parents, their teachers, coaches, and leaders. I have thought about boyfriends, about my first boyfriend, and my first long lasting true love. People who have hurt me and I forgive and one I am still working on trying to forgive. Those I have hurt and I am so sorry I did, hoping that they have forgiven me. Every person I have thought about has made some type of contribution to how rich I really am. All those contributions...made me who I am today. I have thought about those I have met recently and would like to get to know better. I have so much more to learn and to do. I have thought about those who I have really wanted to reunite with and some I may never have the chance...like my firstborn child, that I placed for adoption when I was seventeen. Wondering if we will ever get a chance to be together again.

So I am driving home from this awesome day with my friend and I pass a banquet hall as I am thinking about all of this. The "what ifs" creep in again and I think, "If the doctors tell me that there isn't anything they can do to cure this...and it looks like they are just giving me a little extra time, I am going to take the time and money to throw a huge party, while I feel well."

There are at least four people above that are in bands, and I want to hire them all for my party. Why not see people while I am alive to celebrate life, why do we have to wait until the people we love die to get together? I want to be there and I will invite everyone I mentioned above and then some....and you are coming, okay? Can you also invite and bring those who you know that know me and I didn't get an invite to? Everyone needs to be there because you and them are the reason I am so rich and it would be like a "this is your life" kind of thing. You all should know each other because you are amazing and so are all my other family and friends. I want my kids to see a huge party with all the people who have affected my life, even if it was for a short time, I think of you. I want my kids to really know how rich I really am, and how rich they are because of the people in our lives, not the things in our life.

I didn't want to go straight home because of the tears so I went to my brother and sister-in-law's house to settle down some. Steve and Patti only live a mile away. As I was getting out of the car there was a woman and her teenage daughter walking in preparation for the Susan G. Komen walk... I met her the day I had the mammogram, I interviewed with her! She is one of the people I would like to know better. She shared with me that she is also a breast cancer survivor. Our boys go to school together. I know there are things we can learn from each other.

Our lives are all intertwined for a reason, those reasons may be short and our time together may be brief but it is all meaningful to me. I plead with you not to underestimate your contribution to my life. There are people I am Facebook friends with from early school years that I didn't know well but they are so supportive. Some I have gotten together with when I wouldn't have been able to do that outside of my small group of friends in school. It makes me wish I had done some things differently, yet at the same time I feel so lucky that they have given me a second chance. We grew up and know what matters now. Thank you for taking the time to express to me that I matter and that you are rooting for me, it helps more than you know.

I hope you don't take this as a down post because it is quite the opposite. I am so grateful for all the people I have had in my life and am trying to spend more time with them, there are so many I need to get together with. Let's make a date sometime. I know I can't be in three places at once but the scheduling efforts are paying off.

Love you all, Marcy

P.S. Tomorrow is my last chemo, you can be sure I will be thinking about all of you over the next week, while I am getting through it, thinking of you all really does help.

EM: July 19, 2012

From: PH

To: Marcy

Hurrah!!!! Wow! Amazing and so are you.

You always seem to find the right things to say and of course the right words!!!!

There are just no words that I could say to add, comment or even think to say. You have said it all and how you do it?

God put you here for a reason!!

You are and have always been *one very special person*!!!!

Love!

From: Alan

To: Marcy

Hi Marcy,

I read your journal posting a couple times. The paths we cross and the relationships we have throughout life can be amazing. It's never the way you plan it. It leads me to a story I hope you like.

I didn't grow up with dogs but I married a "dog person." About ten years ago I became a dog person. Over the years we've done a lot for dogs— it's become our cause. Seven years ago we adopted Simba. He gave us a million smiles. We loved him so much, and we think he appreciated the home we gave him. We lost him in February at the age of seventeen. It was in Simba's memory that we donated to the Relay for Life. He is the beloved family member we lost to cancer. This was before we knew you had breast cancer.

Last week we were looking at Simba's bed and his blanket and we both knew that he would want us to give another dog a good home. A few days ago I made a wrong turn in Highland Park and we accidentally found Tails of Hope—a relatively new shelter. We fell in love with a roughly ten-year-old Pomeranian named Teddy. He was found wandering without tags in Waukegan. We brought him home yesterday. He's awesome. I think Simba would be pleased.

I hope the next few days aren't too bad for you.

From: Marcy

To: Alan

Awesome story. Congratulations on the new member of your family. What does Tommy think? I wanted to ask who the donation for Relay for Life was for, thought about it and don't remember if I did ask or not. I think both things you did, the donation and adoption, are great ways to honor Simba!

Dreading Sunday and Monday the most but *this* time I know when I start to feel better I won't have to go do chemo again. I can just start feeling better and get stuff done before surgery. Working some will help, funds are getting low but I do have some resources to tap (with tax penalty of course).

How are you feeling tonight?

From: Alan

To: Marcy

Tommy is a little put off by the attention Teddy is getting but he'll be glad he has a friend eventually.

I'm still in pain but it's a little better the last couple days. One day at a time and just trying to budget what I can do. Saturday night we're going back to Racine for a BBQ with my old office (the community health center). Good people still working there.

I'm constantly worried about what we'd do if I can't work. I have a disability policy but you never know how that will go. And primarily, I'd have zero self-esteem if I couldn't be a doctor. It's kind of all I have left.

I'm not an accountant but I have three pieces of advice that, off the top of my head, I believe are fairly accurate. I believe if you use retirement funds for medical hardship you can avoid certain tax liabilities. I believe you can also access retirement funds as a loan to yourself that you never really have to pay back. Finally, I'd keep a detailed record of all out-of-pocket medical expenses. You will likely qualify for a greater tax refund based on the ratio of income to allowable medical expense deduction. Have a good day. Take it easy.

From: Marcy

To: Alan

Thanks for the medical/financial suggestions. I am trying to keep records on the medical expenses and I worked with an accountant last year. I think he will be able to help. I will have such a low income this year (worse than last). I have not taken out a ridiculous amount from my retirement, only what I feel I need to get by with a little bit of quality-of-life activities to keep myself sane. I wonder if I will live long enough to retire. I think it will all be okay and once I am better I will eventually be switching to home health which will double my annual salary with a higher hourly rate and all-year-round work. We will be okay. Even if this gets terminal my life insurance will let me have 40 percent if needed to live on, if I am diagnosed with less than twenty-four months to live. Morbid I know. But reality.

As far as self-esteem if you couldn't be a doctor: I can't imagine there wouldn't be something valuable you could do like coaching/counseling those struggling with chronic/acute pain or other medical illnesses? We'd find you something to do I am sure of it. I am sure you have other interests that could be turned into a job. If you think it is a real possibility that you may not be physically able to make it to retirement is there anything you can do part time to explore interests that could turn into a career? I would love to go back to school and might but feel like I have to give both my kids a chance first before I go back for my second chance. But it is something I look forward to. Exciting new possibilities, maybe social work? Not journalism, LOL.

Have a good day.

From: Alan

To: Marcy

I always wanted to be an escort for the ladies, but I suppose I'd have to get hair transplants first, and then big muscles and perhaps some strategic hair removal. Maybe I should rethink that.

I'm at work until three. People are starting to come in. How rude.

Be good.

CB: July 20, 2012

I Feel Good Today

Wow, feeling pretty good this morning, I think I slept 8 hours without interruption, which is a minor miracle. Got some filing done, laundry put away, before 7 a.m. Gonna see how much I can get done today because I know I will have some days in bed soon. Those are a little easier when I don't go into it with a lot of things I didn't get done from the days before. Now it is time to let the steroids work *for* me instead of against me. The other good news is that this time when the pain and fatigue sets in I will know that when I get through it, I won't have to do chemo again, I'm done.

Hope you have a good Friday and enjoy your weekend.

NR: Hi Marcy, I just logged on. Been post-op myself, day eight. Love your blog, you've always been forthright and honest, a character trait I like in you (one of many). I am glad you did the memory journey and gave me a call. One of the greatest highlights at the office was getting to know you and the kids. We have much in common besides nursing, kids, birthday. Wanted to let you know I am thinking of you and keeping you in prayer. May you have complete healing, quick recovery, ease of pain/discomfort, and peace. I want to be on the "let's get together" list! Love you!

P.S. Eat Ben and Jerry's Chunky Monkey ice cream.

Jade: Hi Marcy, Sounds like you are doing really great right now. I know I am a latecomer to your journey through the joys of chemotherapy. I hope the cocktail has improved since I had it but there were no steroids then. Just keep on keeping on. You are a strong and smart woman. We are keeping you in our thoughts and prayers.

FB: July 20, 2012

Going to call this my most productive day in weeks. I hope I still feel good tomorrow so I can take the canoe out in the morning with Riley. I haven't had it on the lake all season.

Laurie: "Trooper" comes to mind every time I think of you!

I am going to learn to ride a motorcycle when my kids are both grown. I am going to get a Harley. Just watch me, they don't believe I will.

FP: Get a sidecar and I'll let you take me for a ride.

Marcy: FP, don't you trust my driving skills?

ST (my stepmom): You were seven the first time you rode as far as I know, right behind me.

Marcy: Motorcycle vacations, YAY! I remember!

FB: July 21, 2012

Dusting the house with very few eyelashes makes for drippier eyes than usual, so I am not going to "sweat the small stuff," no more dusting today.

I have double the amount of teenagers in the house...all still asleep. I love having them here.

Side effects of the last round of chemo kicking in. Soon Norco, my bed, and the fan will be the only things I want. Just too bad I know I am going to feel even worse on Riley's birthday, which is Monday. Hopefully I will be better on Tuesday and feel much better for the pool party on Wednesday. This round will not beat me, but I think I will wait until the count of nine before I bother getting up. Productivity, not for a few days anyway.

EM: Jul 24, 2012

From: Lucy

To: Marcy

Hey lady—I hope you are doing well and that we will still be on for a Monday visit next week.

Love you.

FB: July 24, 2012

Today proved to be as physically exhausting as I thought it would be! Really don't want to do another thing.

Clara: Then don't! Put your jammies on and cuddle up with a blankie and watch some good old TV!

Marcy: Riley just had me in hysterical laughter. He comes into my room, sits on my bed, and says, "So, what's the plan for the day?" I motioned to my laptop and bed and said, "This is the plan." LOL! Are you kidding me? What's the plan?

FB: July 25, 2012

Gonna have to take today's activities in small segments and rest while I am short of breath. Will try not to be a perfectionist or sweat the small stuff and hope that the teenagers rise to the occasion if they want to have parties. They did pretty well after they had Dani's party when she got her culinary certificate. I worry because this party it is at Harrison and Grace's house so I have spent a couple days and several visits to the store to try to get everything together. I am tired and I don't think the kids always get that. The anemia has its effects on my energy level.

Marcy: They did all chip in. I crashed at about 6 p.m., the older kids are still there and will clean up and bring everything home. Exhausted. I will get labs tomorrow, hopefully my levels are coming back up.

FB: July 26, 2012

Really wish I didn't have to wait until August 13 for my surgery, just want to get it over with and move on.

Considering staying in bed for the next couple of days. Any objections?

FB: July 27, 2012

I keep wet washcloths in my mini fridge. Wanted one for my swollen eyes. Riley got it out but it was dry. I set it aside and we continued to talk about how much he loves his new computer game and the part he just finished. Before leaving my room, without being asked, he soaked my washcloth and put it back in the fridge for later. Seems like a little thing but I was impressed that he thought of and did it without being asked. Yes, I have hope!

Kady: Thanks for training him to be a thoughtful future man for his generation of future women!

Laurie: It's the little things in life!

EM: July 28, 2012

From: Marcy

To: Alan

Hi Alan, How are you doing? I haven't really felt much like updating the CaringBridge lately. I have not been doing much of anything except lying around. Short time out of the house today to get Riley some new shoes. I am going to go to the amusement park tomorrow to see my friend and her brother who is playing in a band there. Riley and her kids can do the rides while we just sit and visit, it should be okay. Still ridiculously tired.

I have a question, I could ask oncologist or look on the net but thought you might know, don't see oncologist for another week.

I think I did develop some peripheral neuropathy from chemo. Mostly numbness in fingers and some weakness in my grip. I previously had cubital tunnel on the left and had an ulnar transposition, pretty successful but I can tell I am losing some sensitivity and strength in my fingers and hands. Will this get better? I know my hair will come back and my fingernails and toenails will eventually be normal but I am afraid the fingers and hands will have lasting symptoms. When I am done with surgery, do you think I should see my neurologist? (I used to work for him...love the guy.)

Anyway, over all, I know each day I will get better and hopefully will be feeling really good before surgery. I hope you are doing well today,

From: Alan

To: Marcy

Hi Marcy,

You are literally on the top of my list for things I planned to do tonight. I was wondering how it was going. Sophie asked me about you today as well.

As for me I continue to have a lot of back pain, which physical therapy always makes worse. I don't go back until Thursday so I'm hoping some of it is just soreness that gets better. They make you do things in PT that hurt and sometimes you wonder what you should and shouldn't be doing. I put my faith in a specific therapist and I'm still in a "trust and see how it goes" phase.

I'd suggest B complex vitamins that contain B12, folate, and thiamine. Specifically, Nature Made Super B-Complex (I know it sounds goofy) is a very good product and is certified by USP—a trusted independent organization. Nature Made is one of only three to four companies that submit to independent testing and is easily available.

I'd ask about B12, folate, magnesium, and zinc levels, which can all get messed up by chemo. You might need large doses of folate or B12 to get caught up. Nevertheless, taking a B complex daily could only help though it could take a few weeks. I do believe some of the neuropathy can be long term unfortunately.

The amusement park sounds fun. I think they've worked really hard to make it a nice park. Just being there would be nice because of the atmosphere. We keep talking about going.

I do hope you feel better every day.

Be good.

From: Marcy

To: Alan

What a ditz am I? I don't think I have taken my MVI, B12, or calcium in a couple weeks, just haven't filled the night time med container. I am sure it will help.

From: Alan

To: Marcy

You're not a ditz. You might consider 1000 mcg of B12 daily and 800–1200 mcg of folic acid daily. I'd ask about thiamine, magnesium, and zinc. I wonder if chemo has affected those.

I'm working today. Hope it's quiet. Enjoy.

From: Marcy

To: Alan

Ha! I like Nature Made. I specifically take B12 because my levels were low years ago when my headaches and restless legs were bad. It helped. I will add the B-complex to it. *Thanks!*

Maybe I will go see the neurologist at some point, and ask about the other levels. Not like anything can be done now besides supplements. I just worry if it gets worse about going back to home care and doing blood draws. It's hard to open packages right now.

The other annoying thing is the swollen drippy eyes, even fluid seeping from the skin of my eyelids. I am hoping my vision gets better when my eyes aren't swollen and drippy because right now my vision is so much worse in the past couple weeks.

I know what you mean about PT, there was only one PT that ever really helped me, everyone else made things worse. I told her I was afraid to go back to PT because of past experience. She was gentle but effective.

Tell Sophie thanks for thinking about me. I think about you all too. How are the puppies? I got to hold a soft fluffy golden retriever puppy on Thursday! Now *that* is therapeutic!

The outfits are crazy at the amusement park. Also women my age wearing four-inch heels. There is definitely a lot of people-watching to be done.

You should go during Fright Fest when they have costumes and shows, even cockroach-eating contests.

Thanks for the free advice! I value your opinion, you are smart and funny too.

Take care.

CB: July 29, 2012

Hissy Fit

The reality is, it's not over. I tried to be a "normal" mom, person, friend today. Ten days after my last chemo, thinking it is had been long enough and I can join the real world again and make a day of it. Now, my feet are burning, my legs are achy and restless, it is difficult to type because my nail beds on my fingers hurt and the ones on my toes hurt also, my eyelids are still swollen and seeping fluid from the skin. What am I complaining about? As long as it keeps me alive, and I never have to do chemo again, it'll be worth it, right? Well, maybe reality is finally setting in and I am afraid that they haven't been as aggressive as they could be and it won't be enough. Then I think, "Stay positive, it will be enough," but then I wonder, will I ever be the same? I guess how can I really expect to be the same? I know my hair will grow back and even my nails will go back to normal even if I end up losing these disgusting-looking ones that are pulling away from the nail bed. But will the neuropathy get better? Will I develop worsening numbness in my fingers and decreased hand strength or will it get better now that chemo is done? When will I feel like "me" again? I look at the outward signs of what the chemicals that were needed to kill the cancer have done to me physically and I wonder what the damage to the inside of my body is, what will recover and what won't. Every new ache, pain, symptom, I wonder if it is from the chemo and if it will go back to normal someday. Will my vision start getting better, because it has really gotten worse the last couple weeks? I feel guilty for not being positive again but honestly...sometimes I am awake at night and am still in disbelief. In all of my years of thinking I had "this or that," even thinking I had breast cancer a couple times. I ran to the doctor for exams, mammograms or ultrasounds and now I don't believe it. These past 4 months don't seem real, yet the effects of them certainly do.

Today, I took Riley to the amusement park. Remember a long time ago I said one of the things that would bother me the most is him being around and me being in bed. Well after a few days of him lying around because

I was lying around, it was time to do something. We got there early like usual. He rode Superman, I sat out. We rode Batman together. I was holding my doo-rag and sunglasses. The guy checked my harness and said, "Sir, you can't hold those on the ride," and took them. I don't think he ever realized he was talking to a woman. We rode a water ride together. All the stairs made me short of breath and by that time I was done with the amusement park and it was only 11:00. I was there to see a band and some friends. Riley and I had lunch and we made our way to the stage. PG, my high school friend, came with her two boys and they all went to Hurricane Harbor. I felt guilty I didn't go with them and that I didn't visit with her also. I couldn't be in two places at once and really was out of energy, although I tried not to let it be known. I enjoyed visiting with my friend SV while listening to the band and meeting some new friends. That felt great because it felt "normal" but at 5 p.m. I had to go. I should have gone earlier but I was trying to convince myself that since my last chemo was ten days ago, I should be better now. What was I thinking? I wonder what I am going to feel like in two weeks when I have surgery. I have a lot of work to do both at home and at my job in the next two weeks.

I am getting impatient. The reality is, we have been working on getting rid of the cancer for four months but I still have surgery and radiation to do. I want to be done. So my little hissy fit is done now…waaa-waaa-waaa and that is all. At least I can write it down here and let it go. It really does help to vent.

EM: July 30, 2012

From: Marcy

To: Lucy

Lucy,

So nice to see you and Hope tonight. I really enjoyed it. I hope I didn't upset you about the pictures. I am usually all about the pictures, it isn't really the hair thing. I just sometimes feel like people who I haven't seen in a while want a picture because they think it may be the last time they ever see me and I don't want pictures like that. My eyes are puffy and I am bloated and I just don't feel like any would look good. I know I will see you again and we can take pictures then. I hope you understand. I don't want you to look at any pictures and say, "That was the last time I saw her." I know it sounds crazy.

With that said, can you send me the picture of the kids.

I love you,

Marcy

From: Lucy

To: Marcy

Marcy—Not a problem dear friend—I understand. I truly do expect to see you again, so yes we can take pics then. Love you and thanks for suggesting Melting Pot—we loved it!! I wasn't sure you received the pic when I sent it from my phone the other night, so I'm attaching it again for you.

Yes, I guess I was pretty shocked when you got on me for taking the photo of the food with you and Riley in the background. I really didn't think about it—was actually just taking a pic of the food, but included you both in the background. I did bring my camera in case we wanted to take pictures later like usual, but wasn't sure if you would be up to it or not. The photo in the restaurant was just a reaction to the food. I guess it hurt me and took me off guard the way it happened. I didn't know what I had done wrong.

I truly understand that you weren't feeling well and didn't feel up for pictures, so don't worry, pictures were definitely not that important. I love you and wanted to visit with you to support you through this and celebrate your birthday. I in no way wanted to have a picture of us together for a final time—not even on my mind. I've been thinking the doctors were very optimistic about your cancer and I like the way they have been so aggressive with your treatment. I know it is hard on you, as I went through this with my brother—the very aggressive chemo, surgery, radiation. It was extremely hard on him too. I wanted to see you before school started, as I knew I couldn't get away after that and couldn't come for your surgery. It was so nice getting to spend some time around Riley. He is a sweetie and has a great sense of humor—seems to be all boy! We loved the Melting Pot experience!

Take care and know you are in my prayers daily dear friend! Love you,
Lucy

From: Marcy

To: Lucy

Yes, I know and I am sorry, it snuck up on me too. I had taken pictures in the recent past, not sure why this hit so hard and taking pictures of the food was not the issue. I hope that those few moments don't dominate an otherwise fantastic visit. Thanks for the picture of the kids.

From: Lucy

To: Marcy

Thanks, I love you. Maybe we can come down for a visit over the holiday again. We shall see how it all plays out.

CB: July 30, 2012

Pictures

I feel bad for not allowing a friend I don't get to see often take pictures of me. I totally enjoyed dinner with my friend and her daughter tonight at the Melting Pot but I realized I have been avoiding pictures. I am a big scrapbooker and usually document and take pictures of everything and everyone. Shortly after I lost my hair I didn't mind pictures but now I do. Maybe because of the changes in my face with the puffiness that probably most people don't notice anyway. But when I really think about it, I know it is because I don't want pictures of me when I feel sick or pictures that others look at and say, "That was the last time I saw her," or "This is when we went and saw her because she was sick." I know it happens because I have those pictures. I remember all the people in and out coming to see my Grandma and taking pictures when she was dying of cancer. When I get better we will take more pictures, until then we have some great pictures from past times together. If things don't work out with the cancer treatment, remember me the way I was before I got sick. I am hopeful we will see each other again. I will be strong and healthy again and will take tons of pictures. I can't have you thinking this is the last time we will see each other. Lucy, I am sorry I freaked out on you and I am glad you took a picture of the kids. I didn't realize the camera bothered me. Am I crazy?

Alan: People who are crazy don't ask if they're crazy. If you're no more quirky than me (and that's a lot) then you're not crazy. Hope you have a good day.

CP: You're doing great Marcy! It was good to see you and spend some time with you! Love ya!

Liza: Hi Marcy, I just read your journal update and wish we were chilling at a coffee shop together to catch up. I hope the pains and aches subside in the next coming days. You totally deserve the break! Miss you lots and always thinking of you and your kids. Love you.

EM: July 31, 2012

From: Alan

To: Marcy

Hi Marcy,

After PT I'm beat up and hurting. Then I spend the next week trying to decide if I'm getting better. Every morning I wake up and try to determine if I'm better than yesterday in the first five minutes of the day. At 3 p.m. I tried to decide if I'm 8 percent better or 3 percent worse than the morning. Will I feel better tomorrow or will it take three more days? I get obsessed with it.

It's no good to focus on how you feel every moment of the day. I'm sure each round of chemo has a slightly different action on your body. I suspect at this point it will take significantly longer to "recover" than you think or would like.

Get the big picture—you're killing the cancer. Or stop thinking about it at all for a few minutes. Give your mind a break. It takes time to recover from rounds of chemo and perhaps each interval improvement will take days. And it's OK to be crabby when things suck, and let it out. I'd agree that drippy eyelids and diminished vision both suck not to mention all the other things.

I'm still cheering for you (although the skirt has gotten tight over the years).

Be good.

From: Marcy

To: Alan

I get what you are saying. One of the risks of blogging is people think because I express my thoughts those are my only thoughts. I try to mention good and bad but maybe I'm not expressing both lately.

Today I see my counselor, change my oil, lunch with friends, then have a friend over in the afternoon, she will have dinner and play cards. I won't be thinking about everything I feel today.

From: Alan

To: Marcy

Glad to hear it. Enjoy lunch! I'm off to work—oy vey.

CB: July 31, 2012

Thanks—Moving On

Feeling better. Saw my counselor today, visited by email and in person with some friends and was reminded that we will get through this. Focusing again on what I need to do, which is go to work tomorrow and try to prepare my office for the first 3 weeks of school when I won't be there. Will meet the nurse who is going to take care of "my kids" (students at HHS) and give her the "ins and outs." Thursday I have my pre-op appointment with my primary doctor. I will then go to my follow-up appointment with my oncologist. Thanks for letting me vent and not losing faith in me. Moving on.

CB: August 2, 2012

Doctor Visits

Hi,

Met with both the oncologist and my primary care physician today. They both agree with bilateral mastectomies and no reconstruction. Although they both said reconstruction is available they both think that I made a good decision.

Oncologist: Said that the puffy eyes and fluid from them was because the tear ducts atrophied from the chemo and fluid can't drain down into my nose like it normally would. When my eyes stop draining, if the vision is still bad, see the eye doctor. He suggested Vitamin B6 300 mg for the neuropathy, numbness in my fingers, and burning feet. The neurologist (I used to work for him) called today just to check up on me. I will call him back tomorrow to chat, maybe he will have other suggestions on the neuropathy or will address it in an office visit if the B6 doesn't work. I know that will take time, like everything else. Had my pre-op labs drawn;

the CBC I got results immediately and things look okay, my hemoglobin is still low at 10.4 (normal 12–18) but that is up from 9.4 so it is going in the right direction. When it came time for his exam though, I wasn't sure how to read him. Last couple exams he seemed encouraged and pleased. I see him every other visit, so I haven't seen him in a month. This time he said he felt what was probably scar tissue from where the cancer was? His demeanor was a little different. How can you tell the difference between scar tissue and cancer from the outside just palpating? I tried to clarify the whole thing about what if there is still cancer in the lymph nodes, why wouldn't he do more chemo (not like I want to do more chemo!)? He said because there is no evidence it would help. The chemo first was to kill any cancer that had moved to other areas of the body. He said radiation would be next and he wanted to see me in three weeks to go over the biopsies from surgery to make sure radiation was still the plan. I guess I thought that was the plan, no matter what. Maybe it is just so there is one main doctor controlling the treatment plan. He kind of confused me this time. Guess I will figure that all out later and just focus on doing what I need to do before surgery, which is now a little more than a week away.

Primary Care Physician: It was so good to see her. I had not seen her since my physical when she noticed "skin thickening," the last week in March. I don't think I talked to her since she called me the day after the mammogram and said, "You have an invasive and aggressive breast cancer." I have seen her partner and talked to her over the past four months, which is just the way it worked out with their schedules. Now I know both of them. She cleared me for surgery. Told me I would probably be in two nights. All is well and she will see me when I am in the hospital.

So that is where things stand. Going to try to do some fun things, get some rest and get some work done next week. Will start with going to see *Total Recall* with Riley and my nephew, Parker, tomorrow. Have a great weekend.

EM: August 3, 2012

From: Alan

To: Marcy

Good morning,

I'm at work—again. I refreshed my knowledge of B vitamins. The B6 sounds like a good idea. I can't see any harm, and I think it's a good idea to add B12, thiamine, and folate.

Usual good doses are thiamine 100 mg daily, B12 25-100 mcg daily, and folate 800 mcg daily all for a couple months.

None are harmful and all three are generally used for diabetic and alcohol-related neuropathy.

Be good.

FB: August 4, 2012

I had no idea how much fluid eyes produced until my tear ducts atrophied from chemotherapy. Now it all just drips out and down my face, instead of draining down the ducts. It's like I am crying all day long.

Riley just burst into my room saying, "You and me are going to play archery on the Wii." How could I say "no"? Just glad my fourteen-year-old wants to do things with me.

FB: August 7, 2012

I want to go into work today to get more organized before I *have* to go in Thursday but I am still running a low-grade fever and my body disagrees with my head. Maybe in a few hours?

Clara: Only if you are feeling okay.

Marcy: I scrapped that idea. It will be more pressure Thursday when I do have to go in, but I don't feel well and tomorrow will be my last day to do something with Riley before my surgery.

Clara: Rest up so you can enjoy your day tomorrow. I love you.

Can't stay upright and keep my eyes open. I guess someone will have to come get me when they need money to order Chinese food. If I ever died in my bedroom I know it wouldn't be long until someone found me, they always need my wallet for something.

GC: Isn't that what having kids is all about? Oh, by the way, I'll take a shrimp egg-foo-young to go.

Marcy: Yeah and sometime in the not so distant future I will be complaining about being an empty nester.

GC: Don't worry, I'll be here to remind you.

Marcy: Maybe I will have the time and money then to deliver your Chinese food to Colorado.

FB: August 8, 2012

It is one of those days that I am in tears from feeling bad that I feel bad. Riley understands, I think. We are going to a movie instead of the water park, but I feel awful because I feel awful. GGRRRRR! It will be our last day to spend together until I get home from the hospital and I wanted it to be special and a good time for him.

Salvaged the day. Time with Riley: A little shopping, lunch and saw the movie *Step Up Revolution*, which we both enjoyed. I am doing what I can but Riley is no fool. He said to me at lunch, "You look sickly today." Wish I could hide it from him better.

Shelby: No need to hide it, honey. It is what it is! Riley obviously loves his Mom and would see through anything you tried to do to hide feeling icky. Hoping you feel better very, very soon.

Hannah: Why do you feel you have to hide it? Everyone wants you to actually BE well. If you're not, you're not.

Marcy: Well, I know I can't hide it entirely. I try because I don't want him thinking that I am going to die! I know it crosses his mind, that is why I try to hide just how sick I feel and how much I hurt sometimes.

Reflections

As much as I tried to hide the cumulative side effects of chemotherapy from my kids, friends, and family, there came a point when they saw through me. I guess the poker face I thought I was exceptional at didn't work with those closest to me.

Looking back to the days before my surgery, I can't really say I was worried about the actual surgical procedure. My main concern had more to do with the effectiveness of chemotherapy that had passed, the result of which I would only know long after. I knew I could learn to live without breasts. I knew I could still feel attractive without breasts. I knew there was no longer a functional need for breasts. What I didn't know was if the poisons I had been given had killed the cancer or just my vivacity.

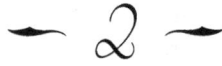

— *2* —

Surgery

Filet of Breast

Preparing for surgery by eating as many superhero popsicles as possible between now and 4 a.m. Monday!

PO: You go girl... *You are my hero!!!!!*

Marcy: You are my *hero*! You are an amazing woman! I will share my superhero popsicles with you any day!

Penny: See ya in the morning! Get some sleep tonight!!! I'll make sure you get great care!!!!

Miriam: Mega bunches of prayers being sent your way! Please let me know when you're up for a chat. Love you!

EM: August 11, 2012

Subject: No Response Please

From: Sasha

To: Marcy

Hi, I don't know what to say to help for Monday, if anything at all. I hope that you will heal well, physically, emotionally, spiritually. You have courage and wisdom and I gotta believe those qualities will stand you in good stead. Whenever you decide to post again on the online journal I'll be watching and I'll be keeping good thoughts for you, Dani, Riley, and your mom. Take care. Your friend always.

From: Marcy

To: Sasha

Hi Sasha, I know it says "No response please" in the subject heading and I accepted that the first couple times but when you do this all the time it isn't fair. That isn't how relationships work, one-sided. You say something, I communicate back, etc., that is what it is supposed to be like in a friendship.

Don't ever worry about not being able to find words "to help," sometimes there just aren't any. I know you are there and that is nice. Sorry we weren't able to get together this summer.

Take care.

EM: August 11, 2012

From: Marcy

To: Alan

Hi Alan, How are you?

I am a bit nervous. Not about the surgery itself but that this cancer is too aggressive. It seems like some of the progress made in chemo may not have lasted in the past three and a half weeks. My right breast has the orange-peel appearance coming back and feels dense again. I also have a small lump behind my earlobe, that is on the left side though, maybe a small cyst? Are there lymph nodes there? I will point it out to the surgeon on Monday morning but I am worried that the chemo didn't do enough. Trying to keep this to myself and between us. Don't want anyone else to worry but I know what my breast looked/felt like before, during and after chemo and it looks like the lymphatic vessels are getting blocked again.

I guess I won't know until all the biopsy results are done. Not worried about the surgery itself, just worried that as usual I will battle low blood pressure and no one will do anything about it, except tell me to drink, which I do and it is never enough. I am also worried about biopsy results.

Talk to you later,

Marcy

P.S. I felt warm and have a 99.7 temp. I know that isn't high but since I normally run in the 97s I wonder if they will make a big deal if I have a temp tomorrow. I assume that they wouldn't postpone surgery, just give me antibiotics and something for the temp? Maybe it is an inflammation fever?

From: Alan

To: Marcy

Good evening,

The bump behind the ear is likely nothing and a temp in the 99s is not really concerning for infection, perhaps some nonspecific inflammation.

As for the breast finding hopefully it's just confined to the breast. I'm assuming the chemo was intended to rid any cancer that had been in the lymphatic system, and that the surgery will get rid of what is in the breast. I don't think the breast finding is necessarily a bad thing as long as you can't feel abnormal nodes in the armpit or neck.

You're right. The pathology report will be the key. I'd tell you not to be anxious about it but that probably wouldn't have much effect. I'd be anxious too, to say the least.

Good Samuel is a good hospital. My mother-in-law has gotten very good care there. Be good. Sleep well.

From: Marcy

To: Alan

Thanks for calling after you sent the last email. Sometimes talking things out is the most helpful.

Yes, the chemo was to rid the lymph nodes and prevent it from spreading. But he kept saying the change in the breast was so good that I feel like it is bad that it is like that again. But as long as she samples or removes as many lymph nodes as needed to remove it, I will be fine.

It was a cyst behind my ear and I cleaned it well. I think all will be fine in the morning. I think it is a low grade temp from inflammation too, not as worried about it now.

I will like Good Samuel, so far they have been good. Both the kids had tonsils out there *and* one of my grade school classmates that I reconnected with on Facebook is a nurse in the surgical department! She works on Monday too. Looking forward to seeing her.

Thanks for all your help Alan, through all of this. Being able to talk/email with you has been more helpful than I can ever really explain. Good night.

Marcy

P.S. I will be good and if I can't be good I will try not to get caught.

From: Alan

To: Marcy

Any time—seriously. I'm back at work—it's busy on such a beautiful day. Hope you're feeling OK today.

CB: August 12, 2012

Surgery Tomorrow

Surgery is at noon tomorrow at Good Samuel hospital. Dani asked if I was scared about surgery. Honestly, the answer is no. Not the surgery itself. She said she was and I asked her if she was scared when I had surgery in December and she said no. Why is this different? I have had five surgeries, my jaw surgery was much riskier and longer. She told me she did want to cry after that when she saw me but didn't because of her brother... awwwww. I don't know if it is just the diagnosis that suddenly people are worried about the surgery or what, no one ever made a big deal before about surgeries or coming to see me in the hospital. Sometimes I think the safest place to be is in the operating room at the hands of skilled doctors and nurses. Really the actual surgery will be fine. These are the things that I want to happen.

(1) Keep me asleep during surgery and wake me up when it is over. Priority number 1!

(2) Take as many lymph nodes out or samples as needed and I want them all to come back clear of cancer. Take as much off my chest as needed and even a little more if that will keep it from coming back.

(3) Manage my post-op low blood pressure that I always have and nothing ever helps. If they aren't going to manage it with a fluid bolus or some other way, I may have to set up a coffee pot in my room to see if caffeine helps.

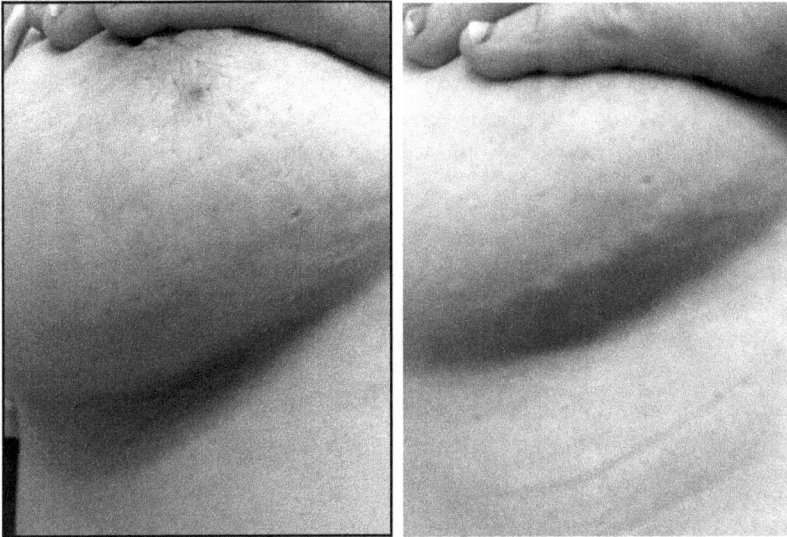

Figure 2-1. (Left) My right breast with the pitted skin visible with an "orange-peel appearance" (peau d'orange) that is caused from swelling in the breast from blocked lymph vessels. (Right) Appearance of blocked lymph vessels and damage to nail beds from chemotherapy.

(4) Put me back on an anti-inflammatory ASAP. I had to go off of it for surgery and my arthritis is so much worse than it was four months ago. I stand up, bend over and walk, like I am 90 years old! My neck, back and hips hurt a lot right now.

My mom or I will let you know when I am up in a room. Not sure if I will be up for technology Monday night but surely by Tuesday. Thank you everyone for your support and kindness.

Love ya, Marcy

Many messages of support showered down on me from email, Facebook comments, CaringBridge comments, and phone calls. It was a little odd to me as I didn't think this surgery would be a big deal. I'd had multiple surgeries in the past; in fact, this would be my sixth surgery. Having a five-hour corrective jaw surgery for developmental defects and having my jaw wired shut for six weeks, *that* was a big deal. Yet the support for this surgery was profoundly more. I suppose it is because of the cancer diagnosis, the reason for the surgery. I honestly did not care about the loss of my breasts, my major concern was the pathology. Did the chemotherapy work? Would there be cancer in the lymph nodes? When I thought of the fact that the oncologist told me that we couldn't do more chemotherapy, the fear of still having cancer seemed insurmountable. It did make sense though. If he gave me the most aggressive chemotherapy and it didn't work to clear all the cancer, why would we do it again?

FB: August 12, 2012

This was at the bottom on an email I just got. I think this quote by Randy Armstrong is perfect to say good night with. "Worrying does not take away tomorrow's troubles: it takes away today's peace."

Too many emotional conversations today. Thank you everyone for the compliments and encouragement but I am going back to watching *Criminal Minds* now.

HC: You are in my thoughts.

Miriam: I won't call. I know you are overwhelmed right now. But I will be there with you in spirit and if you want to talk, please don't hesitate to pick up the phone and call me. Love you.

Marcy: I know sweetie, even some of the messages I get tear me up. I have so many loving friends and family. So grateful but it is a bit more emotional that way. My mom will post to my wall as she can and I will be back on Facebook as soon as I can. You know me.

PO: You got this.

Marcy: Wow, even some nice texts from Dani's friends, the teens I have watched grow up. Great kids. Nice to know my daughter has such a great support system.

When I walked into the hospital I felt like I had a posse of supporters. In that moment I was more concerned about my mom and Grace than I was about myself. Once again, I could see the concern in their eyes. I knew my sister Becky and Harrison would give my Mom and Grace all the emotional support they needed in the surgical waiting area. In a way, it felt like old home week, which was comforting. I had been in touch with Penny, a grade school friend who was also a nurse and happened to be an admission nurse for the surgical unit.

Having a mini reunion with Penny took the focus from what was about to happen. After I was prepared for surgery, my support team crowded into the small curtained presurgical holding area. There was very little room between the stalls separated by curtains. I wondered if the other patients could hear us and what they were thinking as we tried to ease the tension with humor and distraction.

Penny and I showed each other pictures of our kids from our phones and learned about each other's families. We reminisced about grade school and discussed who was on Facebook, whom we kept up with over the years, and whom we were curious about. I glanced intermittently at the dry erase board that had my name and my surgeon and anesthesiologist and the surgery I was scheduled for on it. Seeing "bilateral mastectomies with right lymph node dissection" in writing caused me to have silent moments of worry. I tried not to stare at the board as I was sure they all would notice my grief. Grief not for the loss of my breasts but for the person I was before the cancer diagnosis and for what my family was surely going through as well.

Old home week was interrupted when the doctors came in. I told the anesthesiologist that I had issues with low blood pressure and dizziness after surgery. He was confident that extra IV fluids would address that concern. When the surgeon, Dr. Campbell, came in, she gave the opportunity for my family to ask questions. I asked them to step out just for a minute as I didn't want to worry them more. I showed Dr. Campbell my breast, which (to me) appeared to be getting larger again, had the orange-peel appearance, and had what I suspected was a swollen lymph vessel. As she looked at my breast I studied her face to see if I could read any concern from it. She attempted to assure me that if there was still cancer in the breast, it would be gone soon. All the tissue would be sent to the lab and her goal was to have clear margins, meaning there would be no cancer in the edges of where she cut. Clear margins would indicate that she removed all the cancer when she removed the breasts. I quietly nodded but wasn't comforted. I was ready to get the surgery over with.

Things started moving quickly as Penny brought my family in to wish me well. Hugs and kisses all around. I wanted that part to go quickly as I knew any one of us could easily start crying. Penny instructed them where to wait and then gave a report to the surgical nurse regarding my history and the pre-op medications that were given. She confirmed the surgical procedure yet again and asked if I was ready to go as she put the surgical hat on my bald head. Sometimes the medical field's rules and procedures don't make sense. I chuckled as I said, "Make sure you get all my hair tucked under the hat." She chuckled too as she unlocked the bed to push it down to the operating room.

From the moment I woke up in recovery and heard my surgeon say that I had flowers already and that she had not seen flowers delivered to the recovery room before, I felt the outpouring of love and support. Family and friends expressed messages of hope and encouragement and reminded me that I was strong.

My mom told me later that when they informed her I was going up to my hospital room from recovery and they could meet me there soon, Grace and Harrison left and told my mom to tell me they would check in on me later with a phone call. They walked in my room and I was already on my laptop posting on Facebook. My mom and sister were shocked at how alert I was after surgery.

They were getting ready to leave for the night when my mom stood up and yelped like a puppy who'd had its tail stepped on: it was her hip. I raised my voice at her, telling her to call the doctor. The arthritis in her hip was progressing and we knew she needed to have a hip replacement. She did call the doctor, but only got a steroid injection to control pain and delay surgery. This was something I didn't want her to postpone. I knew I was the cause of much emotional and mental anguish. I couldn't help that. But I didn't want to also be the cause of increased physical pain because my disease held her up from getting what she needed to have done.

FB: August 13, 2012

So, in thinking about some of today's events, one stands out a little more than others right now. Not sure why I got a little emotional at that time but when they moved me from surgery to recovery, I was in and out of awareness. The only thing I remember was a nurse telling me before she walked away to "keep fighting." Those two words got to me. I couldn't open my eyes, speak or respond to her but I heard her. Keep fighting!

Willow: That just brought tears to my eyes. I admire your strength and courage! You are an amazing woman.

Kitt: I love that nurse! She's right on and she somehow knew you had it in you! You're a fighter!!

Marcy: I love her also. I wish I was with it enough to know who it was or could have responded to her.

Many years later this story and how those two words made me feel came to be the example that I used with the families of my hospice patients. I encouraged them that if they had something to say and didn't get a chance to say it before, they should say it, even to an unresponsive, dying patient. The medical field does not know for sure which senses shut down in what order and I knew from this experience that I could appear out of it and not be able to respond but still hear what was going on. This experience made it possible for me to teach families to say goodbye and provide them with some closure and peace when their loved one was dying.

FB: August 13, 2012

Thank you Penny for the awesome care. You and your coworkers are fabulous.

JP: Hey, how are you doing?

Marcy: Very good. I am surprised I feel the way I do. Just had dinner, pain is minimal with the medicine. My blood pressure usually is low post-op but I told them how much it bothers me when I get dizzy and can't get up. They gave me extra fluids and I have been able to move around. All is good, very pleased with how things are going so far.

JG: Hey Marcy, Hope you're resting and you have pleasant dreams. Heal up! God bless.

Marcy: My mom, and my sister, Becky, were witnesses; the nurse actually said I was being a good patient, LOL. As long as they let me sleep tonight it will stay that way.

JP: I know it's hard to get rest in there *but* they are just doing their job. So kinda go light on them! LOL!

Marcy: I know. I was a night nurse at a hospital. Because of that I know that the good nursing staff at night "cluster care" to minimize waking up patients.

Laurie: You are a trooper. You make a great Wonder Woman!

Penny: You're the best. Such a tough day, but you did amazing. What a nice family!! I loved seeing the pictures of your children. I wish our lives were a little less troubled, but we can do it girl!!!

CB: August 13, 2012

Doing Well Post-surgery

My blood pressure is better, so I am not lightheaded. Up to the bathroom without problems, pain is under control, thank you morphine! No nausea, so I am waiting for dinner to be delivered. Very pleased with the care I have received. I will not know until maybe Thursday on the biopsy results. Just want my lymph nodes to be clear. More information later but for now, things look and feel good. Thank you all for your support.

FB: August 13, 2012

Friends don't let friends Facebook while on morphine. Really though, feeling good. Pain is controlled, no nausea, much better job controlling low blood pressure. No catheter to cause problems. Considering I said goodbye to the "girls" today, I am doing great!

Shelby: You are like Wonder Woman! Can't wait to see you.

Harrison: Glad we were there and what a surprise to hear from you. We love you.

My hospital stay was short and I really had time for only one visitor. Surprisingly, she was someone I went to high school with but had not been in contact with until somewhat recently when we found each other on Facebook. Shelby was such a calming presence. It made me think that even friends who haven't been close recently can be the best support, as I knew she cared or she wouldn't be there but I didn't feel responsible for her feelings and wasn't worried about her being worried. Those two things made her a great hospital guest.

Maybe there was not as much postmastectomy teaching regarding prosthetics as I expected because they knew I wouldn't be getting them for months, after my incisions healed and radiation was done. The educator from the breast center came up to see me the day after surgery. She gave me a halter top with foam inserts for breasts to wear if desired after the drains came out in a week or two. I was shown how to empty the drains as protocol but already knew this from being a nurse myself.

I saw Dr. Dunkin and Dr. Campbell as well the day after surgery. Dr. Campbell replaced the large bulky dressing with a chest binder and a smaller dressing. They indicated that if I was ready to go off morphine and would have adequate pain control with oral narcotics I could go home the next day, Wednesday. That was music to my ears.

When the time came, Dani and Nick came to the hospital to pick me up. Physically I felt good. I was anxious to be home, anxious to have some type of return to normal. Anxious to be in my own bed.

Not Done Yet

CB: August 16, 2012

No News....

The surgeon said to call for pathology reports Thursday morning, which I did. Just now got a call back saying the report isn't available yet. Hmmmmmmm. But maybe they will know something when I go get the drains out in the morning. This is the hard part for me because being a nurse, I know there has to be some information. A preliminary report of some sort, but they will make me wait and go insane anyway.

Pain is minimal, numbness in my arm and nerve pain shooting down to my elbow. Hopefully that will all get better as inflammation subsides.

Yum, *Pizza*!

Got an awesome delivery from Lou Malnati's from SS. I know three people with initials SS. Who can I thank for this?

Alan: Lou Malnati's is not only good, it has special healing powers. I think it's the secret tomato sauce. Have a pleasant evening. Feel better!

Sasha: Go figure that you know three people with initials SS. From the one that doesn't cook much herself hence sends somebody else's cooking or meets you at Bakers Square. Take care and enjoy!

FB: August 16, 2012

Dani wanted to know how my life will change now that I have no breasts. I'm not exactly sure yet but at least I never have to buy and wear a sports bra again.

CB: August 16, 2012

Call from Surgeon

Call from surgeon just now, she said she wanted to wait to check for the close of the pathology day to see if results were in. If they are not in when I see her in the morning she will call the pathologist and get a verbal result of what they have ready. Just the sound of her voice calms me, even if she doesn't have anything new to say. For now, I am chilling...literally, with ice packs on my chest, and that seems to help with the inflammation and swelling.

FB: August 16, 2012

Dani's birthday is tomorrow and although we had a party with her friends, we are going to have a small celebration dinner at home. I feel guilty though, for sending her to the store with money to buy stuff to make lasagna and to buy her own dessert. She will be making the dinner tomorrow also. She doesn't seem to mind. I just feel a little guilty about the timing of it all.

CB: August 17, 2012

Hard Not to Cry

Hi all,

Sorry I can't talk to everyone on the phone or in person, sometimes this format is best because when I hear your loving and concerned voice it is hard not to cry. I have spent the better part of the day trying to put things in perspective after talking to my surgeon. The things she said that were encouraging are 1) there was no sign of cancer in the skin—which there was before chemotherapy—and 2) the "margins" were clear. The area she cut didn't have any cancer, so it appears she got all of the cancer that was in the breast when she removed the entire breast. There was no evidence of cancer in the left breast, which is gone now too. The lymph nodes are another story and she tried to be encouraging, but to me the lymph nodes either have cancer or they don't. I can't comprehend what it means to have "a little cancer" in six out of twelve lymph nodes. I rely on two doctors I worked with to help me sort through this stuff. I know they will be hopeful but honest and I trust and respect them. This is what one said: "The positive lymph nodes are somewhat concerning. Don't freak out." Both doctors agree that a second opinion is appropriate and there are several that I could go to. No one physician is the perfect one, so I have a few names, will look at them online and make some appointments. I am not saying I am not getting good treatment but I told myself that after four months of chemo if there was any cancer in the lymph nodes I would get a second opinion just to make sure we are being as aggressive as possible. As my surgeon said, "We aren't done yet, we still have radiation and hormone-targeted oral medication." [Hormone-targeted oral medication reduces the circulating estrogen to keep those levels low, as the biopsies showed that my type of cancer grows in the presence of estrogen.] So that is the update. Sorry it couldn't be better news but we will still beat this. Sometimes I just need a little time in the corner of the ring before I can come back out swinging at the bell again.

Surgery post-op is going okay. I have numbness and shooting pain in the right arm but that will get better when the swelling goes down. The drains weren't taken out today because there is still a moderate amount of bloody drainage coming from the surgical sites. Overall, in comparison to the five surgeries I have had previously, three were much worse. Recovery from the surgery itself will be fine. It almost seems like the easy part, if there is such a thing.

Have a great weekend, I hope you get to spend it with the people you love.

EM: August 17, 2012

From: Marcy

To: Alan

The surgeon is focusing on the positive result of clear margins and no cancer in skin as previous. I am concerned that there was still "a little cancer" in six of twelve lymph nodes. Do you think I should go for a second opinion at this point? How would I find a doctor who specializes in inflammatory breast cancer?

From: Alan

To: Marcy

Hi Marcy,

The positive nodes are somewhat concerning. If it were me I'd get a second opinion.

Dr. Gradon was one of my teachers in med school. He's a breast cancer specialist.

He's a good guy. I know they also have ongoing study protocols. I wouldn't freak out.

I'll ask around specifically about inflammatory breast cancer.

Hang in there.

From: Marcy

To: Alan

Thanks for the honesty. I will go for a second opinion. I just want to get to the right person... Talk to you later.

From: Marcy

To: Alan

There have been several suggestions for physicians who specialize in breast cancer for a second opinion. It is hard to decide.

From: Alan

To: Marcy

A reasonable strategy would be to call and schedule a couple appointments for another opinion. You can always cancel if you find someone you like right away. I'd say something along the lines of "a friend referred me to Dr. X and I'd like to get her/his opinion on my situation." I know it's hard. Hang in there.

From: Marcy

To: Alan

I'll make some calls on Monday. It really takes time to process this stuff.

How are you doing?

From: Alan

To: Marcy

I know what you mean. Sometimes it's hard just to make phone calls and deal with the person on the other end of the phone and answer all the same questions again.

It's probably a good idea to take it easy this weekend and get back to business on Monday.

I'm ok. My back always hurts. I just keep going. My physical therapist is gone for two weeks.

Have a good night.

EM: August 17, 2012

From: Liza

To: Marcy

Hi. Please tell Dani Happy Birthday from the Izzys. Maybe we can find a day where we can celebrate her birthday and certification sometime soon. I'm so proud of her.

I just read your journal update, and I would love to go with you when you do a second opinion with another doctor. If that's okay.

Love you, sweet dreams.

From: Marcy

To: Liza

Thanks, I was actually going to ask you if you would come with me. I have a couple names that I looked at online.

Both names were given to me by the neurologist I worked for who called around to get those recommendations. The female looks like she does a lot of research and clinical studies as well. Both physicians would probably be good. Just want to make sure I am doing all I can.

I was really disappointed today... Love ya.

FB: August 17, 2012

Sometimes I just need a little time in the corner of the ring before I can come back out swinging at the bell again.

FP: Get 'em Rocky!

Marcy: Just so long as I don't have to drink (or eat) eggs in any form.

CB: August 19, 2012

Herceptin?

The doctor that I was thinking about doing the second opinion with, Dr. Colby, worked a lot with Herceptin when it was first being used.

Honestly, the predominate feeling I have right now is rage! I am thinking but won't know until I see the oncologist on Thursday that Herceptin infusions may be done with radiation since there was cancer in the lymph nodes still. I thought this was orally, but it is by infusion, either once a week or every three weeks, not sure. If he doesn't recommend this, I would question how we are treating any systemic cancer since radiation targets only the local area.

FB: August 20, 2012

Really going to have to get some endurance back if I am planning on going back to work full time after Labor Day. Did a little bit today and I am drained. Maybe I can start walking a bit after I get these drains out.

CB: August 21, 2012

Sad, Angry, Frustrated...Grateful

Hi all,

I am not as angry anymore. Man, I really have to go through the range of emotion to get through this. Spent some good time with my brother Steve, sister-in-law Patti, nephew Parker, Riley, Dani, and my mom over the weekend and that helped a lot. Especially being with Patti, she is so good at letting me feel and be wherever I am, at the moment. Dani celebrated her nineteenth birthday Friday night. I felt guilty she had to cook her own dinner but I couldn't have made a better lasagna than she made. She didn't mind. Both the kids have been very helpful during this surgical recovery time. I am so lucky and grateful for my family and friends who help me process all of this emotion and information. I really cannot do this without all of you. Do not underestimate your contribution to my health and sanity.

So the frustration is trying to get appointments made. I got the surgical drains out today and I am happy about that. I am still using cold packs for the swollen areas. Already the lymphedema has started, just slightly but I can tell there is swelling in the arm of the side that the lymph nodes were taken out. I am going to have to call around to find a place that treats that for physical therapy because the place my doctor recommends can't see me for at least two weeks and by that time I am supposed to be back to work. I don't know now how I am going to work full time, get radiation after work, get physical therapy scheduled and possibly infusions, if they can even do them at the same time as radiation. I am hoping it can happen. I don't want any stray cancer cells setting up shop in my lungs, liver, brain, or bone (most common sites of metastasis from breast cancer). I have to work. I need to support my family and have medical insurance and I am almost out of FMLA [Family and Medical Leave Act] time if not already. But sometimes I wonder if I can do all these medical appointments and work full time or if I will have to see if they will agree to part time for a while.

I haven't heard from the Rush Medical Center specialist yet; if I don't hear from them tomorrow I will move on to another health system, Northwestern or North Shore. My mom did fax over thirty-five pages of my treatment/tests/reports to the specialist at Rush and I left my message on her voice mail, explaining why I wanted to see her. Kind of weird that this is how you get an appointment with her. The doctor listens to your story and then decides when the receptionist can schedule an appointment for you. I feel like I have to beg sometimes to get help: am I sick enough? Is my case interesting enough? Blah, blah, blah, what does it take? I hate being the patient and I hope I never made any of my patients feel that way.

The appointment with my medical oncologist is on Thursday and I am anxious to hear what he has to say. I am going to be my usual nice self but honestly, I think he needs a little push to convince me that he is doing absolutely everything that can be done as quickly as it can be done. I don't feel like we have a handle on this quite yet and that is not acceptable to me.

My kids don't believe we have a handle on this. At least that is the perception I got the other day when we were walking in the parking lot to go register Dani at the community college. A car was going to back out, and it would have hit me first had it not stopped. Then she said something like, "At least it would have hit you first and you are already dying."

Really? Do my kids think I am dying? Ah, no no no! I will not have that. "Dani, they never said I am dying, if I ever get to the point that they can't do anything else I will let you know, until then, do not even think that way for a second." It hurts so bad that my kids think this way, they shouldn't have to. This, people, is why I have tried so hard not to "act sick," why I want to do as much as I can, even if you think it is over doing it. If I don't, my kids think I am dying and that is what actually kills me, or at least kills my spirit.

Wow, do I ramble or what? I didn't intend for this to go on so long. So that is the update for now. I will let you all know what I find out on Thursday.

Feel free to tell me about your weekend, did you get to spend some time with your loved ones? It helps sometimes to hear what other people are doing. Love ya.

PO: Marcy, I am sure part of it is society. Cancer is still seen as a death sentence. They still teach it that way in school and give them statistics.

Marcy: Unfortunately, she has heard conversations. She is very smart and looked up inflammatory breast cancer and knows it is rare and one of the most aggressive form of breast cancer. I have told her that rare and aggressive does not mean that it isn't curable. I know though sometimes when they see me sick that is hard to believe, for all of us.

PO: I know you want her educated, but not that much. She still is a kid and hasn't learned to read without convincing herself that the worst is the only way it goes.

Marcy: Yeah, nineteen-year-olds know where to get information on the web. We have discussed which sites are more reputable and not to put too much stock into those numbers. The medical field is getting better every day and a lot of those statistics are from ten years ago. We talk about future stuff all the time. That helps. We have been watching *Say Yes to the Dress* and talking about that.

SV: That's a good thing they talk to you about it.

Marcy: I wish Riley would talk more but it usually comes out in bits and pieces, with comments here and there, and then that is my cue. Dani is very straightforward and blunt about what she thinks and feels, easier to read.

BJ: Marcy, your posts are *so* inspirational. Your kids are great, smart and *so* love their mom! You are strong. You will kick this stupid, incompetent inflammatory asshole called cancer in the ass, but first it will drag your ass around in the mud a bit! It did that to my mom, but then it got what it had coming! Fight on girlfriend!!!

Marcy: BJ, how old were you when your mom had cancer? Would love to talk to you about what you were thinking and what I could do better for the kids from a person who went through it with their mom. Call me when you can some evening.

Krystal: Marcy, I was sixteen when my mom was diagnosed and nineteen when she died. Even though she was so sick in that last year I always thought she would get better. I didn't believe she was dying until my sister called me at school to tell me the doctors were giving her six weeks. It only sunk in then. I guess I'm just trying to say that you may not know what your kids are really feeling. Perhaps Dani was throwing out one of her fears to see your reaction and maybe learn some insight. It may not necessarily be her belief. I don't know, but I do know I love you. I hope this helps.

Marcy: Thanks Krystal, it could be that she goes back and forth with the thought but doesn't really believe it and that was a way of opening the door to the conversation instead of saying, "Mom, I am afraid you are dying." I know it crosses her mind but she may not really believe it and I hope she doesn't. Thank you for your insight. You were at an age between Dani and Riley when your mom was diagnosed.

My surgeon gave me an order for the evaluation and treatment of lymphedema. When the lymph nodes are removed, the body has less ability to move cellular debris and infection throughout the lymphatic system for processing. There are three levels of lymph nodes and two levels were removed. Already there were signs of edema (swelling) in my right arm. Physical therapists have to have special training in the treatment of lymphedema. It involved lymphatic drainage to move fluids across the lymphatic system and compression wraps placed on my right arm. Multiple calls were made to multiple area hospitals and physical therapy clinics to find a location I could get into later in the afternoon after I got off work at the high school. I also knew I was going to have to work radiation in to my daily schedule.

FB: August 22, 2012

I just want the people I know and love to be healthy and happy, this includes you!

Thanks to a call from a friend who is a doctor to the specialist at Rush University, the receptionist called this morning and scheduled an appointment for me next week on Wednesday. I would have never asked him to call in a "professional courtesy" request, but he read my online journal and could tell how frustrated I was. Ah, the benefits of my life and feelings being an open book. Thank you for extending that offer and making a call.

I Think I Understand but I'm Not Sure I Buy It

Hi all,

I saw the medical oncologist today. Mixture of good and bad news. I am still trying to process it. By the end of the visit I literally said, "I think I understand but I am not sure I buy it just yet." I also told him, "Since we are dealing with my life, I wish I had some more definitive answers." I don't know if definitive answers are realistic but am hoping the consult with Dr. Colby will help me with that.

As far as the visit...Herceptin infusions are not an option. [When they do the biopsies they check the cells' receptor status to see what the cells feed on and that determines what treatment can be given. If I was HER2 positive, Herceptin would be an option.] I thought I was HER2 positive but I am not, so giving it would not help at all. The plan remains radiation therapy and after that I can start hormone therapy. There are two options on the hormone therapy, which I will research and decide on later. Although the radiation oncologist isn't the one in the health system my oncologist is part of, my oncologist had only good things to say about him. He came highly recommended by 2 physicians that I respect and trust and I feel very comfortable with that choice. I will see him on Monday.

I asked the medical oncologist when the PET scan is repeated and he said unless I had problems or symptoms he wouldn't do another one. How do you know when I am cancer free? He says he considers me cancer free now. This is the part I don't buy just yet. How can he guess at that? The cancer was in 6 lymph nodes; how does he know there wasn't any cancer in the ones that weren't taken out or are there any cancer cells starting to set up in other places in the body? How can we take the approach of "wait and see if I have symptoms" before scanning again? He is going by the assumption that because the PET scan was good if there were any small cancer cells circulating in the body that the chemo would have gotten them. But we know the chemo didn't kill all the cancer because I still had some in my breast and 6 lymph nodes. Maybe I am unrealistic because I am afraid of the aggressiveness of this type of cancer. There may not be a definitive answer but I think it is worth looking at some point. Maybe not now, maybe after radiation is done. I think I should have another scan... not just if I have problems. By then, you are trying to catch up again and are never really ahead of things. These are the things I will talk to Dr. Colby about.

I finally got an appointment for physical therapy but since I will be going back to work full time and doing radiation after work, the soonest I can get in is September 19. That seems like a long time to me considering my arm is starting to swell already but there is nothing more I can do on that I guess.

So that is the news from my appointment today. Frustration again. I would like to celebrate and think I am cancer free but again I don't think I can make that assumption with the information I have. Maybe I am wrong, I hope I am wrong. Until next time...

EM: August 23, 2012

From: Alan

To: Marcy

Hey Marcy,

The medical system can be frustrating to plow through, can't it? I sometimes think a good strategy is to put aside today's visit, get a good night's sleep, and then formulate your opinions tomorrow. Sometimes you have more clarity the next day.

This is just my opinion: I think it's reasonable to be suspicious of a cancer cell remaining here or there. You're not wrong to think that. I doubt a PET scan would pick up such a thing at this point.

The thing to do is get the radiation and go on the hormones and get on with life. The unknown is so hard to deal with but the Zen thing is to not worry about what might be.

You can buy an arm compression sleeve at medical supply stores or online for $25–$40. You can buy a very similar item at sporting goods stores for less.

Near me is a drug store. It's not actually a drug store. It's like a superstore of medical products. Over the years I've gotten ankle and wrist braces there and have bought all kinds of catheter and ostomy supplies, dressings, and podiatry stuff for my elderly neighbors. They have every home medical product you can imagine. They take insurance.

Glad you're still posting on online journal. Glad you're honest and open too.

My thoughts are with you.

From: Marcy

To: Alan

You are awesome as usual. I started my journal with "I am still processing" because I know if I put it out there I will get some thoughts like yours that will help with that processing. Thank you. A night's sleep is always helpful.

You are probably right. I didn't really know if a PET scan would show anything now, but at some point I think I would like to do it, maybe after radiation. I may change my mind about that later.

I am glad to hear I can buy a sleeve anywhere. I didn't know if it was something I had to get measured for. Maybe I will check out the medical supply store around here. I think there is a ma and pa pharmacy/supply store nearby.

I do like the online journal. It helps me get all kinds of opinions without calling all kinds of people individually. Your thoughts have always meant a lot to me.

Thanks for that. Take Care.

From: Alan

To: Marcy

Thanks Marcy, my guess is any medical supply place could help you. I send people for pressure stockings a lot too. I usually advise finding a place close to home because most such places are helpful.

Your writings on online journal have been special. I think all medical providers should know more about what a person really goes through when faced with something like this.

It can't be put into words at times but you've done a heck of a job. Get some rest.

CB: August 23, 2012

More Thoughts

The thing I love about this site is that after I post my raw, rambling thoughts I sometimes get feedback in the form of a guestbook entry, email or phone call. I do realize a PET scan right away would not be the answer and I am not really suggesting that. But in my mind if I had the option of a lumpectomy the doctor wouldn't say, "You don't need a mammogram unless you have problems." A PET scan will not show something minuscule, but it may show something prior to when I would develop symptoms from a problem. Wouldn't it be nice if there was a blood test to detect breast cancer? I think they are working on it. At some point I will have to trust, let go, and get over the fact that I feel like a time bomb. I don't think I will be confident that I am cancer free until after radiation and after a follow-up scan of some sort.

As far as the lymphedema, it was suggested I go get fitted for a compression sleeve at a medical supply store. I guess my head isn't on straight because as a nurse I should've remembered I could do that and not have to wait for physical therapy. I will look into that tomorrow.

Thank you all for your feedback, suggestions and support...it is always welcomed.

Love, Marcy

EM: August 23, 2012

From: Marcy

To: Alan

LOL, you should read what my tired mind just wrote. I'm trying to decide if I should post it. I probably will. Some of my better things are when I am tired, not specific health stuff but just what I am thinking. Good night my friend.

P.S. Been hanging out watching *Scrubs* on my laptop most of the evening, will call it a night soon.

CB: August 23, 2012

Warning Tired Personal Rant

I am warning you up front this is a personal/political rant; you have a choice not to read this. It is about who I think I am as a healthcare provider and therefore what I want as a patient.

When I care for patients, I look at the elderly and see my grandma and I love them. When I go into their homes, when I work home care, it is like seeing Grandma and Grandpa. I want to do my best for them. When I take care of the high school kids, I see my teenagers. I am tough on them when I have to be and when I don't have to be tough they get every ounce of TLC I have. Treating people my age, I see my friends, brothers, and sisters. I see my nephews and nieces. I see my patients as friends and family and I think what would I do for them if they really were my friends and family, and I guide myself that way.

As a patient I want to hear, "If you were my wife, if I were you, if you were my daughter, this is what I would recommend." Those physicians or nurses who can't do that are the ones that I think are thinking, "What does administration want me to do to cut costs?" or "What does the insurance company want me to do?" Maybe that sounds cynical but I can really feel the difference. This is why I will not have an HMO [health management organization]. I want my physician to decide what is best and not the insurance company. I want him/her to fight for me, just like I would fight for you. This is what makes me a "difficult" patient. I know I am judgmental about the care I receive and that is why if I recommend a physician to you, you know it is because I believe in them, I trust and respect them. I want you to see someone I am confident in, not just anyone my healthcare system may be associated with or to make the administration happy. I really felt like the care I got at Good Samuel Hospital was from my brothers and sisters, my mom or dad. I felt like they cared. When the one nurse wheeled me into recovery and I was too drugged to open my eyes or speak, she told me to "keep fighting" and I remembered those words later. She touched me. That is something you do when you see your patient as your loved one.

This is the kind of care I want to provide, this is the kind of care you and I deserve and this is the kind of care I will get; if not I will go somewhere else. I have choices and I am in control of my body. You have choices too and you are in control of your body. Thank you to those who didn't let me forget it and I hope you never forget it either.

So this is the kind of post you get right before I need to go to sleep. Good night.

"You know that before medicine ever became a business, the only rule was to do your best to help the patient." -Dr. Cox, *Scrubs*

Dr. Douglass: It is always a difficult balance between being a strong advocate for your own health and having faith in your physicians, but in my opinion, ultimately it is your body and if it makes you feel more secure there is nothing wrong with pushing hard for additional safe noninvasive testing.

FB: August 23, 2012

Post on my wall

Joe, DJ at Star Radio Station: I signed the Pink Breast cancer awareness truck for you! "Marcy! Keep Fighting!" Joe

Marcy: I am truly touched. Thank you so much Joe! My 19 year-old-daughter also says, "Thank you."

For the last year or so I listened to Joe and Tina in the morning on Star 105.5 when I drove to work and often on my computer during the work day. I was very familiar with Joe's story of his mom having breast cancer multiple times. He was and still is active in the community and very accessible to the community. I must have been friends with him on Facebook for some time prior to the post he made about signing the pink breast cancer awareness truck to encourage me.

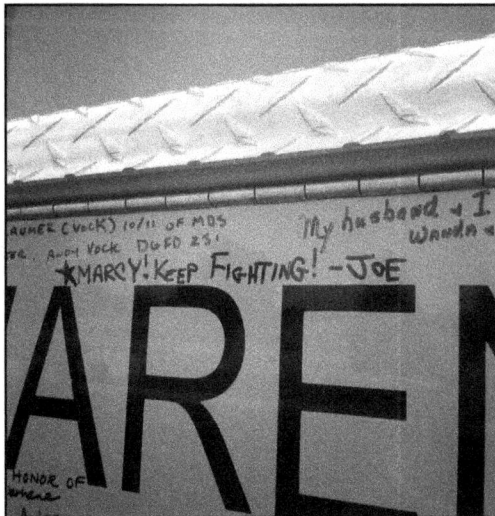

Figure 2-2. A photo of the pink breast cancer awareness truck that Joe signed

CB: August 24, 2012

Feeling Pretty Good

So my friend who encourages a good night sleep after I get overwhelming news is so right. I feel pretty good today and am going to ride that wave as long as I can.

I found a little medical supply store across from the big one that was locked in the middle of the day. I was fitted for a compression sleeve. Not the most comfortable thing to wear, in fact in hurts a little on the upper arm, but it will help keep swelling down. He also showed me some foobs (fake boobs), silicone and foam for when I am ready. I am thinking that I will just wear what the hospital gave me until my incisions heal and until radiation is over because if my skin gets to where it feels sunburnt, I am not going to want to wear much, clothes will need to be loose.

Da Bears play tonight and I am just going to play it by ear this weekend and rest. I am also going to explore some of the exercises for lymphedema that are in the breast cancer book the hospital gave me.

I think I am in a good mood because I am grateful to have such wonderful people in my life to follow my ranting and writing. You step up to help in many ways. How can life be better than knowing how loved you are (no matter how long or short life is), isn't that what we all want, to love and be loved?

Thanks for being there for me, Marcy

EM: August 24, 2012

From: Alan

To: Marcy

I read all 1,400 pages of Harrison's *Textbook of Internal Medicine* today. I couldn't find any mention of foobs. I was laughing out loud when I read that. There's really nothing funny about all you've been through but I guess sometimes it's just good to laugh. Sleep tight, whatever that means.

CB: August 25, 2012

Compression

I have a better understanding now. I know why patients are noncompliant with compression sleeves, and compression stockings. I try to tell my patients the rationale for why I ask them to do something, to try to get them on board with me. I understand the rationale for the compression sleeve but man it is annoying. I wish all this was on my nondominant side. I will get used to it but I think I will have to work my way up a few hours at a time. Maybe if more of us medical providers had to do the things we asked our patients to do we would have a better understanding and more patience with our patients.

EM: August 26, 2012

From: Sasha

To: Marcy

Hi, I got your thank you note and I am really glad that the pizza works. A small apology before the big apology: I am sorry that I didn't send you this message sooner than now. You'll understand when you read below.

I am the one who signed "your friend" [for the pizza order]. I realize now that if I'm not comfortable posting in the guestbook I should just send you a private e-mail instead of using stupid sign-offs like "your friend." I did not mean to upset you. When I composed that stupid note I was trying for some semblance of normalcy in a really abnormal situation. I was trying to connect with the Marcy who introduced me to tube socks, the one who could paint the rooms in her home phenomenal colors, the Marcy who despite all the information and decisions right now is much, much more than a cancer survivor; a spectacular mother, a good and loving daughter, and a caring friend.

Whatever the opinion, I hope that you find satisfaction with the consultation with Dr. Colby on Wednesday. Something came to mind recently.

You are doing an amazing job of handling this illness and the bad days don't change the truth of that observation. Again hope that this week will give you some clarity. Take care.

From: Marcy

To: Sasha

Thank you Sasha, no worries. I know your schedule is rough, hang in there.

I met Sasha in 2008 while training for the Avon Walk for Breast Cancer—the one where I hid away my white sash. Afterward, Sasha and I kept in touch via email, telephone, and a couple of in-person visits when I was in her area. She was a person who followed my CaringBridge journal for updates consistently yet did not feel comfortable posting in that type of public forum. I understood that and had no problems responding to emails from family and friends outside of the public forum. What became frustrating for me was continually seeing emails from her that she labeled "Do Not Respond" in the subject. I let that go for awhile but there came a time when I had to address this as it felt like she was trying so hard to connect, but those connections are impossible when you only have one side.

The emails back and forth talking about this and even calling her as I wrote this book proved to be healing for both of us. We shared feelings of disconnection and powerlessness but experienced them in different ways. I learned that those in a supportive role often feel guilty reaching out to a person who is ill. She didn't want to trouble me with composing an email back to her, but I needed to. I needed as much of my communications with others to continue as it was before I had cancer. I would have replied to her emails before I got sick; I needed to continue to respond to them. Communication as usual made me feel more normal and more myself. The less I had to change the less impact I felt like cancer had.

Other email communication worked more transparently. I continued to use email as a primary method of communication with Alan, Lucy, and others.

EM: August 26, 2012

From: Alan

To: Marcy

Doctors should have to go through all the stuff they advise and prescribe. I too treat people the way I'd expect to be treated. I think compression sleeves come in a variety of compression gradients. Perhaps you need a lighter one.

Hope you enjoyed the rain today.

From: Marcy

To: Alan

I know when you give me advice it is what you would do for you or Sophie, you would recommend the best you could regardless of politics and such.

I have heard you say, "If it were me." The other doctor that I worked with, Dr. Douglass, you may have seen a comment or two by him, he is like you in that way. He was never offended and often encouraged his patients to get a second opinion. I know if he recommends something it isn't based on who he is employed by; it is what he would do for his family.

I really am not sure what gradient this sleeve is. I haven't worn it today. My underarm and arm have been hurting more than I really expected it to. I feel like something is wrong but I can't put my finger on it and it could just be the healing process. It feels a little warm too but it isn't red or anything.

I am in bed now after eating too much. I really enjoy the rain, breeze and birds. I like rain and the cooler, darker weather makes it easier to relax.

FB: August 27, 2012

My leg hair is growing back much faster than the hair on my head. That stinks!

Laurie: Life is so cruel! Murphy's Law.

PG: Yay! Congrats! (Your body is working.)

Quote. "Maybe she laughs and maybe she cries. And maybe you would be surprised at everything she keeps inside." —Author Unknown

Reflections

Looking back on this period of time and looking ahead as well, the thoughts are very similar. It was becoming more and more challenging to trust what I was being told by the medical field I'd spent my career being part of. All I asked from my medical team from the beginning of this ordeal was that they give me honest and complete information. I could process things in time but I had to have the information to begin with, which is one of the reasons I relied heavily on other nurses I worked with and the physicians I was close to on a personal level. Doing this helped tremendously to calm me when "panic mode" encroached and often stifled "survival mode." My learned ability to search reliable websites often provided resources and the words needed to help explain to my family what was happening in layman's terms, but it is possible that by doing so I made survivorship more difficult after treatment was over. My family and nonmedical friends looked to me for answers that I was not always confident in giving them.

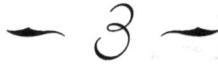

— 3 —

Radiation

On Track with Treatment

CB: August 27, 2012

What Cancer Cannot Do!

Hi all,

Today I saw Dr. Jacoby, the radiation oncologist. The first thing I saw when I walked in was a printout on the counter of things cancer can't do.

Cancer is so Limited...

It cannot Cripple Love

It cannot Shatter Hope

It cannot Corrode Faith

It cannot Destroy Peace

It cannot Kill Friendship

It cannot Silence Courage

It cannot Invade the Soul

It cannot Steal Eternal Life

It cannot Conquer the Spirit

I think he is a physician that will be honest with me, good or bad. He will spend more time trying to figure out how to cure me and give me a long life vs. trying to tiptoe around my feelings. That is what I want in a physician, complete and honest information. I have always said I can handle almost anything as long as I have the truth. On Thursday, they make a mold so I am in the exact same position every time I get radiation. They will put me through a scanner and make markings so that the radiation will go where it is supposed to. I will go after work Monday through Friday for thirty treatments. That may change by the response and total dose required once they have all that calculated but at least it is a starting point. Overall I left his office feeling okay about the plan.

I had some time so I treated myself to lunch and then bought myself a Pandora bracelet and a breast cancer awareness charm to go with the birthstone charms I got for my birthday from my friend Liza.

The highlight of the day was meeting my niece and sister for massages and facials. My niece's husband flew her in from Texas to visit family and he scheduled massages and facials for her, my sister, and myself. We had three hours of pampering with a little champagne to go with it. The massage felt good. I knew my muscles were sore but it really identified where I was achy and worked on it, very relaxing. It also identified how many areas of numbness I have. We stayed away from my right arm due to the lymphedema and nerve irritation but again, it was great.

The timing was good too, between surgery and the start of radiation.

This week is going to be a busy week with appointments. Tomorrow I am going back to the surgeon. I am not sure if the swelling at the edges of the surgical site, near my arms, is normal two weeks post-op or if it is too much fluid buildup after the removal of the drains. The office was good about scheduling me so she could take a look and say, "Yep, that is normal and will get better," or "Nope, we need to aspirate the fluid out." I will also go see if I can get a different compression sleeve, I really can't wear this one. I don't know if I bought the wrong size or just got that much more edema to make it not work for me. Hopefully he will exchange it; if he doesn't I will have to buy another for $90. I also will have to figure out how to submit it to insurance to see if they will even reimburse me for it. Wednesday I have the second opinion at Rush with Dr. Colby. Thursday it is back to the radiation oncologist.

Friday, there is absolutely nothing on the calendar and I am going to try to keep it that way.

So, I will let you know what the doctors say after my appointments. I will be really glad to go on Wednesday and get a little clarity because honestly, ever since my last appointment with the medical oncologist I have been very unsettled and not sleeping as well.

So, I think after the massage, and nice visit with my sister and niece and having a plan for the week, I may get a little better sleep tonight.

Here is to hoping you are getting all the rest you need to enjoy your life and the people in it.

Clara: After my surgery in 2000 on my knees when I was fifteen they had me wear the compression hose and let me tell you I hated them! Lol...I did wear them but not as much as I should've and I blame my big cankles on not wearing. So take it from me...it sucks but wearing it will be better in the long run. Love you, Your always-inspired niece, XOXO.

Lucy: Sounds like you have a good radiation plan in place. I'm so happy you had the opportunity to get a massage—that must have felt wonderful. I'm glad to hear you have a charm bracelet—thanks for the tip! Love you.

JY: Hi Marcy, Thanks for the update... So glad you got a chance to pamper yourself. This is such an awesome tool to be able to check for updates and saves you from telling the same story dozens of times! I think of you often... Hang in there!

CB: August 28, 2012

"I Can Fix That"

Hi,

Update on the extra visit with the surgeon. I told her I wasn't sure if this is normal post-op two weeks. I was feeling like I had mini boobs growing under my armpits. I guess it wasn't her intention to take the originals and replace them with side boobs. For a change, I heard a doctor say, "I can fix that." She drained 30 cc of fluid off the left and 40 cc off the right and then wrapped me tight with an ace bandage. Hopefully after wearing it for twenty-four hours things will be okay. It didn't hurt a bit. I am so numb in so many places, including the chest that I didn't even feel the needle or numbing medication. Was nice not to feel the stick and burn. I did ask her about the lymph nodes again. I am starting to think that everyone expected them to be positive except me. That is fine, but I guess I wish one of the physicians (surgeon or medical oncologist) would have prepared me for that, because cancer in the lymph nodes has such an ominous reputation. She tried to assure me again that it doesn't mean that things aren't going well. I think I will be able to get on board with that way of thinking after the second opinion tomorrow. I just need to hear it from someone who is looking at my case for the first time, with specialty background and fresh eyes.

I think other than the itchy ace wrap, I will sleep better without the lumps there. Still need to get the right compression sleeve for my arm and I still need to research my choices for medication after the radiation.

I'll update tomorrow after I see Dr. Colby. A big shout out to Liza for picking me up at 6 a.m. and taking me to the appointment. It is nice to have someone else drive and be there to help ask questions while we have the opportunity. What do you think I should ask her?

EM: August 28, 2012

From: Alan

To: Marcy

I'd ask what the real significance of the positive lymph nodes is. I'd ask if it's reasonable to expect the radiation to eradicate any remaining cancer cells.

I'm working again tonight. I wish people would stop injuring themselves. We should all just sit on the couch and watch TV.

FB: August 29, 2012

Fun night with my family eating and playing Farkle, singing and dancing in the kitchen. Love to let my hair down like that—oh wait—never mind, LOL.

RH: Sounds fun! Watcha singing?

Clara: LOL yes ma'am, it was amazing!!! We will have to do it again soon!!! Love you.

Marcy: RH, we sang: "Play That Funky Music," "Sweet Home Alabama," "Another One Bites the Dust," "Jack and Diane," and whatever came up on the radio.

CB: August 29, 2012

On Board and Confident Again

Hi all!

Going down to Rush University Medical Center for a second opinion is just what I needed to be confident in my treatment plan and my medical team again. More hopeful on my prognosis for the future. It was almost like after reviewing my records and talking to me, Dr. Colby was like a mom, shooing her kids outside to go play after their homework was done and telling them the hard part was over...go have some fun.

So here are some questions and answers.

Q: What is the significance of the positive lymph nodes? Could there be cancer cells in other places in my body?

A: Of course we would have loved it if there wasn't any cancer in the lymph nodes but the pathology report shows that if there are still any microscopic cancer cells they will be extremely responsive to Tamoxifen; it will be as effective or more so than the chemotherapy.

Even if there is cancer in other lymph nodes or in my body the radiation will get any remaining cancer cells that are in the local area, and the Tamoxifen will catch up to any that are systemic when I start it after radiation is complete.

Q: There were two options for endocrine therapy: Tamoxifen and Arimidex, which is slightly more effective. Since I still have ovaries, if I took Arimidex I would have to take a monthly injection, to keep the ovaries shut down (they shut down during chemo and possibly could recover). Working ovaries makes Arimidex less effective and since I had hysterectomy it is harder to know for sure if they are working or not. Should I have my ovaries removed? Which medication would she recommend?

A: No need to have ovaries removed. I am not at any higher risk for ovarian cancer—we know this from the genetic testing. She would recommend the Tamoxifen for five years or so and then I would switch to the other, Arimidex, when we are sure my ovaries won't recover and start working again.

Q: How do we know when I am cured?

A: They believe the remaining cancer was removed during surgery and there is "no evidence of disease."

Q: Does she agree with no routine follow-up scans?

A: She agrees with my oncologist and surgeon about not needing follow-up scans. (But she was able to explain why.) Studies were done taking two groups of people, one group had routine scans and the other didn't. There was no difference in outcomes. The people scanned that had a cancer recurrence were identified three months earlier than the others that were only scanned after symptoms appeared, but when treated, the group who was scanned after symptoms started did catch up with the ones who started treatment sooner and those patients had the same response to treatment. (I don't think I explained that as well as she did.) She also explained that there is an added risk to the scans with radiation exposure and false positives that could move a person to get unnecessary invasive testing, and suffer complications from those unnecessary procedures.

Q: If you don't do routine scans how would you monitor for recurrence?

A: Physician exam and labs every three months for a year, every six months for years two to five, then yearly.

Q: Is there anything else I should be or could be doing?

A: Continue to be aware of my body, if there are significant symptoms see the doctor right away, if there is a mild symptom, e.g., cough, headache, pain, give it a month—most issues will be better in that time. If not, see the doctor. Take care of myself by eating healthy, exercising and get back to my ideal weight.

Here is a side note from my friend Liza who went with me and asked some great questions. From Liza:

"Basically, at the tail end of the visit, I asked something to the effect of how do we know that the cancer is gone and isn't coming back? The doctor replied that we can ask her that when we see her in her office in thirty years. I'm good with that."

I know I must be getting healthier now because when I was going through chemo, and gradually gaining back the weight recently lost in Weight Watchers, all the doctors were telling me not to worry or think about my weight during treatment. Now it is an issue again. I know I must be better since they are bringing up my weight. I was planning on going back to Weight Watchers this weekend and I know getting into my normal routine at work starting next week will help.

Bottom line summary from second opinion: My medical team has done everything the way she would have. I have received excellent care. They are confident (and now I am also) that with radiation and endocrine therapy (Tamoxifen) I will not have to deal with a recurrence of breast cancer.

I am very glad I went for a second opinion and feel like the shakiness of faith I had in the effectiveness of my treatment plan is gone. I am so relieved. How about that for good news from me for a change?

How can you help me? Help me with eating healthy again, help keep me on track. *Don't feed the bear!*

Thank you all for not giving up on me, for being patient and loving, especially during the moments of doubt and discouragement from the time I got the surgical pathology report until today. I think emotionally it has been the roughest couple weeks since the original diagnosis.

I will keep you posted on how radiation goes. I will see him tomorrow for the markings.

Love, Marcy

I received many calls and messages from family and friends who confessed that they were relieved I went for a second opinion and shared the answers to some of the questions they have had as well. I encouraged them to ask me questions when they were concerned and if I didn't have the answers I would find out. I felt it was important for them to get as much reassurance and be allowed to have questions and doubts. I know they have them, who wouldn't. I think at times caregivers and family and friends don't get the support they need because they are also trying to be positive and encouraging for the cancer patient.

FB: August 30, 2012

On occasion I don't tell people how I feel because I know I will hear, "What would you tell me to do if I called you with this problem?" I don't want to listen to my own advice.

CB: August 30, 2012

Beam Me Up Scotty

Hi, I really like the folks at American Cancer Center in Athens, which helps because I will be seeing them Monday through Friday for about six weeks. Today I was put in the scanner but first a mold was made so I could lay in the exact same position each time I was there. They did a simulation scan to determine positioning, the sounds made me think of "Beam me up Scotty" transporters from *Star Trek*. Then she gave me three needlepoint tattoos. Okay, yes, I have six tattoos and thought, no problem, but *wowza*! It is a good thing they were less than a minute each. I can do almost anything for less than a minute. The left side one was first and I was a bit surprised that it hurt so much. She said the sternum area would hurt the most, so I said, "Do it last then." The one on the right I didn't feel at all. Thank God for postsurgical numbness! The one over the sternum hurt a lot and she had to remind me to stay still. I didn't realize I was shrinking my chest in, away from the pain. She said that the ink was hard to get out of the needle and she has to twist it. I then understand why it's wickedly painful. It is done now. In between working, we talked, smiled, and joked around. She gave me two hugs before I left. Too bad my radiation treatments will be in the afternoon due to work, I really liked her.

I went back to the medical supply store. He measured me again for the compression sleeve, and it is the right size. Bummer. I guess I am just going to have to deal with it. Going to have to work really hard to be compliant with it to treat the lymphedema. I know it will get better when I can get into physical therapy on September 19.

Now that the doctors are starting to point out my weight again...I rejoined Weight Watchers. I know what to do, what to eat, that I need activity. The biggest reason I go to Weight Watchers is to keep my head on straight and keep motivated. Right now the motivation is from my understanding that estrogen is what the cancer cells feed off of. Not only do ovaries release estrogen, fat and skin cells do too. The Tamoxifen will help that but I don't start that until after radiation. So it makes sense to me, to reduce estrogen I need to reduce body fat. I know overweight women have an increased risk of breast cancer. If I can beat cancer I can beat obesity, with your help of course. I have not done any of this without you. So today, I ate healthy and tracked my food. I am trying to get as many people as I can around me to focus on eating healthier, not perfectly, but healthier. Want to join me? Feeling so much better and in control. Have a great weekend.

CK: I'm with you!!! You can do it...*all* of it. I'm glad you rejoined Weight Watchers. Like going home, right?

Lucy: Yes, I will join you and I am so happy you feel the need to eat healthier now. You know me—I'm convinced we need to get back to nature—eating what God gave us to eat—not all this processed food. We get enough toxins from our environment. I'm so proud of you and your positive attitude! Love you! Have a good weekend.

DA: Too bad I read this after I ate that last cookie!!!

EM: August 31, 2012

From: Alan

To: Marcy

Enjoyed the *Star Trek* reference although I never was a "Trekkie." I hope you get a cool tech to do the treatments. It makes a difference to have someone who's nice and informative.

I'm working again today and Sunday. Happy Labor Day Weekend! Don't overeat.

From: Marcy

To: Alan

Hi, You're awesome. Labor Day is filled with food but I do feel pretty in control again. Besides I am tired of eating Twizzlers, ramen, and popsicles. Eating healthy feels better.

I was never a "Trekkie" either but the line is so well known and it really did sound like a plane or UFO warming up for takeoff while I was in the scanner.

I hope it isn't too busy at work. When I worked in the emergency room and immediate care, this is the kind of weekend I remember getting drunk people who do stupid things and hurt themselves. Which is where the line that I so frequently tell the boys/men in my life comes from. "Stupid *should* hurt." Good luck at work.

FB: September 3, 2012

Nervous about returning to work full-time. I already know that I have to call the surgeon and get in to have this fluid buildup taken out. I hope she can see me after work.

Dad: We have been blessed since way back when to know you and watch you grow. There isn't anything you can't do, you are special. Love you.

Marcy: Thanks Dad.

FB: September 7, 2012

Can't decide whether I want to eat breakfast or go back to bed.

GC: Bed. There's always time to eat later!

CB: Eat, then bed. Never a good idea to skip breakfast, young lady!

Marcy: I ended up doing neither, started cleaning, then sat down with my computer. I guess I should eat something. The back-to-bed moment has passed. I honestly couldn't tell if I was hungry or tired. I still am not hungry.

CB: September 7, 2012

Random Updates

It's been a while. Right now I feel very good in mind, body and spirit. I know miracles do happen. Much has happened recently so I will just do random topics and try to keep it brief.

Work: I returned to work on Tuesday. I was nervous about going back, not only worried about physically pushing it but being behind and overwhelmed.

Mind: I was able to give myself a break and not expect myself to be caught up with work in the first week. The substitute nurse that covered for me worked with me my first day back and helped me get oriented to what was going on.

Body: The first day after I got off of work I had to go back to the surgeon so she could aspirate the fluid buildup again. I tried wearing the compression sleeve a little more often. Other than aches and pains it was manageable. As far as energy, I can't complain.

Spirit: The love and support I have received this week from coworkers, students and their parents has been overwhelming. The energy and hope I have from being around loving people is priceless. I still have a lot to catch up on but my expectations are a little more realistic.

Radiation: Wednesday I went in and got more markings, kind of like sharpies with tape over the markings to keep it from coming off. Lying in the machine I was a little panicky, no idea why. Thursday I got my first radiation treatment. I was in and out in less than fifteen minutes. Today the doctor came in to the treatment room, changed a couple markings, and met with me afterwards. We discussed possible side effects and how to handle them. He also discussed the treatment plan. The area he is going to radiate will be larger than we thought. I accept that, I want to make sure we are as aggressive as we need to be so I never have to do this again. I feel less panicky. I almost don't care about the process anymore. Let's just do it and get it done. Maybe part of this is trust in the treatment plan again since the second opinion. Maybe it is because I really like everyone at the radiation oncologist's office. Whatever the reasons, it feels more peaceful and hopeful than I have been ever since the biopsy results from the surgery came in.

I feel more energetic and positive than I have in the last few weeks. I feel healthier. A big part of that is going back to work. During the summer I don't work at the high school, so being off work wasn't as big of a deal but when my coworkers went back to work and I didn't, I felt useless. I am not sure if it makes sense, but now that I am back to work I don't feel sick and I am not as tired, even though I get less sleep and expend more energy. The radiation may catch up with me like the chemo did, the cumulative effect. For now, I am going to enjoy the energy I have when I have it. It also helps to be eating healthier again—okay I still had my donut binge and dessert at Applebee's but overall I am eating healthy food again. Going to continue to work on that.

I am glad the weekend is here, plan on going to some football games, watching Da Bears on TV, shopping for a new bed and going to a birthday party. Maybe some rest in there somewhere would be good.

I hope you enjoy your weekend. Thank you all so much for being with me through the highs and lows. Love, Marcy

P.S. Saturday morning, very tired and my back hurts, going to skip the football games outside for now but plan on seeing the little tykes play at some point soon. Weighed in at Weight Watchers and even with my binges lost one pound. Slow but sure is how I want to lose, the healthy way. Going back to work and moving more plus eating healthier 95 percent of the time makes a difference.

Alan: Read your journal. Great to hear things are going well. Sometimes going to work is the perfect remedy for restoring normalcy. I know it helps with with my self-esteem. The thing is though, after reading your journal I really really want a donut or three. I'm thinking double chocolate, rainbow sprinkles, and maybe a jelly-filled. I hope the drive through is open.

Lucy: So glad to read you're very positive and encouraging report—sounds so good! Congrats to you for getting back to work, getting started on your next step (radiation), and feeling better mind, body and spirit. I pray all that continues for you. Love you!

Having had back pain for the past thirteen years and often sleeping in a recliner, on the couch, or in my bed with large pillows for support, I had been considering buying a Sleep Number bed. After I priced them, I knew they were well beyond my reach. There were things that I thought I would like that could make me more comfortable, but I was honestly afraid if I died that my family wouldn't have the resources they need. I did make sure ever since Riley was born in 1998 that I had a separate independent life insurance policy not associated with work. In fact, I had just updated it early in March, merely weeks prior to my cancer diagnosis. When I met with my life insurance agent to sign updated documents I told her of my diagnosis. She did inform me that if the physicians ever thought I had less than two years to live I could withdraw up to 40 percent of my life insurance for living expenses. This was good to know but yet I still felt that I couldn't spend money on me for a new bed.

The school nurses at the district I worked for presented me with money they collected for me. This came as an emotional shocker. The generosity of my peers was overwhelming. Monica, my coworker, stressed that I could use it in whatever way I saw fit. So I put a down payment on a Sleep Number bed with the type of frame where I could elevate the head and feet to different positions. I spent some time consulting Alan on medical expenses and if I could deduct the cost of the bed as a medical expense. After talking to my tax preparer it was determined that I didn't have documentation recommending that specific brand in my medical records. However, it was totally worth the cost of the bed to have that comfort and I often regret not allowing myself to have that earlier in my treatment.

EM: September 9, 2012

From: Marcy

To: Alan

I wonder if I will ever find balance between denial and minimizing symptoms and anxiety and worry about symptoms. I really don't trust what my body tells me anymore and that scares me. I know I can't change the past but I really minimized the significance of the nipple discharge I had.

So much so I don't even remember how much earlier it was before my mammogram. I thought it would get better and it did, so I forgot about it. I guess it doesn't matter because it wouldn't have changed the outcome and treatment most likely, but it just makes me trust myself less.

Sorry again to share so much detail but this isn't the kind of stuff to put on the online journal and I don't want other people to think if things go bad that I could have done or should have done something different, even though that may be true.

Grrrr, overall I really am okay, not sure why I went off like this but maybe it is meant to be, so I am going to send it instead of deleting it. You don't have to respond to the ramblings of a crazy woman if you don't want to.

How goes things by you?

From: Alan

To: Marcy

I totally understand the ongoing battle in your head. Eventually your brain overloads like a computer and crashes. Been there. Sometimes it's hard to read your own body. Is what I feel at this moment something or nothing? Is it a good sign or a bad sign? I also understand trying to relive the past, including trying to remember the sequence of things and wondering what I was thinking at the time and why. I wish I'd never had foot surgery and I try to undo it in my head or justify my thought process at the time. You can't change the past but lord knows I've tried. Don't blame yourself for what you thought in the past.

I'm doing OK. I go back to PT tomorrow. We're gonna take Tommy to the park and then catch the rest of the Bears game. I'm doing four shifts a week now. The shifts go fast because we're busy and most of the people are nice. When it's slow I like to chat with patients—all kinds of lives, interests, troubles. Sometimes there's something therapeutic in knowing that a lot of people struggle with a variety of things, just like the rest of us.

Enjoy the day!

FB: September 9, 2012

All that cancer treatment and I just may die of a heart attack on the first Bears game of the season!

CB: September 11, 2012

"All I Want for Christmas"

Hi, four radiation treatments done. Tomorrow I will get my lab test. A complete blood count. My guess is that this will be like chemo: if I am going to have side effects, they will be cumulative, over time.

Although yesterday when I was caring for the teenager with a temp of 103, I did think about the upcoming flu season and was hoping my white blood cells don't go down too much.

I am getting a little tired of the weekly trip to the surgeon and having fluid drained. Although it was less fluid than last week on the left side, there was still enough there to make it worth the needle. She didn't touch the right side due to the radiation treatments. The right side is swollen in my armpit, and also the area to the side of where the mastectomy was done. My arm is sensitive. I just remind myself in a few months radiation will be over, everything will be healed and I can go get measured for my prosthetics (foobs = fake boobs). In my mind I am singing, "All I want for Christmas is my two fake boobs".

I can tell that work is going to get most of my energy and when I get home, it will be dinner, maybe a short walk and couch or bed. That won't seem so bad once my new Sleep Number bed is delivered. I can't wait. I finally decided I could spend that money on myself. I even got the adjustable one, so I can elevate my head or feet when I want to. Wish I had done it months ago.

How are all of you doing? What are you looking forward to this fall season?

Have a good rest of the week, Marcy

Four Weeks after Mastectomies

I'm not sure why there is a crease on the incision line of the right side and why there is the extra skin.

CB: September 12, 2012

Radiation Plan Update

When I went to radiation I had a moment of fright. The radiation oncologist, his tech and student were scanning and marking me for yet another area they are going to radiate. I was in the machine waiting for it to

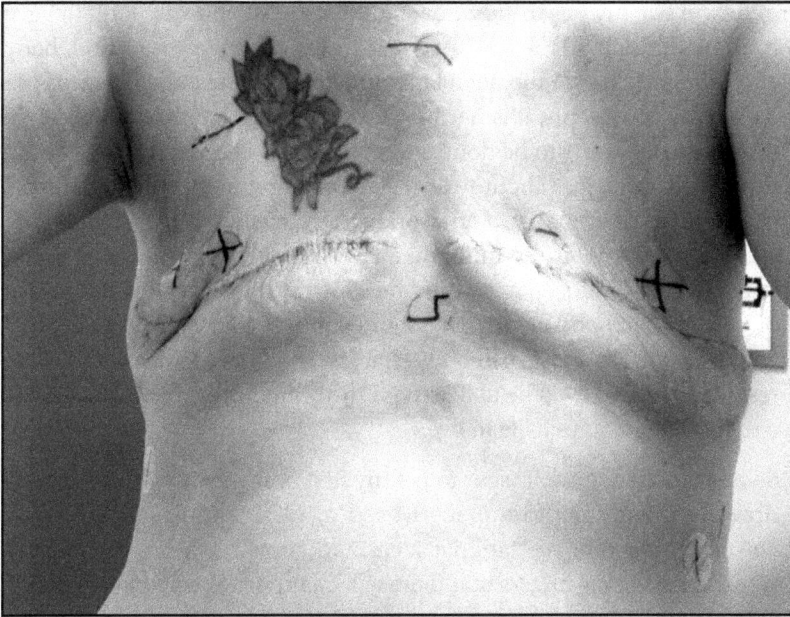

Figure 3-1. Postmastectomy photo of incisions with a
crease on the right and extra loose skin

be over before I could talk to the doctor about what was up. My mind
took some weird turns. I thought, "I was just at the surgeon's, did she
see something concerning and call him?" He is going to radiate around
the clavicle (collarbone) now too. Last week he told me he was radiating
a bigger section of the ribs than he first thought. I wondered if things
were worse. After my radiation, he took me into the computer room and
showed me the images. It is very complicated and I don't understand all
of it, but I probably don't need to. He showed me why they shoot on an
angle to get to the chest wall, this avoids radiation to most of the lung. I
asked him if he saw anything concerning on the scans. Although they are
not "diagnostic" scans, he says to him everything looks good, and that is
good enough for me.

Now is the part you need to sit down for. Are you ready? Instead of trying
to learn his job in six weeks I am going to try something new and trust
his twenty-some years of experience and knowledge. If he says things
are going well, I am going to believe it. When a person is diagnosed with
cancer, or at least when I was diagnosed with cancer, I knew it on a deep
level but at the same time couldn't believe it. Sometimes I look at myself

in the mirror, my peach-fuzz head and flat chest, and still don't believe it. Then, through all the treatments, your life changes, your mind, body and thoughts change too. People around you even change. Towards the end of the treatments, it is hard to start believing that things are better, that it is really going to be done and over soon. I keep telling myself that it is almost over, just about twenty-five radiation treatments left, then I can go on a pill every day. I am working on convincing myself treatment was successful. Weird to think that a person would be in denial about being healthy, huh? That it would be so hard to believe. Just this phase of treatment left and a daily pill, then I can sort out which side effects I will recover from and which body changes I will have to live with for the rest of my life. To even be able to type "live with for the rest of my life" is a reminder I do have a life to live.

So after the radiation, I went to get my first of the weekly blood counts drawn. I went back to a place I used to work and got to see some coworkers. Nice to see familiar faces and know I can see them every week. Crossing my fingers that there will be no issues with blood counts. I am also hoping not to have skin burns. I am using gels and creams that are specifically made to prevent or treat problems with skin from radiation, especially since they are radiating the skin on purpose, which is not done for all types of breast cancer, but mine was in the skin so that has to get zapped. It will be worth the $75 out of pocket for the creams, if it prevents or minimizes the radiation burns on the skin.

I hope you all are well and happy, Marcy

FB: September 12, 2012

"Never apologize for being sensitive or emotional. Let this be a sign that you've got a big heart and aren't afraid to let others see it. Showing your emotions is a sign of strength." By Brigitte Nicole

EM: September 12, 2012

From: Alan

To: Marcy

Hey Marcy, I read your post. I know the feeling. It's hard to trust somebody else's opinion when it's your body, especially when you're in medicine yourself.

Good work today. Now stop worrying and visualize your continually improving health.

Once again, I'm at work. A patient with ankle pain is next followed by the dreaded "boil on butt."

Sleep tight.

From: Marcy

To: Alan

"Boil on butt" reminds me of a story my Grandma used to tell me: when I was about two and my brother was three, I wouldn't give him a toy he wanted. We were playing tug of war, fighting over it. I suddenly let go. He fell and broke the boil on his butt. Funny what old folks "remember." It was probably the only time in my life I came out on top with a power struggle with one of my three brothers.

[...]

I am going to try to think of a way we can earn money without working on our feet as much. I'll keep you posted.

From: Alan

To: Marcy

Yeah, this working for a paycheck really gets old. I'm happy to report a successful drainage procedure and I was not hit in the face with any pus. Enjoy your day!

FB: September 13, 2012

My mom is hiding in her room because she doesn't feel well and doesn't want to get me sick. Riley said he didn't feel well today. I woke up not feeling well, I just want to make it through a full week of work and I am close. One—more—day!

CB: September 15, 2012

Thank You

Don't really have an update. I just saw this quote, it made me think of all the love and support I have received. It comes in many different ways and I thank you all for that.

"We all hit a time when we've lost hope and need someone to put their arms around us and say, 'I've got you right now. I won't let you face this alone.'" —Brigitte Nicole

GG: Hi Marcy, I am thinking of you and sending a hug your way. You are such an amazing person. Just had a memory of stopping at the bank when I was driving you to the hospital to deliver Riley. Also, no more double chocolate cake for you when you have a bad day at work. Just a single chocolate cake (maybe a brownie) when things get tough.

Love you.

Invisible Fight

CB: September 19, 2012

Although I can see the light at the end of the tunnel, I am still in the tunnel and there are some dark areas with some potholes.

I saw my surgeon yesterday. She said she doesn't need to see me again for three months. There was some fluid buildup still but my body should take care of it, there wasn't as much as in the past few weeks. It appears like there was more skin remaining on the left than right. If that becomes a problem when it comes time to get fitted for prosthetics we may have to go back to surgery and remove some excess skin.

I have not been feeling well the past few days. It is really hard to sort out whether it is just fatigue from radiation or if I am sick with something else. I did take the day off work and went to the doctor today (nurse practitioner). She gave me antibiotics for a sinus infection.

I kept my physical therapy appointment for today even though I didn't feel well, because it took me over four weeks to get in to see someone who manages lymphedema. I liked her but then when it came to schedule more sessions, she couldn't do it to fit my work and radiation schedule. If she can't rearrange some other patients, I am back to square one. I will have to start calling around to get into someone who manages lymphedema. I am a little annoyed: if the schedule was too busy to provide the follow-up appointments, why did they accept me as a patient? Couldn't they have told me a month ago they wouldn't be able to accommodate me? It is really hard to manage a work, radiation, and physical therapy schedule, in addition to the kids' schedules, especially with Riley being in high school now.

The compression sleeve I bought probably isn't the best idea right now, the swelling is too great and it is too tight and uncomfortable. So I won't be wearing it until I do get some treatment for the fluid buildup. During the session, we also discovered that part of the reason I have discomfort in my right shoulder and underarm after radiation and decreased range of motion is from axillary web syndrome [also known as cording]. From what I understood from the physical therapist, it is common when lymph nodes are removed. That contributes to the pain, tightness and decreased range of motion. It is manageable with therapy, which I can't work into my schedule. So frustrating. I feel stuck.

Tonight Dani is getting a breast cancer ribbon butterfly tattoo; what I didn't know until tonight was that she is adding "Mom" to the tattoo. I saw the drawing and placement; she is getting it now. I'll post a picture when I can. We were going to get them together but she apparently couldn't wait and I will have to wait until all the treatments are over.

As frustrated as I am with my schedule, not feeling well, and some minor complications, I know that I am closer to the treatment finish line and then I can return to a "normal" schedule.

I hope you all are doing well. Thanks for being here and taking an interest in this ongoing battle.

EM: September 19, 2012

From: Alan

To: Marcy

Hi Marcy, Last week I went to PT and the guy adjusted my S-I joint. Then I spent the weekend in the grandstands at the NASCAR races. I've been miserable for the past few days. I'm really down.

Naturally, I'm working my second of eleven shifts in thirteen days. It's slow right now but at dinner it will pick up.

So how are you? How's the radiation going? There's light at the end of the tunnel right?

Nothing fun planned for me this weekend. I'm working Sunday. You're always in my thoughts.

From: Marcy

To: Alan

I really wish I could do something for you. I don't know how you work so much with the pain you have. Distraction must be your most effective tool. I'm doing okay. Frustrated. Just updated CaringBridge.

I don't have anything fun planned this weekend either. I have to go to the Apple store on Sunday and have them help me figure out an external hard drive and restoring photo issue. But most of the weekend will be trying to figure out what Riley is doing. It's homecoming weekend. Driving him back and forth to the parade and dance and whatever else is going on in his teenage world. I don't like running him around sometimes because I am always tired now but I am glad he is getting involved.

I hope you feel better and you don't have many butt boils to contend with in this next stretch of thirteen days.

From: Alan

To: Marcy

It's like I always say, well not always, it's better to stab a boil on butt than have one. Have a good night.

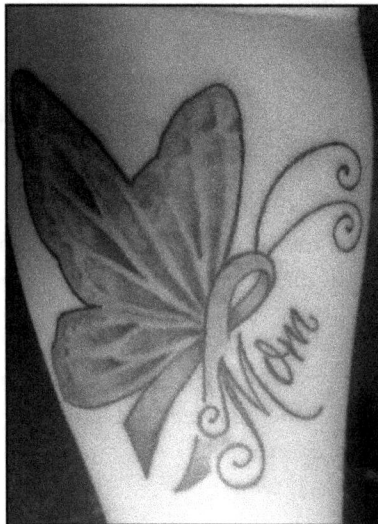

Figure 3-2. Dani's breast cancer awareness tattoo by Nikki Harris

CB: September 20, 2012

Update

A few things: Dani's tattoo is beautiful. Whether you like tattoos or not, it is an amazing feeling that she wanted to get it and put "Mom" on her body forever. I guess she likes me a little bit.

I did get my CBC and my white blood cell count did go down in the last week as well as my hemoglobin. Again, not dangerously low. I am glad I went to get antibiotics yesterday and hope that will make the sinus headaches better soon.

Feeling very grateful for the physical therapists who both adjusted their schedules to accommodate me on Tuesday and Thursday after radiation. So very nice of them to do that for three weeks so I don't have to wait until radiation is over to get help for the lymphedema and axillary web syndrome. Truly they are such caring people.

So, onward we go. Have a good night, Marcy

Alan: That is an extraordinarily nice tattoo. Nice work. Great to hear about caring people once in while. Hang in there!

EM: September 22, 2012

From: Marcy

To: Alan

Riley will be in a homecoming parade in about thirty minutes. I feel like I should leave now and go to the school and take pictures of his first homecoming experience. He doesn't care about pictures now but I know both kids love their scrapbooks. They don't always like the moments I take the photos to go in the scrapbooks. It is cold out, I'm tired and have a headache. Don't want to go sit outside. I feel like a bad mom but really he probably doesn't care...but I do. Grrrr. Dani didn't do any of the homecoming stuff her freshman year, but she did the years after that because her friends talked her into it. I did manage to take him clothes shopping after work and radiation yesterday. That kid grows too fast. He got dress slacks, a purple shirt and yellow tie. School colors are purple and gold... Couldn't find a gold tie but I think yellow counts.

Well, gotta go lay around and feel guilty for it. I am imagining you have felt that way before.

FB: September 22, 2012

There are many moments that I can forget that I have breast cancer, but Monday through Friday at work when I place my hand on my flat chest while doing the Pledge of Allegiance is *not* one of them.

PO: I for one am so grateful that you are still here to say the Pledge.

Marcy: Me too. I love saying it and I think about my nephew who is in the Marines. Thank you PO.

Lucy: I think of you now every morning when we say it.

FB: September 24, 2012

Can't wait to get in my new bed tonight. Thanks to the Dist. 601 nurses.

Hannah: I'll never forget the time Trent fell asleep on my sister's Sleep Number bed after letting all the air out. He looked like he was in a coffin. Dislike!

PO: I am tired. Maybe I need a new bed. Do I need to rob a bank to get one?

Marcy: Don't rob a bank because then you'd be on a prison cot. I did the free financing but then you have to pay it off in eighteen months.

CB: September 25, 2012

The Little Engine That Could

Hi all,

This week my chant is, "I think I can, I think I can." I feel like the Little Engine That Could struggling up the mountain this week so that I can get to the fun downhill this weekend. I am planning on taking Riley and my nephew to Fright Fest. I am fourteen treatments into radiation, sixteen or so to go. The radiation oncologist reminded me (yes, I needed to be reminded) of the importance of using the skin gels and lotions he gave me. So far the skin has been okay, just has had slight redness. There was a brown discolored area under the scar that I was starting to worry about but he said it was radiation related. Of course I was worried because the cancer was in the skin and I was scared it was rearing its ugly head. I wonder how long it will take for me not to be as paranoid. How long will it take to find the middle of the road between denial and overreacting? I imagine it may take a little while.

Tuesdays and Thursdays for the next three weeks I will go directly to physical therapy after radiation. Today my arm was wrapped to help reduce the lymphedema. I will then be able to go get the appropriate compression glove and sleeve soon. It makes for a long day: work, radiation and physical therapy. Thank goodness my kids are older and my mom lives with me. I am spoiled. Dinner cooked for me and my laundry even done by my mom.

I am starting to eat much healthier and I am sure that is helping fuel the little engine. I just hope to be consistent with it. I also got my new bed, a Sleep Number bed with the adjustable head and foot controls. I am hoping this helps with my back which has been hurting so much more the past couple weeks, not sure why exactly, but will talk to the rheumatologist about it in a couple of weeks.

The generosity and support of my coworkers is never-ending and I am blessed. I really am so glad to see the people at HHS every day, staff and students. There are some great things going on for October's Breast Cancer awareness month. Today I had to call the paramedics for a student. (The student was okay and went home with his mom.) The paramedics came in with their pink breast cancer shirts on. I realize how much community support there is for people fighting cancer. Not just breast cancer. Many of the proceeds go to American Cancer Society, they help people with any type of cancer. Again, sometimes we hear all the negatives of society, especially during this political time of year, but I am seeing such loving and supportive people. That in itself gives me hope for myself and for our younger generation.

So, tomorrow is only Wednesday but I will keep chugging along. I think I can, I think I can.

I hope you all have a good week, Marcy

EM: September 25, 2012

From: GG

To: Marcy

Hi Marcy,

What a great thing CaringBridge is. I am thankful that you directed me to this site so that I can hear how you are doing. I wanted to tell you that it is very important that you use the lotion or gel and best to start now. My sister had radiation and they told her to use the lotion and at the end she realized its importance. I'll call her to help her refresh my memory of it.

Marcy—there is hope for this ugly thing called cancer. It is funny how until it affects your life one way or another you don't realize the hope. But there is hope. My husband had appendix cancer and he is back to normal (which really isn't normal at all but for him it is normal). He did go through the neuropathy from the chemo but is now back to typing. Two of my sisters-in-law have had breast cancer and they are doing well. Marcy—as far as the "Little Engine That Could" goes, you are a survivor and I know you can! You are an amazing woman.

My prayers are going out to you. Love,

GG

P.S. Would you prefer I write in CaringBridge or in an email? And if ever you want to talk please call anytime.

From: Marcy

To: GG

Thanks.

People will write short notes on CaringBridge but you can do either. If it is longer or personal info, you can send email. Love ya and we will have to talk more or get together sometime maybe next month?

Love, Marcy

P.S. I am using the gel and lotion like I should now, no worries.

EM: September 25, 2012

From: Alan

To: Marcy

As the great philosopher Bob Marley said, "Don't worry about a thing, 'cause every little thing is gonna be alright."

Be good.

From: Marcy

To: Alan

How are you doing tonight? Really busy?

My mom is going to the ortho doc tomorrow. I guess she will be scheduling her hip replacement, sooner than later. She checked out a rehab four miles from here, so that should work out okay. I think she wanted to put it off until I was done with treatments but she is in too much pain. I don't want her to be in pain waiting for surgery because of me.

Take care, Marcy

From: Alan

To: Marcy

The rehab place is key. Gotta find a place you like. It's good to be close so you can visit and bring stuff.

Work has been nutty. We had three IVs going earlier. Then back-to-back patients with paronychia with abscesses. Then a student from Barcelona, Spain, who broke his ankle. It's not even a full moon.

My coworkers are fun.

I hope you're feeling good. There is light and health at the end of the tunnel.

Be good.

FB: September 26, 2012

Two months after chemo is over and I lose my big toenails. I guess they couldn't hang on anymore.

FB: September 27, 2012

Not a huge citrus fan, unless it is a lime in a margarita, yet I am craving grapefruit. Last time I craved grapefruit was when I was pregnant with Riley. I wonder if it is because of low immunity that I am craving Vitamin C?

PG: Or, you're pregnant, congrats.

Marcy: The baby-making factory has been gone for years, the workers left long ago, and I don't even have the milk machines left. Baby-making days are long gone. Now I just have to wait for grandkids. I can wait a little while for those.

FB: September 28, 2012

I am so tired and my back hurts, I could cry. At least I managed to get to the grocery store so my family has the food they like.

Willow: Oh NO!! The Sleep Number bed?

Marcy: The bed is great. It helps my back. I wake up without pain for a change. It starts hurting about 11 a.m. and it is worse when I am at work. Maybe the chair?

FB: September 29, 2012

Just got called "Sir" at a restaurant.

Shelby: You are *beautiful!*

Willow: Seriously!! That person needs glasses. Agree with Shelby, *you are a beautiful woman*!!

Okay, I hate that I look so yucky without makeup and I am not even sure why I would take a picture and post it on Facebook, but wanted you to see that my hair is growing back. My eyebrows are growing back and maybe my eyelashes will come back soon too. It isn't growing back evenly but it is as soft as a peach.

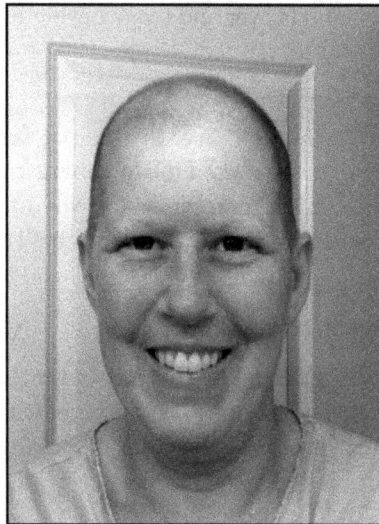

Figure 3-3. My new hair growth

FB: September 30, 2012

At the amusement park but have already had enough of it after riding Raging Bull, X-Flight, and Superman (why I rode that one I have no clue). Just waiting until Riley and his friend will agree to go home.

FB: October 4, 2012

"A friend who understands your tears is much more valuable than a lot of friends who only know your smile." By Sushan R. Sharma

PO: You know it, cry all you want. The river could use the water!

Marcy: Had one of those days too. Sometimes it gets to me when I feel so bad physically and emotionally and people tell me that I "look good." I don't care how I look. I want to feel good.

CB: October 5, 2012

Trying to Manage

It's been a while. Guess I have been a little down lately. I always strive to be honest and again, since I have an issue with not bringing other people down with me, sometimes I avoid the journal until I know I can balance the honesty with positive thoughts too. So I will start and end with positive and put the messed up junk in the middle.

The people in my life are incredible. Today I sat in a nurses meeting. Usually I am the only nurse in my building but once in a while we all are in the same room for a meeting. I felt so much support and encouragement as usual but what impacted me most today was acceptance. I didn't have to be well, or feel good, or look good. They seem to be okay with just me. I am privileged to belong to such a caring group of people.

Kids have also always had a powerful effect on my mood, not just my kids either. I got a random phone call from a young friend of mine. He is almost 10 years old. His Mom, Lola, said it was his idea to call me. Hawk and I chatted about what he was up to and for moments I was out of my head and smiling. How can I not be in a good mood when I am talking to a child or with children?

A couple things are frustrating me; the things that are making going back to work difficult are lymphedema and my back pain. The back pain is new and different than the chronic arthritis pain.

When I wasn't working in the summer it was okay because I am a school nurse and none of my other coworkers were in school either so it didn't feel bad, when school started I had surgery but it was okay to be on leave because it was for surgery. When I went back to work I felt pretty good, radiation was just beginning, had some energy and felt useful. But since I started work again I have called for a sick day two times...that makes me feel bad again, because I feel like I need a bail out. I am starting to feel run down and when I get sick I feel guilty. It is very difficult to work with the lymphedema bandages on so they often get taken off. Sitting in my chair hurts, standing too long hurts, and then I have to "lie down on the job." That is not "me." It takes away the positive feeling I got from going back to work. I hope I am making sense. I was hoping for some normalcy when I went back to work but at times it is such a struggle. Then on the weekends I want to do something fun, but I physically pay for it later. So it seems like work gets the best of me and my loved ones get the leftover mess.

The lymphedema treatment since I have started physical therapy is trial and error and it seems like it isn't helping or at least not consistently. I know I could be more compliant but it is really hard to be compliant at work. I had a student put a chisel part of the way through his hand—if I was wrapped from fingers to armpit, it would have been difficult to care for him. It would have been more difficult to assist the student who had the seizure to the floor and protect him had I been wrapped up. We are trying the Kinesio tape that the athletes use. I just took off the wrap that was done last night because the fluid was being pushed into my knuckles and the finger bandages don't seem to work. So I take that off and use the big blue Caresia thingamabob [compression wrap], but that is only partially effective. There is cording now in my armpit and forearm.

See what I mean? I complain and complain. At least the lymphedema is not painful, it just makes fine motor activities more challenging. My bigger concern is the back pain. I was braiding Dani's hair and could barely finish, I was almost in tears and had to lie down...could not sit one more minute. Is it arthritis? Is it something else? I will be seeing the oncologist and rheumatologist on Monday...I hope one of them will figure it out for me because I can't continue with my lifestyle with this kind of pain. Complain, complain, blah blah blah. I hate the way I sound. I should be happy. So now I am going to try to end with some more positive things.

Radiation will be done in about two weeks and considering I have had four weeks of radiation and they are targeting the skin along with lymph nodes and chest wall, I have very little skin side effects, minimal redness, and minimal discomfort.

October is breast cancer awareness month. I am blessed to be a part of Hamilton High School. They are doing so much for breast cancer awareness and fundraising for the American Cancer Society. The students and their parents, the staff and faculty continue to be loving and supportive. I wish sometimes I could give myself the same love and compassion that others give me. I would never say to others what I sometimes think about myself. I would never be hard on them or put such high expectations on someone in my situation. I think I will try to work on giving myself a break more often.

Didn't mean to transition into the negative again but this is my life...up and down, positive and negative, hard and easy...maybe that is just life itself and I can learn to accept it.

Have a great weekend,

Marcy

Lucy: Marcy—everything you say makes sense to me and I'm sure I would feel the same. Feeling bad, whether sick or in pain, is just no fun and those of us that like to be busy, productive, and positive, just have a hard time with it. I'm sending positive prayers your way. I pray you get some relief after the radiation is finished. Maybe more rest right now on the weekends will help you get through the work week —at least for a couple more weeks. I think of you every day—love and prayers.

P.S. You are allowed to feel bad and complain when you do.

GG: Marcy, you are such a special person and mean the world to me. Kids are amazing and have such a way to make you smile. So glad that Hawk was able to do that for you. Love you.

EM: October 6, 2012

From: Alan

To: Marcy

Hi Marcy, read your journal today. Battling several things at once is tough. Hang in there.

Be proud of yourself for your determination. Keep finding the strength.

I'm at work again today. Are we on for Monday? Be good.

From: Marcy

To: Alan

Definitely on for Monday lunch. I'll call when I leave the oncologist's office. Hard to type when I am being a good little patient and wearing the Caresia.

See ya in a couple days.

From: Marcy

To: Alan

This may sound neurotic but I was looking at the nutrition info for TGI Fridays and wondering if you wouldn't mind Potbelly's or Chipotle instead. I know I can make better choices. Did you know that a Turkey burger at Fridays has 45 grams of fat and 93 grams of carbs. Sheesh!

From: Alan

To: Marcy

Potbelly's rules. See you Monday.

Alan and I met at Potbelly's. He brought a couple of his scrapbooks. It was a different type of scrapbooking than I did; my scrapbooks were mostly photos with journaling and a few pieces of memorabilia while Alan's were almost all memorabilia, sprinkled with an occasional photo. We flipped through the pages of his scrapbooks as he recalled all the places he has been and the things he has done in his life. He saves matchbooks, ticket stubs, airline tickets, napkins, brochures, name tags from conferences, and even horse track bet tickets. It was good to see him smile as he told those stories. Although I value big, exciting events and activities in my life, I learned that those "smaller" events in my life were fun and had purpose, even if that purpose was just helping me remember that I took advantage of life. The times spent in bed or on the couch from cancer treatment or chronic pain don't seem as impactful if I can actively reminisce via scrapbooks.

We updated each other on family and he updated me on his dogs. We talked about sports. He is a White Sox fan and I am a Cubs fan, but we both can agree that we root for Da Bears and whoever is playing the Packers. I wore an NFL breast cancer awareness cap. It had a pink "C" on it for Chicago and a pink bill. Alan complimented it. I wanted him to have it, and gave it to him readily. The very next Bears game I received a text photo of him wearing that cap for luck. This began a tradition of sending selfies to each other before games wearing Chicago Bears caps or other attire.

Our catch-up time was coming to an end, not only because a guitarist was beginning a set and we couldn't hear each other, but also because I had an appointment with a rheumatologist to look into the back pain I was having, thinking it was a flare-up of my chronic arthritis. We said goodbye in person, but traded words again just hours later.

EM: October 8, 2012

From: Marcy

To: Alan

Hi. Thinking about you and wondering how PT went, did you let him do anything?

The rheumatologist gave me a choice of Lidoderm patches or gel. The gel is $15 and patches $50. Don't really think either will help but I filled the gel to try it. He also mentioned a Dexa scan [bone density scan], maybe I will do that before the end of the year.

It was really nice to see your scrapbooks. You have been a lot of places and done a lot of things and that is so cool. Thanks for lunch.

From: Alan

To: Marcy

Hi, it was truly great to see you. The guitar player was good but it got a little loud in there. The hat is awesome. I'm still wearing it. Thank you.

PT went ok. They did a little heat, ultrasound and "therapeutic" massage. I'm sore but functional. What doesn't kill you makes you stronger right?

I don't think the topical lido products do much for deep pain but it's pretty easy on the skin and for $15 it's worth a try.

I really enjoyed lunch. Thanks.

FB: October 9, 2012

The radiation tech said he was concerned that the doctor may hold the radiation to the chest wall because the skin is looking so scorched. They would still do the clavicle area to zap the lymph nodes there. I don't want any delays, just want to be done with all of this. If the skin broke open it would delay radiation more. I just hate the delay in starting the systemic treatment of the Tamoxifen.

Clara: I love you! Haven't told you lately.

Marcy: I love you too and I know you love me. You're the best!

Miriam: It will be done soon enough and then you can move on. *You are loved!*

Marcy: Thanks Miriam, Love you. Tomorrow would not be soon enough.

Lola: I am happy to inform you that my almost-ten-year-old was telling our friend about you yesterday because we were talking about breast cancer. In his words, "Her cancer is almost gone, just a tiny bit more"— coming from a boy who has a direct line to the spirits. I say *you got this*!!!!!

Marcy: Thanks, that made me cry.

Looking back at this five years later I wonder why I thought radiation would be the easiest of the cancer treatment phases. I had seen cancer patients in the endoscopy unit when I worked there with radiation burns on their throats and to me it looked terrible. I knew early in nursing school that my weakness as a nurse would be in treating burns; I clearly remember being in the operating room as they were debriding the burn of a two-year-old boy and I had to excuse myself before I passed out. The treatment of burns always caused pain and there were not medications that could combat that pain adequately. I quietly hoped when those patients came in they would be unconscious so that they would be unaware of what was being done to them.

I had not thought much about radiation being actual burns with black, peeling skin. They were targeting the skin on purpose; after all, the cancer had been there. The effects of the radiation, like the chemotherapy, were cumulative. I was pleasantly surprised that I wasn't as tired as I thought I would be and my skin held up as long as it did. But it was catching up to me. I guess the beauty of extensive postsurgical numbness in my chest and underarm area was that I didn't feel pain for the singed skin as it peeled away from my body. I just wanted to be done with treatment. I wanted to get away, run away if I could. I didn't want to talk to anyone, really, or visit with anyone. It was one of those odd situations where I had dozens and dozens of people who would be with me, yet I felt deeply lonely and didn't want to be with anyone. I couldn't be good company and didn't want any company.

FB: October 10, 2012

I'm running away and I am not taking anyone with me.

Lucy: I have a cabin you can hide out in, but I would want to visit you!

Hannah: You can hide here.

FP: After the last few days, take me along. I will sit quietly and split the gas money.

Shelby: We have plenty of room.

CC: Excellent! Where are we going?

When I started to get comments coming in from people who invited themselves to run away with me or invited me to their place to hide I was dumbfounded. Did they not understand that I wanted to be alone? Didn't they get that I didn't feel I could be enjoyable to be around? Later as I realized they were attempting to make me laugh and they were offering an escape plan, a small grin inched its way across my face. Sometimes the moment you want to be left alone is the moment you need company the most.

CB: October 13, 2012

Medical Updates

Since my last post, the radiation skin side effects started to show, to the point that the radiation to the chest wall and skin was put on hold. I still go to radiation but they only do the clavicle area to target those lymph nodes. On Monday my skin will be reevaluated to see if we can restart the chest wall radiation but the bolus [a large dose of radiation] to the skin will not be done anymore. The good news is there was so much nerve involvement from the mastectomies, I am pretty numb over most of my chest and it looks worse than it feels. I understand it is better to delay treatment for healing than risk open sores to the skin and infection because that would delay things longer. I am just ready to be done with this treatment phase.

The oncologist ordered an MRI of the thoracic spine, although my pain is off to the left. No cancer there, but that wasn't what I really was looking for. Nice to know what it isn't but really would like to know what it is and what to do about it. By the time I get home after work it hurts too much to sit at the dinner table. I am going to explore this with my primary care physician because the pain is getting worse.

The lymphedema is better only when I can wear the Caresia and short stretch bandaging. I don't even bother at work anymore. When radiation is done and things are healed the lymph nodes that are being radiated can do their job to make up for the ones that are gone. It will get better, but until then I will be puffy on the right side and my fine motor skills will be lacking...as evidenced by all the things I drop or can't hold on to.

Gonna get going for now and put the bulky dressing on to at least minimize the swelling; even if I can't completely remove the swelling right now I can keep it under control.

Have a good weekend, Marcy

EM: October 7, 2012

From: Sasha

To: Marcy

Hi, *stop*, *stop*, *stop* beating yourself up! Honey, you are surviving a diagnosis of an aggressive cancer, two different chemotherapy treatments, a double mastectomy, lymph node removal, and radiation. You are coping with the side effects (if the first thing doesn't work you explore and try something else). You have returned to work. You worry constantly about your family and friends. You are amazing and you damn well better start thinking that way!

Marcy, I keep good thoughts for you constantly even if I don't write. When radiation ends in a couple of weeks I hope that your schedule will not be as demanding as it is now, that you will have a chance to build up your strength, that you will once again experience what you feel is "normal." The life that you describe right now doesn't sound very "normal"; for Heaven's sake don't put yourself down because you don't feel that way.

I'll follow your online journal blog and keep you posted about stuff here. Take care and be kind to yourself.

EM: October 13, 2012

From: Sasha

To: Marcy

Hi Marcy,

I have been thinking about my last e-mail and worrying that I may have offended you. In your online journal you mentioned the meeting with the nurses where you could be yourself on that day, whatever kind of day it was, and they just accepted and supported you. I didn't mean for you not to be honest. But, "I'm tired, I'm hurting, I'm scared" are very different statements than, "I'm not doing things properly." I just didn't want you to be so hard on yourself. You are living the life that you have right now, even on the bad days, and your courage deserves admiration and support if it can be given. If I didn't convey that message in my last e-mail I am sorry.

Weekend is supposed to be warm but wet. Hope that you have good rest, good food, and good company, not necessarily in that order. Take care.

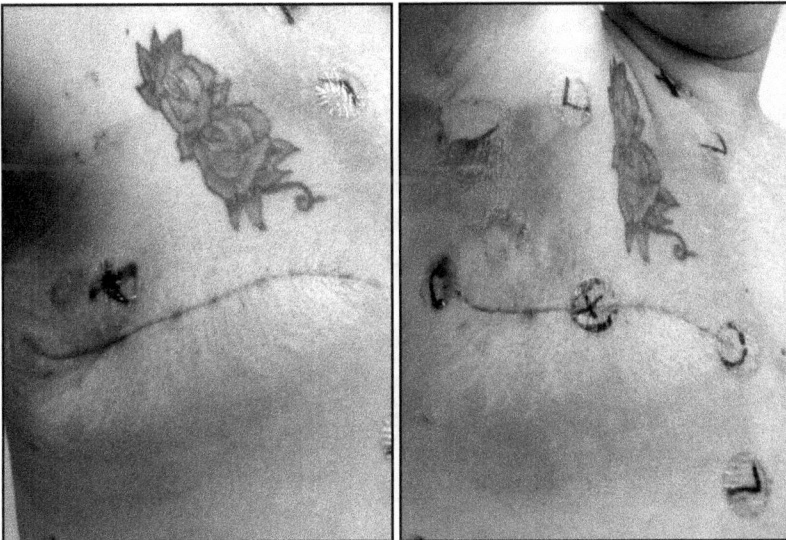

Figure 3-4. Swollen burned skin with puckering
incision (left). Black peeling burns (right).

From: Marcy

To: Sasha

Totally not offended. No worries, I understand. Would type more but just had eye exam and my eyes were dilated, can't see well.

FB: October 20, 2012

I have always wanted to take Riley to Fright Fest at the amusement park. Thank you Kady and Mimi for going with us. I can't believe the crowd! Have NEVER been here when it was this busy.

FB: October 21, 2012

KO, thank you for walking in the Care4Breast Cancer event in support of me.

Bought "Real Bears fans wear pink" shirts for my three sisters, daughter, mom, and me.

GC: You are a badass! I want one of those shirts.

Marcy: I wanted "one" too but I couldn't order one, the minimum for delivery was six.

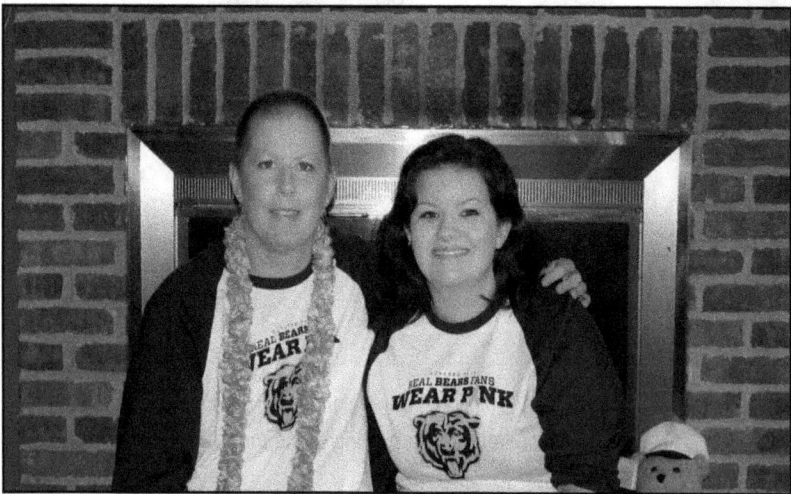

Figure 3-5. Dani and me in "Real Bears fans wear pink" shirts

Reflections

This was such a difficult time for me. Mostly because like other phases of the cancer treatment, chemo, surgery, and now radiation, the "survival mode" focused on doing what was in front of me and not looking forward. By looking forward in this case, I mean being prepared. I thought I was going to be that one person who wouldn't have burns. I thought I would be that one person who wouldn't have fatigue. I thought I could manage a full-time job at a high school, radiation Monday through Friday, physical therapy for the lymphedema, and home and family responsibilities. I thought I was Superwoman; after all, the people who loved and supported me told me I was strong and a hero. I was starting not to buy it.

I did have a successful second opinion visit with my friend, Liza, helping me process the meaning of the visit. I had some fun times with friends and family, I even got a new bed. Heck, I enjoyed the radiation team and felt very supported there, but I was starting to wonder if this would ever end. I had to deal with delays in radiation, delays in starting the oral, systemic treatment. I finally got the answers I needed on why Tamoxifen couldn't be started to target cancer cells that may be circulating beyond the reach of the radiation. It was explained to me that antiestrogen therapy slows down cancer cells that are estrogen-receptor positive. If those cancer cells are slowed down, they are less vulnerable to the effects of radiation. Again, once I understood this rationale I was better able to be on board with the plan. I still felt like I couldn't trust that my body didn't have cancer cells setting up shop in a distant organ while we were treating the cancer locally with surgery and radiation. Bottom line is, I just wanted this to be over so that I could take a pill a day and move forward with my life.

$$\sim 4 \sim$$

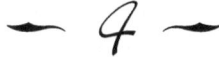

Complications

Burning Up while Drowning

FB: October 22, 2012

Woke up with a fever. I really should have found out the results of my last lab work before being in crowds this weekend. Going to eat soup in bed and go to the doctor soon.

CB: October 23, 2012

Sick...Not Sure Why

Home from work since Monday. Headache, achiness, chills, fever. Fever not terrible but now even with Aleve and Tylenol on board went from 101.8 to 102.4. I am sure the radiation oncologist didn't like me canceling the last clavicle and scar treatment. I only have five treatments left and they were going to give me off until Monday if I did the treatment today. I didn't have a fever at the time I cancelled but would have by the time I got there due to the timing. It seems like these last five treatments are kicking my ass, but I have a lot of padding in my ass and in the end I will prevail. I called my primary care physician; she ordered more tests which were done at the lab, so I didn't see the doc. Blood work results should be available tomorrow and the urinalysis and culture will take a few days. We shall see what happens. I only have one treatment for clavicle and scar left, which they want to do tomorrow or Monday if the skin of the chest wall is healed enough that we can do the last four on it. Why do I feel like this? Nothing makes sense? Viral? Temp is 103 now. At what point do I call or go to ER when Advil or Aleve alternated with Tylenol doesn't work? I should have asked the doc when I called. If my scale is right, I lost five pounds in the last three days, even with amusement park food. Please don't tell me to get in the tub to reduce the fever when I have chills. I am drinking a lot of water...Grrrr.

SS: You know there is so much sickness going around, perhaps you just caught a bug or something. Try not to panic. Rest and fluids are always good. I'm praying you are not on the way to the hospital. We lost our friend Judy and we are not losing you. Take care.

Lucy: Marcy—So sorry to hear you have a fever and are not feeling well. I'm hoping by now your fever is down and if not, that you have gone to ER. I can't see me giving you, the nurse, advice; however, I'm hoping the fever doesn't go any higher. Sending love and prayers your way.

EM: October 23, 2012

From: Alan

To: Marcy

A chest x-ray might not be a bad idea as well, even if you're not coughing.

Any skin redness? GI symptoms?

I'm working tonight. Call me if you like.

From: Marcy

To: Alan

Thanks, skin is not red but warm. It actually looks like it is healing although it feels more swollen. I am still numb there so there is no pain but when I accidentally roll over on that side, my arm and hand go really numb and get tingling. The doc saw my skin yesterday and said it looked "normal" for what he is doing to it.

No GI symptoms. I think I will wait until tomorrow and if I have a fever not budging with medicine, suggest a CXR [chest x-ray] when the doc calls with results of labs? Its better now at 101.3, just have to stay on top of it I guess.

From: Alan

To: Marcy

Sounds like a reasonable plan. It's an impressive fever but it can still be viral. A CXR is never a bad idea. Get some rest.

Hey, I wore my new pink Bears hat last night. I had intended to email you earlier today. The Bears haven't lost a game since you gave me that hat. Superbowl here we come!

From: Marcy

To: Alan

That would be awesome if they won the Super Bowl this year. My sisters, Mom, Dani, and I had a group photo with our "Real Bears Fans Wear Pink" shirts. We were missing my nieces though.

My guess is it is viral, but it just feels so crappy. Even through all of chemo, my fever never got high, just hovered in the 100s sometimes.

You know that we will have to send selfies with our Bears attire before each game now, right?

CB: October 24, 2012

Burning Up

Haven't heard back on blood tests yet. With very consistent use of medicine I can keep the temp at 101 and below; if I am late on a dose from sleeping it can be 102–103. I have been in bed all day and haven't even felt like watching shows on my laptop. I will call for results tomorrow. I was a little lightheaded when I got up last night. Maybe I am a little dehydrated, I am focusing on fluids. For those who offered suggestions; don't ever worry about giving me advice just because I am a nurse. When I am sick I am just me and not always thinking straight.

EM: October 25, 2012

From: Marcy

To: Alan

The fever is more manageable. I feel weak and like I got hit by a truck.

If I feel no better than this soon I'm gonna have to take tomorrow off too. No pay for five days. I want to be checked out by the doctor but don't want to leave my bed.

From: Alan

To: Marcy

Hi Marcy, I hope you turn the corner today. I don't like to use the term 'you should' but I think you should get checked out today. And stay well hydrated. I know being sick like this is the last thing you need but you still gotta be an advocate for yourself.

From: Marcy

To: Alan

Tried to hold off on Tylenol but I am up to 102.2 again. Maybe Motrin instead but then I have to get myself out of bed and I have only been doing that when I have to pee. If I was a guy, I might keep a coffee can by my bed. I know, gross huh? Don't think I'll write about that in the online journal. At least I can assume if the tests were run they aren't critical because lab policy would be to call the doctor with critical results.

From: Alan

To: Marcy

400–600 mg of ibuprofen with food is a good idea. At least keep some water, Gatorade, 7-up, ginger ale, etc. with you. The blood tests should be resulted today. Call them again this afternoon.

CB: October 25, 2012

Doggone

By my mom (Dorothy)

You know Marcy must feel pretty doggone lousy when she doesn't argue with the doctor about being admitted to the hospital. After reviewing some lab work results, her primary care doctor called her and asked her to come into the office, which she did at 4 p.m., and by 5 p.m. she was in her private room at Good Samuel Hospital. She took her laptop with her, knowing that a hospital stay might be in the works, so she'll probably update you more tomorrow. They were getting ready to start an IV of antibiotics when I left. In addition to her primary care doctor, her oncologist and surgeon will also be seeing her. Her favorite nurse from her surgery was admitting her when I left...like old home week.

Thanks everyone for all your support and care for her. After all, she is my baby, you know. (Boy, is she going to kill me for that one.)

All Shook Up

Now that I am not shaking with chills and hiding under the covers I can post a quick update. Yes, everything my mom said is right. The oncologist and surgeon's resident have been in and they all talked and decided to start the antibiotic Vancomycin. They are thinking this is cellulitis, an infection in the skin. Really wish I identified it sooner but the skin was red from radiation already and on Monday he said it looked okay. Maybe I scratched it during the night or something. It gradually got more red and swollen even though I had not had radiation since Monday. There is so much numbness that the pain is only when they press in certain spots. By the time the primary care doctor got my labs (a day late...I should have followed up with them yesterday but I didn't) the skin symptoms were more obvious. Honestly, I thought I was probably getting the flu because I was around a lot of crowds over the weekend but I never developed respiratory symptoms. So at least I am here and it won't get worse, right? Please tell me it won't get worse?

I met my oncologist's partner today. I might like him a bit better than the doctor I have been seeing. Would it be bad if I switched? After all, the man has season tickets to the Bears games, maybe I can work out a deal sometime!

The steady stream of support came in through many avenues during my hospital stay. I had visitors, emails, texts, flowers and phone calls. That support was my life vest that kept my head above water.

FB: October 25, 2012

Direct message

GC: Oy vey—I'm just catching up! Feel better! Are the kids okay?

Marcy: Yea, I think so, who knows what goes through Riley's mind, right now he is focused on a Halloween party tomorrow night, which is good. Dani worries but holds it together. I have great kids.

CB: October 26, 2012

Rest in the Hospital, I Think Not

Get rest in the hospital, ha ha. I was just about to go to sleep, and the teeth-chattering, shaking chills set in. I knew it was a matter of time because the Tylenol was being spaced too far apart. My IV infiltrated after multiple sticks to begin with. Was given a Norco, got warm, chills stopped, fever up to 103.4. Call to doc, blood cultures ordered, and IV restarted. I love the nurse Joan for being so skilled with that. Got orders for Advil to alternate with Tylenol. I think they were avoiding the Advil because of kidney function being stressed on IV Vancomycin. Still warm but I feel better warm than I do shaking. Bacteria like warm too, so that is not a good thing. I hope we can control the fever better now with alternating meds because I am afraid if the chills start again, my IV will infiltrate again. They said if the IV continues to be a problem they will put in a PICC (peripherally inserted central catheter) line. They will be in again to recheck temp in an hour, then I will try to sleep for a couple of hours. I would get more rest at home but lack of sleep and taking care of the problem is better than lots of sleep and getting sicker. I really like the nurses at Good Samuel Hospital.

Alan: Good morning. I know you're up already from the 5 a.m. blood draw. I hope you got a little rest, which is not easy in a hospital. Look at it this way—you get to watch *The Price Is Right* instead of working so it's not all bad. May the sun shine through your window today. Thinking of you. Hang in there!

FB: October 26, 2012

Sleep deprivation + emotion = crabby and exhausted. Proved that to myself yet again. Putting in my sleeping pill request right now and have my ear plugs ready.

CB: October 27, 2012

Pothole

By mom

Looks like that little "bump in the road" has become a pothole. The doctors withheld the 12-noon Advil to see if the temp would stay down. It went up to 104 with shaking chills and a whole bunch of other nasty symptoms.

They've also done a chest x-ray but don't know any results yet. Her sister and daughter, Dani, are with her. I'll probably go down later. When you see her posting on here you'll know the "pothole" is under some control and she's feeling better. Meanwhile, she asked me to post this update so you'd know why she hasn't added anything. Again, so many thanks for your care and concern. Dorothy

Respiratory Issues

My mom said it well. The temperature is down now. Still short of breath when I talk too much and I cough when I take a deep breath. I had no respiratory symptoms until today. Skipped lunch because of the shaking and I'm going to try to eat soon. Anxiously waiting to see what the CXR showed if anything. I wonder if after four doses of the Vancomycin they'll change the antibiotic, as nothing has really improved. I hope they learned it is wise to listen to the patient. I don't have to do those experiments to prove I am not ready to go home.

P.S. Just found out the chest x-ray is normal, will continue nebulizers every once in a while.

CB: October 28, 2012

Ahhhhh Sleep

The parade of doctors must start later on Sundays. It was a much better night, the nurses and I had a plan. [If they had to come in to wake me up for something, they would do everything at once so that I didn't have to be woken up for multiple issues throughout the night. This is called "clustering care," which is what I was taught when I was a new night nurse in a hospital setting.] I got much more sleep than ever since I have been here. Third night's the charm? The fever is down when we stay on the schedule, it has been proven three times now that when off of antipyretics I spike the fever again. So not sure how this is going to work. I am scared now to go off the Tylenol and Advil. Not sure how many doses of Vancomycin they have to give without a big physical improvement before they decide to do some more investigation. I know they don't want to risk puncturing the huge red lump that extends to under the arm, where my right breast used to be but maybe a sample to culture may reveal a more potent antibiotic for this particular crud.

I think my blood cultures were negative, which is fabulous news. My BP is low again. [Generally, 100–130 on the top number is good and mine was

86. The normal range for the bottom number is 65–85 and mine was 49. This would be a problem when I got up and moved around because the BP would drop lower and make me lightheaded.]

I thought that finger numbness and tingling was from wearing the compression sleeves on my right arm but I still have it and my fifth, fourth, and part of my third fingers are getting weak. I have no strength and drop stuff easily with my dominant hand. Will eventually have to figure it out but wonder if it is from the fluid in the chest under that arm. Maybe when this is over it will be time to go see my favorite neurologist, Dr. Douglass. I'll let you know if I learn anything valuable today. I hope they are all done with me before the Bears game. TV hasn't been on yet but will be on later, *go Bears*!

Last update today (most likely).

Dad: Your hope and optimism are fantastic. Keep up the good work. I am sure you will win the battle and the war. Love, Dad

CB: October 28, 2012

Chest Underwater

While I am waiting for the "vein whisperer" to come and restart the second infiltrated IV, I thought I would update you on the activities that interrupted the Bears game.

While sitting and talking to a good friend I suddenly felt and noticed my gown over the red, swollen chest area was wet. Minutes later there was fluid dripping down my side. The nurse took some swabs and covered it but the surgeon's office decided to come in to poke and drain it. My surgical numbness doesn't run that deep. He wanted to remove as much of the fluid as he could. Started out almost pinkish to clear but got down to the thick chicken gravy looking stuff. He took 225 cc out and now I have a huge divot there. He ordered Gram stain, culture and sensitivity, and cytology. That should help them know what this is and the best way to treat it.

I wasn't sure at first what was more painful, the procedure by the surgeon or the parts of the Bears game I did get to see. Hope your weekend went well. Love Ya, Marcy

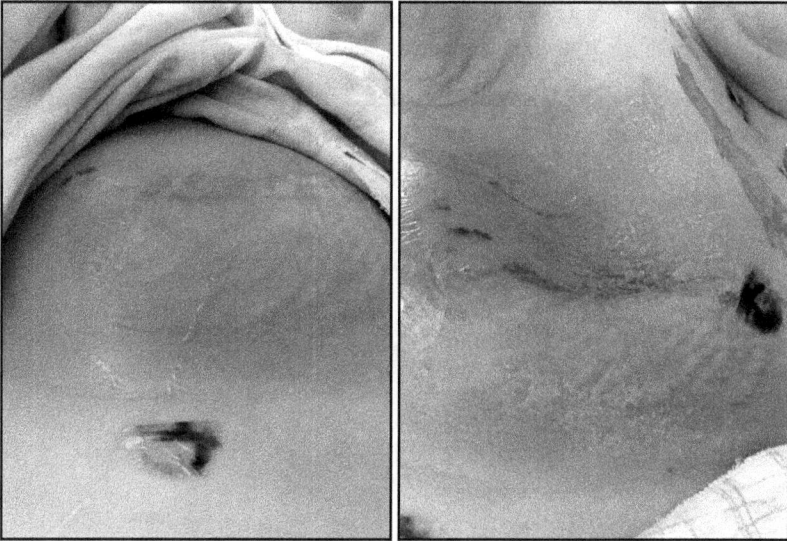

Figure 4-1. My right chest area; red, swollen, and seeping fluid (left). My right underarm and chest area after it was drained by the surgeon (right).

EM: October 28, 2012

From: Alan

To: Marcy

Hey Marcy, I hope you are resting more comfortably. They might have some culture results tomorrow afternoon. Are they planning to open it more and irrigate the area in the OR? Or do they think they drained it fully? I hope the latter.

Bears won, the lucky pink hat comes through again.

I really hope the fever spikes disappear soon. Have a good night my friend.

From: Marcy

To: Alan

I don't know if I will go to the OR, but when I was lying down with a pillow against my chest I got up and the pillow and gown were saturated. I guess that is the fluid in the tissue that can't be drained with a needle. I am anxious to see what all the doctors say tomorrow. I'm still not sure why I am short of breath and cough with a deep breath, but I think the aspiration of the chest was progress.

The Bears cut it so close, watching them is sometimes more stressful than fighting cancer.

From: Alan

To: Marcy

Not to alarm you. Next time you see the nurse ask them to check an oxygen saturation. If it's in the low 90s I'd have them report it to the doc on call.

I think it's unlikely but a pulmonary embolus would have to be considered if your O2 saturation is low. A quick chest CAT scan (no IV contrast necessary) would rule it out.

I know it seems like one thing after another and I don't want to scare you but you're in a delicate situation. You shouldn't be short of breath. Better to be a bit proactive.

Hang in there Marcy.

From: Marcy

To: Alan

They've been about 96 percent. I'll keep an eye on it for sure. Thanks for coming to visit today.

From: Alan

To: Marcy

96 percent is good. No worries. It was really nice to see you. Better days are coming.

Sleep well.

CB: October 29, 2012

Worried Momma

By my mom

A rough day for Marcy. After having so much "stuff" drained yesterday she had to have an additional 100 cc drained this morning. A chest compression wrap was put on and by 3:30 this afternoon the fluid was building up again. Her hemoglobin is 8.9, which is low, and we don't know why that is either. She did take a Xanax and when I called the nurses station a few minutes ago she was sleeping. I thought she might be and that's why I didn't call her directly. I'm sure all this will eventually get sorted out but this momma feels pretty helpless right about now. I just wanted to update you. (And, as if all this wasn't enough, I did beat her at the one game of Farkle that we played about 11:00 this morning.)

My mother was with me as much as she could be during my stay. I didn't know it then, but she was afraid for my life.

FB: October 29, 2012

The fluid that was drained for the second time this morning has completely returned and filled in the divot in my chest. Where is it coming from? I was even wearing the modern day torture device of the compression binder.

Mom: I'm speechless and feel so helpless. Mommies should be able to make their children feel all better.

Lola: Pray Momma, it's all in God's hands and after he hears all of us pleading for her health maybe he will comfort us with her good health.

Mom: I want to come down to see you but I think I can best be of help by being here for Riley.

Kit: Take another Xanax, keeping you in my prayers!

Marcy: I will never take another Xanax.

CB: October 29, 2012

Anxiety?

As soon as you start taking Xanax even after being a great patient for four days the new nurse blames every symptom on anxiety, even the ones that started three to four days ago before the anxiety. They should talk to all the nurses who took care of me before. And again, too busy to do the report in the room. Yes, I am anxious but it is directly related to communication and physical symptoms. My hemoglobin hasn't been normal and this nurse tried to tell me it's "no big deal" to go from normal to 8.7 with symptoms of shortness of breath. She must know best. *Sarcasm and anger*

FB: October 29, 2012

No more talking to anyone until tomorrow morning because being upset makes this staff and some people blame everything on anxiety. So good night. I won't be answering my phone for a while either.

Willow: You have been through more hell than any person should have to take!! Anxiety is not to blame. You are the strongest, sweetest person I know.

Kitt: That's BS and you know it. I know you're strong, don't even have to know why you posted that or the situation but I know you. I'm here! Love you.

Lola: You need to keep calm. I know it is difficult but this is just one small challenge in your journey.

Cindy: Okay Marcy, I have been quiet, but I have *never* stopped having you in my thoughts. Weak is *not* in your vocabulary. Keep fighting!

Marcy: Thanks guys, I have had great relationships with all the nurses and techs here. This nurse sucks and we butt heads. Thankfully my sister-in-law came over when I called and kept me from strangling her. I know I have enough strength for that. I don't think I will be seeing her as my nurse again and she leaves in 1 hour. Just very poor care and condescending. I am a tough stick too and my IV is gone now because she took way too long to take care of an issue in a person who is a known difficult stick. My IV has infiltrated twice before and I have limb precautions (meaning you can't use one of my arms for IVs). My hemoglobin was 13 when I came in and it is 8.9 now and she doesn't think it means anything. Something's going on and if there isn't any concern, explain to me why instead of brushing me off.

CB: October 30, 2012

The Plan (part 1)

Today's plan so far consists of going to get a drain put in so the chicken-gravy-like fluid doesn't keep accumulating. They will also put in a PICC (peripherally inserted central catheter) line for IV access while I am in the interventional radiology department. Will be sent home with that for about a week. Haven't seen any of the doctors yet but that is just what I heard from the nurse who came to take my water away. The worm has turned, as my Grandma used to say.

Sophie: Each day this lady came. She sat by my bed. No words were spoken, she sat silently by my side. One day I looked over and said, "You never speak, but come each day." She replied, "There are no words, I come to let you know you are not alone." There are not always words to say, but we are all sitting by your side every day. You are not alone.

EM: October 30, 2012

From: Marcy

To: Alan

Tell Sophie thank you. Her entry made me teary.

From: Alan

To: Marcy

I will. I'm sorry I've gone all doctor on you the past couple days. I want you to get the best care possible.

I like the plan this a.m. A drain and a PICC line sounds good. I assume they want to avoid opening the area surgically—that makes sense.

Take good care of the PICC line site.

Are you taking iron?—Get that Hgb [hemoglobin] up.

Be good.

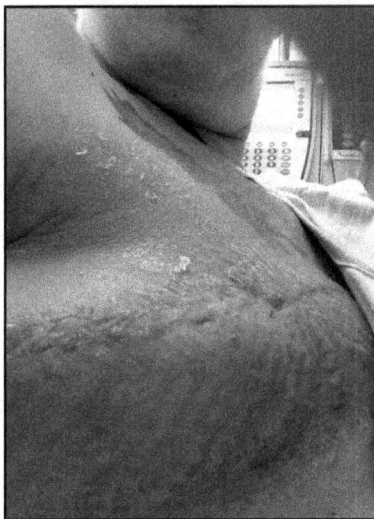

Figure 4-2. My right underarm and chest that filled with fluid

From: Marcy

To: Alan

I really would like to know why it went down. I have been 12-13 all through radiation *and* it was good when I got here. I drink tons and I don't think there were any other indicators of dehydration which is what they blame it on (haven't seen oncologist though). Cytology [lab analysis on the fluid] from Sunday is not back yet. I also don't think they have done that many blood draws to cause that level of anemia.

They aren't giving me iron. Really seems like they are brushing the hemoglobin issue off even though I have some breathing issues. They are not terrible but definitely making me short of breath with any activity. I wonder if it is related to the low hemoglobin (anemia). Oh well.

I'll try to be good unless I get a stupid nurse. Only ran across the one so far, which is pretty good since I've been here since Thursday night. Don't apologize for "going doctor" on me because sometimes it is what I need and sometimes I wish you could be on staff here and straighten them all out. Funny too, no one ordered a CBC to monitor the level. I would have thought when they saw it was low yesterday they would want to monitor it. I asked the lab to draw it when he drew my Vancomycin trough, so that after I discussed it with Dr. Dunkin, I could ask her to order it again. Maybe I am putting too much importance on my hemoglobin value?

From: Alan

To: Marcy

Sometimes when you get a serious infection and you're hospitalized the bone marrow gets "stunned" and slows down for a few days—a weird but common stress response to being rather ill. Also, all the IV fluids relatively dilute the blood and will lead to a lower Hgb concentration.

I don't think there's any reason to believe you are bleeding somewhere, which is good news.

Frankly, I think iron supplementation is a good idea.

If it were me, and I'm admittedly a type-A person, I'd want the opinion of my hematology or oncology person. After all the chemo and radiation, I'd like to know that my bone marrow is capable of replenishing my Hgb. There are some basic iron studies and a reticulocyte count [which would show if the blood marrow has produced new red blood cells], that can provide a lot of information.

In any case, I think it's reasonable to assume that—as the infection resolves, as you get some iron and home cooking in you, and as you get home to your own couch—then all your cell counts will rise. That's probably what Dr. Dunkin is thinking.

In summary I'd ask about iron and ask if they plan to draw a follow-up CBC in a day or two.

Don't let all my science upset you, it's just how my mind is always going.

Hang in there.

From: Marcy

To: Alan

I love explanations. What you say makes sense, I may have to explain it that way to everyone else. As long as I know it is going back up I am better in the head. I just wish docs would acknowledge and explain those things better and nurses would find out answers instead of brushing patient's concerns off.

Thank you!

CB: October 30, 2012

The Plan (Part 2)

I just got back from getting the PICC line placed. No more IV sticks and we can resume IV antibiotics. They have helped but I think things will progress faster now that the extra fluids aren't pooling in my chest. The fluid that came out this time was thin and red. Completely different from before so that is also going to the lab. They kind of did a betadine flush in there to help things along. Now I have a drainage device to keep the fluid from accumulating. It may be in for about a week. As far as I know I can go home when I am not running temps. Last temp was 102 degrees last night at 8 p.m. I had Tylenol at 3 a.m. No temp since then. So I am really hoping I can get home tomorrow. This will heal and I can get my last five radiation treatments done.

The CBC follow-up test I requested was up to a hemoglobin of 9.2 so at least I know it is recovering. As it is on the rise I won't worry about it too much.

Human resources called and I am relieved about what she said. I was afraid I would have to start coming up with the company's portion of the insurance or could even lose my job if I was out too long. She said the employee portion is all I need to pay through November and then we will reevaluate, and I should be all good by then. Also FMLA [Family and Medical Leave Act] will reset December 5. So if I needed it later it would be available for the twelve weeks again. That doesn't solve the problem of not having my income and no sick time but she is also going to check into the sick bank to see if I qualify for some help.

Overall progress can be seen and I feel better in many ways. Unfortunately, the postsurgical numbness doesn't go deeper than they have been poking, so it is starting to hurt, but not enough to take anything for pain. Just splinting the area with my hand or pillow helps.

Thanks for hanging in there with me.

Marcy

FB: October 30, 2012

I wish I was a lefty. All the bad crap from the cancer is affecting my right arm. The pain in the right chest from lifting my arm will get better when the infection is gone and the drain is out. The numbness and tingling, who knows. The swelling will be intermittent possibly the rest of my life depending on prevention techniques and also circumstances beyond my control.

Think of every cuss word you know. The dang fever is back, 101 at 6:30 p.m. So close, so close. I wonder if I can talk them into discharging me if I can keep it 101 or below.

GC: Ooh! I have TONS!!!

Dakota: F#%<, s#i+, d^~n, b*+€h..

Lola: Give it time, you just got cleaned up today and started the PICC line.

Marcy: You're right. I am sure putting in the drain shook up things a little and there was a big delay in the antibiotic schedule. Should get better from here. I am just homesick. I think if you put all my surgeries (seven to eight) together, they wouldn't add up to the number of days I have spent in the hospital for this. Just want to be home. Maybe Thursday?

Clara: I'm sure you're stir-crazy and nothing is like being at home in your own bed.

Who wants to break me outta here? They didn't take my clothes or shoes away. We can do it. Bring a hat and sunglasses!

Miriam: What floor are you on? If you collect bed sheets for a few days, I'll make sure the getaway car is waiting below!

RH: On my way. I'll hurry! We need to come up with a diversion!

Marcy: OMG! I love you all. I am not willing to collect sheets for days but I have a collection of blankets from when I had the chills. Will that work?

Miriam: Sure will! We'll tie them all together and you'll be long gone before they know you are missing. We'll head to Florida. The beach will do you good. They'll never find us.

Marcy: I see hinges on this windoooooooowwwwww. My sneaking out attempts in high school usually failed. I do need some help from those who succeeded.

Clara: It's all good, it's almost Halloween. I'll dress as a nurse and bust you out of that place.

Marcy: Great idea Clara, bring a costume for me.

FB: October 31, 2012

I think today is going to be the day I don't run a fever.

RH: I got a good feeling too.

Lola: Yes! Today is the day. No fevers

Marcy: They are talking discharge tomorrow with home IV antibiotics. The cellulitis and abscess area looks completely different overnight, much better. The housekeeper came in and took one look at me and said, "Ooohhhhh, you feel better, I can tell, you look better!" I think I was scaring her the days she came in when I had high fevers and was chilling in bed and shaking. Up until today, I don't even think she said one or two words to me each time she was here. She was so quiet. She was trying to clean without disturbing my rest.

Had a fun visit with Liza, my mom, sister, and my sister-in-law Patti. No fever so far today.

Hannah: Hurray! I'm hoping there's no more chicken gravy, too.

KB: *Best status of the day!*

CB: November 1, 2012

Going Home Today

Big sigh of relief. Waiting for the discharge plans to be solidified. I saw the doctors and since I have not had a fever in more than thirty-six hours I can go home. You know how much I have been hating these hot flashes since chemo drop kicked me into menopause? Well now whenever I start feeling warm I just chant, "Let it be a hot flash not a fever."

The PICC line is in place and the abscess drain is in place. They are arranging home infusion. I wanted to do outpatient at first but the Vancomycin will be every eighteen hours for two weeks and the timing may change depending on blood tests, so for scheduling purposes it is better to do home care and do my own infusions. Everything will be delivered to the house.

The cytology was negative (no cancer in the fluid they took out) and the culture and sensitivity showed the bad stuff is susceptible to the antibiotics we are using. When I am done with the IV antibiotics there are a lot of oral antibiotic options.

Monday I will come back to interventional radiology and maybe get the drain out and the surgeon will come see me while I am there. I will also see the radiation oncologist after I am out of the hospital. He will decide when I can get those last five radiation treatments done. I have to be well healed first.

Not sure yet about when I will be back at work. The timing of the antibiotic infusions I think is going to make it difficult but I will try to get back as soon as I can... I like paychecks.

Can't believe I was in the hospital for a whole week, Thursday to Thursday. I was a sick puppy! Feeling much better now. I will have to take it easy for a bit... And yes, I will *actually* try to take it easy. My body isn't going to give me much of a choice I think.

I hope everyone had a great Halloween, especially those of you with the little cuties in costume!

SS: Marcy, I cannot believe this all has been going on. I have been praying for you since I read this all. Can't wait to see you back at work. Praise the Lord that there were no cancer cells in the fluid. That may be the only bright spot in this whole thing. Does the swelling in your hand look any better? You wonder whether all this fluid was causing some of the backup in your hand and arm. Keep smiling, see you soon.

FB: November 1, 2012

Thank you to the doctors and staff at the hospital for getting me back on the road to recovery but I have to say it is much better to be home.

Jacey: Glad you are home and in your wonderful bed!

Marcy: Me too, believe me though, it didn't get cold, my daughter slept in it while I was gone.

Why did my daughter sleep in my bed? My gut reaction was comfort; her bedroom was on the floor above and there wasn't a bathroom up there, and the Sleep Number bed was awesome. Both the kids loved playing with it and at times while I was still in the bed would raise the head and feet and try to bend me in half like a taco.

In the next coming months she would spend a lot of time lying in bed with me, talking, watching *The Ellen Show* clips and *Say Yes to the Dress*. Just as I worried that I wouldn't be alive to see Riley graduate from high school, I was also fearful I wouldn't be able to be alive to see her get married. When I asked Dani what she remembers now, almost five years after that hospitalization, she said, "I was worried. It was like you were gone for two weeks." It felt like forever to me.

Many of my family and friends thought I could die of the complications associated with the harsh treatment used to treat an aggressive cancer. Relatives, including my mother, tried to appear strong but could not hide the fear in their eyes. My mom told me later that she almost always had faith that I would survive cancer—this hospitalization was the only time she thought I might die. If my kids were anything like my mom and other members of my family, they were downright terrified.

When I was in the hospital I called the high school Riley went to. I spoke with the counselor. They knew I had cancer from my intentional visit over the summer to update them on what was going on with my health. I informed them that I was very sick and that although Riley would never admit to being concerned, he was. I believe he was petrified. Although he had seen me sick, he'd never seen me go to the hospital for any other reason but surgery. He didn't want to come to see me. I wanted desperately to see him but can't blame him for wanting to keep his distance as it would be easier to deny how deathly ill I had become. I am sure he was feeling as powerless as my own mother. I did find out later that the week I was in the hospital, the school staff did not check in with him once, even after my plea to keep an eye on him. Not one item of homework was turned in that week. When I got out of the hospital, we spent the next week trying to get him caught up. This was how he began his freshman year at high school.

I also spent time with Dani once I had my freedom back. I was out at a restaurant with her when the server called me "sir." This wasn't the first time. It seemed to bother her more than me. I told her that with the hair stubble and baseball cap, it was probably an easy mistake. When the server identified his error, which was almost immediately, he corrected himself and things went back to normal. I convinced her not to mention it to him, even making her pinky promise, as he had his tail between his legs in embarrassment and he had already corrected himself.

Maybe it was good that she oversaw this misunderstanding and was disturbed. It gave her a glimpse of what I'd been going through. I am still unsure why Dani was bothered by this as much as she expressed. She never had any issues with my baldness or my chest being flat. In fact, she too used her sense of humor to deal with stress at times. Once when we were shopping at DSW, she asked me *not* to wear a hat or head covering. She said when we were separated in a store or mall it was always easier to find me when she could look for the "tall bald woman." Likewise, she didn't seem to have any issues with my choice not to have breast reconstruction. When I told her I had found out there were many different types and shapes of foobs—my pet name for fake boobs—she asked if she could go with me to pick them out. We laughed often, we cried often, we loved always. Thinking about that now, I wonder if she was upset because she thought being misgendered upset me. Maybe she was fine with my physical changes but could see others treating me differently, which she knew would bother me.

Derailed

EM: November 1, 2012

From: Marcy

To: Alan

Hey there,

Got a dose of Vancomycin just before leaving the hospital, expecting supplies and Vancomycin to be delivered tonight for the nurse to get me going in the morning.

Thanks for coming to see me and for filling in the monumental holes in knowledge and information I wasn't getting from the doctors. The oncologist isn't at all worried about my bone marrow or interested in other tests. He thinks it will come back up just fine, and didn't think I needed iron either? You guys both agree that my own couch or bed and home cooking will have the most therapeutic value.

How is Tommy doing after surgery?

Thanks again for everything,

From: Alan

To: Marcy

No problem. I recently ordered you something else I stumbled across. Do you hunt by the way? Did you know there's a hunting supply company called Browning? I saw a patient last night wearing one of their shirts.

You probably have good iron stores and will replenish the Hgb on your own over the next couple weeks. Nevertheless, the iron tests are simple blood tests (Fe, TIBC, Ferritin, Transferrin).

Tommy came home today from the hospital too. He's on Dilaudid and he refuses to share. He's doing OK on three legs. The surgical site looks good. He says hello. Enjoy some peace.

From: Marcy

To: Alan

I'm laughing out loud, did I know there was a company called Browning? Of course! They have all kinds of hunting stuff, camping, clothes. I couldn't wait to get a bunch of shirts and stuff with Browning on it when I went back to my maiden name. Quality stuff too.

I think at some point I may ask my primary doctor to order those tests.

I am glad Tommy is doing so well, tough little guy, surprised he won't share with you.

Looking forward to a quiet weekend at home...at least quiet until the Bears play.

CB: November 3, 2012

Healing at Home

Thanks for all the support while I was in the hospital. I don't think I have ever been so sick. Hanging out this morning and letting my home IV

Vancomycin drip. I am grateful I can do this at home quietly with no IV pumps beeping and no one coming in to take vital signs. Things will progress from here. Still not sure when I will go back to work. A lot depends on if this drainage slows down and they can take the drain out on Monday, and if the Vancomycin blood levels are where they want them to be; if I have to have them every twelve or eighteen hours I won't be able to do that and get to work.

Checked in with the radiation oncologist yesterday, will see him again next Friday and when things are healed enough will resume the last five radiation treatments. I only understand a small portion of the radiation treatment and I get how complicated it is to treat exactly what needs to be treated with exactly the amount of juice needed to not damage good tissue. I am in good hands. This wasn't the fault of radiation alone but without working lymph nodes, infections and lymph fluid in that area can't be cleared as well. After radiation is completely done and everything recovers, things like this won't be as much of a problem. I will always have to be careful of cuts and infection on the right side but it shouldn't ever end up like this again.

Overall feeling much better, just a little tired.

Have a great weekend, Marcy

EM: November 4, 2012

From: Marcy

To: Alan

Go Bears! There is no way we can lose now!

From: Alan

To: Marcy

The hat's record remains perfect!

Yep, that was awesome. Almost a little boring that we were so far ahead but then there would be a great play!

From: Marcy

To: Alan

Keep up the hat wearing!

FB: November 5, 2012

Due to the recent hospitalization, I am going to put my family and friends who were nervous about my winter road trip at ease and cancel my Grand Canyon reservations. Hoping to find a deal by train or plane to see the Rizzo family in California still. Have to get out and explore after seven or so months of being sick!

CB: November 7, 2012

Drain Out, Sclerosing Chemicals In

On Monday the drain was taken out after a procedure in which they try to damage the fluid-producing cells inside of the abscess sack by causing sclerosis [tissue hardening]. They did that by injecting alcohol, waiting, taking that out, and injecting betadine, and then waiting and then taking that out. So far I don't think there has been much fluid buildup but I am going to keep a close eye on it.

Home infusions are going well. Had the Vancomycin blood level drawn yesterday, just waiting to hear orders on how many more days of infusion and the frequency. The home infusion pharmacist thinks it will be every twenty-four hours. I am taking the rest of the week off though, still very tired.

Follow up with the radiation oncologist will be on Friday and I am hoping he will say that I have healed enough to get the last five radiation treatments done, starting next Monday. I plan on going back to work next Monday.

Things are gradually improving.

FB: November 7, 2012

As much as I wanted to take Riley to see the Mythbusters' live show on Saturday, I think it would be wise not to overdo it and to stay out of public crowds, so Roger (Dani's Dad) is the recipient of my ticket and will take Riley. They are sure to have a great time and I am grateful that Roger is able to take him. I'm sad I can't go but happy he will be with Roger.

FB: November 8, 2012

Three more days of IV antibiotics were added, then I will go to oral ones. Monday I am planning on going back to work. I am hoping to be done with *all of this* by the end of next week. Wouldn't that be something awesome to be thankful for...the completion of breast cancer treatments? Then maybe I will be healed enough to get my new "foobs" for Christmas.

Kady: Let's hear it for foobs! Can't wait to see you Marcy, we've really missed you!

Marcy: Thanks Kady, other than surgery, I have never been in the hospital for being sick, to be there a whole week, I was sooooo sick. Will be good to be back in the swing of things, even if it's tiring it is what I need. I missed all of you too.

CB: November 8, 2012

Better to Be Sure

I had the fourteenth dose of IV Vancomycin this morning and a visit with my primary care doctor this afternoon. We agreed it was much improved but not quite sure if it was good enough to go on oral antibiotics and remove the PICC line. She called my surgeon, who isn't in the same building but in the same complex, and she came over to where we were... how sweet is that?! I didn't have to get dressed, go there, get undressed and wait for phone calls and decisions. Wish we three were meeting to share a bottle of wine though (my PCP said we would celebrate when I was all done with this). It was decided that I would do three more days of IV Vancomycin to take me through the weekend, then switch to oral antibiotics on Monday. Monday I am going back to work and when I get home the home care nurse can come take the PICC out or I can go back to the doctor to get it out. Offered to take it out myself but the PCP said maybe not...probably would be awkward with one hand. I will see the surgeon in ten days and see the radiation oncologist tomorrow.

So that is the latest. Still a little sore in the chest area, especially when I use my right arm a lot but that will improve quickly. Still a little tired but I am sure when I get back to a normal schedule I will be really tired the first few days but my endurance will build quickly. For now, I am just hanging out and driving Riley back and forth to school for tech crew [for a play].

Have a good night, Marcy

DA: Hi Marcy! I'm so glad to hear that things are improving! Glad you can get to work and more normal schedule. Hopefully radiation will also be done soon. What will you do with all your time when you stop running??? Still in my prayers!

SS: Marcy, this is all sounding great. I can't wait to have you back at work. I miss you terribly and I only see you once a week. Imagine how the rest of the staff feels. I will pray for your daughter Dani. I know how those college kids need a break once in a while. Love you all.

CB: November 9, 2012

Growing Brighter

Hey there, I saw the radiation oncologist today. He was pleased that the antibiotics were working. So pleased I guess that he wanted to restart radiation today, so we did. Was a little surprised but I am glad we are moving on and that there are only four more radiation treatments. As a friend of mine wrote in an email, "The light at the end of the tunnel is growing brighter. Then it's on to good health!"

I can see a lot of improvement from the infection but there is a lot of healing to be done, it doesn't feel right. Although I guess it hasn't felt right since last March. Hoping soon that I will know what my new normal is, so I can believe I am healthy and cancer free someday soon.

This hospitalization scared me. I didn't realize how sick I could get so fast. Scared me into compliance, which is why instead of taking Riley to see the Mythbuster's live at the Sears Center I am giving my ticket to someone else to take him. I was really looking forward to doing this with Riley but don't need to overdo it or be in crowds right now. Thanks for taking him, Roger.

Another big thank you to the medical team I have. Such a blessing to be in good care.

Have a great weekend, Marcy

Lucy: Four treatments left—great news Marcy! Yes, there is a light at the end of the tunnel and you are getting closer. I pray everything from here on out goes well for you. You have done an amazing job with all the treatments. Love you and have a restful weekend.

GG: God Bless you Marcy. I am so glad to hear you are doing better.

CB: November 12, 2012

Derailed

Grrrr, I am having so much trouble getting back on track physically and emotionally. Sunday was my last IV Vancomycin and the home care nurse came and pulled my PICC line. I started Levaquin orally this morning. My stomach doesn't like it much but it's tolerable.

Over the weekend an area over the incision and scar started filling with fluid again; this is the area the doctors were describing as "spongey." I wasn't and am still not running a temp but the area has grown, it hurts, it's pinkish red and tender. I thought, just get back to work and get through radiation this week and make it until the twentieth when the follow up with the surgeon is. When I took a shower the hot water must have done something to the area because after the shower there were pinhole areas in the incision that started dripping fluid. Mostly clear. Still though, I thought I have to get back to work. Saturday I called to get a substitute nurse to work for me on Monday, changed my mind and called back on Sunday saying I would be there Monday, so I had to go. The whole time driving in, I was almost in tears, this isn't right.

Got to work, love the people, missed them so much but knew when I walked in, I wasn't ready. This area of fluid that builds up, is well... building up. Called to ask for someone to come relieve me and someone came. Made it through three hours at work.

Left messages for the surgeon, really thinking this needs to be aspirated. I don't think it is infected but it is getting painful, especially the more I move my arm. I went to the radiation oncologist. Had a mini break-down there, first time I think they have seen me cry. Such compassionate people there. The radiation oncologist, said he won't do radiation on the chest wall until this was taken care of but he wanted to do the last clavicle and lymph node treatment as it wouldn't affect the abscess area, which he believes is a different pocket than the one that had the drain. I think he knows that I want to quit radiation because he reminded me I need to finish even if there is another delay before getting the last four to the chest wall. He told me to call after I see the surgeon and we will figure out when we can finish the radiation treatments.

Came home, rested on the couch while waiting for surgeon to call back. More crying, this time trying to explain what I was crying about to my sister-in-law Patti, who came over to be with me. The surgeon's office called and said to come tomorrow at 4:30. I'm so tired of this. She said if I get a fever or it starts leaking again I am going to the emergency room. I called the surgeon back and left a message too that I won't go into work tomorrow like this and if they have a cancellation to call me and I could be there in twenty minutes.

I think I have held it together for the most part, with a few valleys in there but honestly I am sick of this. I feel guilty for still being sick, I feel tired and less patient and then guilty for being less patient. I snapped at Riley last night and although I apologized, he may never forget that. That was one of my darkest moments. Crying now just writing about it. I will take as much pain as cancer can dish out if I could have those ten seconds back because I know my words caused him pain. I haven't been much more patient with Dani either. One thing I have always been able to tell myself is that I am a pretty good mom and I don't feel like that anymore... all because I am sick and tired of being sick and tired.

So that is the physical and emotional truth. I know many will be uncomfortable with it and tell me to have hope and faith and all that stuff. The truth is I am human and at times weak in body and spirit, now is one of those times. I know it will pass and I will feel better soon but I can't see how pretending and denying my feelings will help me move through them...they will just sneak out like they did last night.

Thanks for keeping up with me, even the tough stuff. I know it is hard for you too.

Alan: It really isn't fair. I don't know why this happens. If there's a higher power controlling this what the heck is she/he thinking? I feel bad for you. I'm sorry it's been an out of control day. Always hope for tomorrow being better.

Personally, I hate "losing it" but sometimes it's good for you. You can't pretend that things are always rosy. Sometimes you just gotta scream. You'll get past it and so will Riley. An apology is a powerful thing. You're a great mom. If losing it on one of your kids made you a bad mom we'd all be in DCFS [Department of Children and Family Services] group homes. When you love and care about your children 24 hours a day you're a good mom. Tomorrow is another day. Keep fighting.

Laurie: Just know I love you. I know that the words don't really help, but I just needed to say that!

PO: That is your life…and you are doing the best you can, and sometimes that is not pretty. Keep going Marcy… Four more…just four.

Lucy: Marcy—Glad you are able to cry, get mad, be impatient, etc. Those feelings make you human and quite frankly with all you have been through, I think it is completely normal. I know you are one strong lady, but let's be real—everyone reaches their limit. It's okay to have a break-down—you are completely entitled. We all hate it when we say things that hurt our children. You will have the opportunity to apologize and make it up to them. This is just a very trying time when you are trying so hard to be a good patient, be a good mom, be at work and do your job, and are trying so hard to get better and get back to your normal health.

You are doing so well, so please don't beat yourself up. We love you no matter what and I'm praying hard for you. Love you dear friend!

SE: It's OK to feel the way you do. That's why you have family and friends who love you. We love all the different and awesome sides of you! Know that you are very much loved no matter what mood you are in. That's what family and friends are for.

EM: November 12, 2012

From: Marcy

To: Rona at YMCA Camp

Hi, Riley will be fifteen on July 23, can he sign up to be a leader-in-training next summer?

From: Rona

To: Marcy

Yes, absolutely! Love this kid!!

From: Marcy

To: Rona

Thanks, I know he will really be glad to be there.

A short story: Riley and I were talking about families having favorite chil-dren. I said something about being his favorite mom, because he only had one. He said, "I consider Rona my second mom." I thought that was so cool.

Things could be better here, he is hanging in there. He is involved in tech crew at school. I have had some complications in the cancer treatment and still am not done. I thought this would be over by October. I was really sick the last week in October and in the hospital for a week.

He is trying so hard and I know it is tough. He really looks forward to camp, and I am so grateful he does. Take care, Marcy

From: Rona

To: Marcy

That is a great story. I would be glad to be his second mom! He really is a sweet boy.

I am sorry things are tough with your health. You can beat this! You are in my thoughts and prayers.

I know I am not supposed to have favorites but Riley is one of my favorites. I am glad camp is second *home* to him. It is a good, peaceful, safe place and we will always be here for him.

You take care and hang in there okay!

CB: November 13, 2012

I Don't Like a Mystery

I saw the surgeon, she aspirated 55 cc of what looked like yellow Gatorade. Feels a little better but really sore. It is difficult to make the motion with my right arm to take my shirt off. She said if it starts filling up I will need to go to interventional radiology to have the sclerosing procedure again. It seems like this is a completely different pocket. I asked why this keeps happening…if you put all the answers together from all the doctors there is a hodgepodge of reasons that put together set up the circumstances for this: empty space in the chest from surgery, reduced function of the lymphatic system from removal of the lymph nodes, damage from radiation, etc., etc.

The focus is to get the radiation complete and reevaluate after that. I am going to try to see the radiation oncologist tomorrow and see if we can restart radiation. I hope we can do it in the next four business days, which will bring me to the follow-up with the surgeon on November 20.

Mentally, a little better today. The exchange with Riley bothered me much more than him. Last night when I asked if he forgave me yet, he said, "Yeah," it wasn't a big deal. My kids are great and I am so lucky that they have handled all this as they have.

I am hoping my next journal entry will be to tell you that radiation is complete.

Thank you for accepting me for who I am. Love, Marcy

DA: Marcy, I for one am grateful for your honesty. It has just been a very tough, long battle. I think you expect yourself to be stronger than those around you expect from you. Even without the suffering you have endured, we all mess up with our kids but love will win that battle. Give yourself the rest you need and the grace to blow it once in a while. Your kids will blow it too, but you are teaching them so much when you show them by example how to truly apologize when we make a mistake. It's a life lesson they will need too. It was great to run into you over the weekend. Hope Riley's project turned out well. You keep fighting, we'll keep praying.

Dad: I know that the ups and downs are very discouraging, may God help you through to your complete recovery.

EM: November 13, 2012

From: Alan

To: Marcy

Just thinking about you. At work again tonight. How was your appointment?

From: Marcy

To: Alan

Just got done, she aspirated 55 cc of yellow Gatorade. The nurse said, "We call that a shitty titty" when I showed it to her. I said, "I'm not supposed to have titties." Follow up on appointment on 11/20.

From: Alan

To: Marcy

I looked up "shitty titty" in Harrison's *Textbook of Medicine*—I can't find it. Did they send it for culture?

Get yourself a donut or two tonight. You deserve it.

From: Marcy

To: Alan

She didn't send it for culture...maybe because I am on Levaquin already? She did confirm I was taking it and told me to finish it. Is it reasonable to assume that it is just fluid based on appearance and if there was infection it would be the same organisms as the other culture? She said if it started to fill up again, it would be back to interventional radiology. Her demeanor was a little weird. I said I just wanted to finish this up so I could get measured and get my prosthetics by Christmas, she acted like that wasn't reasonable and told me to just focus on finishing the radiation. I told her it was frustrating because this was going on longer than I mentally prepared myself for. I wish she would have said, I think we will be able to get your prosthetics by Christmas.

Today while I was home I filed and organized papers that were piling up on my floor. Mentally it feels better to get a little organized. I hope work goes well.

From: Alan

To: Marcy

You're right about the culture. It would not be helpful with the Levaquin on board. I really hope the fluid doesn't reaccumulate. What a pain that must be for you.

Organization is key.

FB: November 13, 2012

Shouldn't having cancer make a person more patient? I just want to get it done and move on.

Mom: That's how I feel about the hip replacement. I want to get it done and move on. Then I think about all you are going through and I tell myself (in the words of my dad), "Quitcher bellyachin."

Marcy: Just because people in your life are going through something doesn't mean your issue is any less real or important. I would like to know you aren't in pain anymore. I hope you can get it done and get on the road to recovery and activity.

FB: November 14, 2012

Appointment today to see if I can restart radiation since the surgeon took 55 cc of fluid out of that area yesterday. Want to get radiation over with! Hopefully back to work tomorrow, the unpaid time off I've taken is ridiculous. I'm happy to still have a job and insurance. If I can't get four radiation treatments done by Thanksgiving I am going to lose it... For those of you who have not seen me "lose it," it is pretty ugly.

AV: No, no please. Don't lose it!

Lola: So did they allow you to make some standing appointments for fluid removal just in case so you don't have to wait an extra day to get seen?

KB: Wish I could give you some of my sick days. Stupid unions.

Marcy: That's okay, cashing in more retirement. I hope after surviving cancer, I don't get killed at tax time.

Called "sir" again, when I was buying sweets for the radiation staff. I'm wearing a feminine hat with a pink ribbon on it too. Five out of six times I was called "sir," it was by a man. I'm going to start wearing dangling earrings.

I am a slow learner. Was sick of the disgusting house so cleaned the upstairs bathroom before going to radiation, got radiation, felt good when I got home so I started cleaning downstairs bathroom, chemical fumes made me vomit. After that was over I started cleaning the kitchen, now it feels like the chest area is more swollen. I'm such an idiot, just want to do normal things like take care of my home.

CB: November 15, 2012

Last Chance

So Tuesday the surgeon aspirated the fluid accumulation. Wednesday I had radiation, three more left.

This morning I went in to work at 7 a.m. and at 9:30 the front of my shirt was wet from that area filling up and spontaneously leaking a steady stream of fluid. Called for help covering my job, covered my draining chest with gauze and called the surgeon while I was in the car. Completely soaked through the gauze and my shirt, changed the dressing a few times before the 1 o'clock appointment. She put steri-strips on it and called the interventional radiologist to do the sclerosing procedure tomorrow with the alcohol and betadine, again!

I asked her if this is going to heal without surgical intervention and she said after radiation if it doesn't heal she would do surgery again, with a primary closure or skin graft. (I think she has known this for a while and that is why her demeanor was different when I mentioned the goal of getting prosthetics by Christmas. In order to purchase prosthetics, my skin needs to be fully healed.)

Here is the part you might not like but I am telling you this is how I feel and no one can change that. I told her if the sclerosis doesn't work and it fills up again before I can complete radiation next week I will quit radiation. I really mean that. I know it is a cumulative radiation dose but honestly with only three left, if they can't manage this fluid first I am not going anymore. Ridiculous, aspirate one day, radiation the next, fluid accumulation the next. I have had it. If the sclerosing works and dries the tissue long enough to get radiation Monday, Tuesday, and Wednesday, that is great. In my gut I know I will need surgical intervention at some point to fix this mess of a chest I have. The question is, can this temporary fix hold me long enough to get the last three radiation treatments? If not, no more radiation, period!

I hope you don't think I am blaming my doctors because I am not, it is my stupid body. I have a great team. Something different needs to be done or the cycle will continue.

Right now that is all I have.

EM: November 15, 2012

From: Alan

To: Marcy

I agree. My gut feeling is you'll be fine with seventeen or twenty radiation treatments. As you know, nothing in medicine is an exact science. There is still light at the end of the tunnel.

And soon there will be Christmas lights everywhere, which always makes me smile.

Be good.

From: Marcy

To: Alan

I know they aren't happy with my way of thinking. He will say the studies show I need this specific dose, blah blah blah.

I'd rather fix my chest and go on the Tamoxifen, but I will give this procedure a shot and try to get it done.

I like lights too, I want to get some hot spiced wine at Christkindlemarket.

Talk to you later. Marcy

FB: November 15, 2012

Post on my wall

Lola: *Keep your eye on the prize!!!* Chin up.

Marcy: What's the prize?

Lola: Your health and wellbeing.

Marcy: Yeah, that's a good prize! I was wanting foobs and a trip to California for Christmas. Not sure that will happen now.

FB: November 16, 2012

Hi ho hi ho, it's off to the hospital I go. Hopefully the sclerosing procedure will stop the fluid buildup where my right breast used to be. Got to get done with radiation treatments.

Dang it! I'm craving Ho Hos now. I asked for it when I said if the sclerotherapy didn't work I was done with radiation because I didn't want any more delays. This is the third time I have had it done and I think he was overly aggressive with the chemicals in the sclerosing procedure. I am burning from the inside out!

Lucy: I'm worrying about your radiation—too much?

Marcy: It'll be okay. The pain and burning just caught me by surprise because the sclerosing didn't feel like this the other two times. It will be better in the morning, I am sure. I trust the radiation oncologist and they want to get to a prescribed dose. I have only had three treatments the last month and am still having trouble. Could be that I didn't heal right from the mastectomy, the effects of not having enough working lymph nodes and radiation. I want them to fix me! I will know more Monday and Tuesday. I have appointments with my primary doctor, the radiation oncologist and the surgeon. Hopefully we can put our heads together and figure it out. It isn't leaking anymore but it feels like it might be accumulating again.

CB: November 16, 2012

Interventional Radiology

Hi all,

What do these things have in common? The book *Eat That Frog*, food shows, unicycles, zombies, government, break dancing, air travel, decluttering, and paranormal activity? If you answered, "topics of discussion during my interventional radiology procedure," you are correct. I love their sense of humor while we listened to Poison, Def Leppard, and Motley Crue. Three times now I have had the "abscessogram and sclerotherapy"; sounds like a singing telegram and spa treatment. What will I do when I don't need to go back and visit with them in the interventional radiology department at Good Samuel? It is the most fun I have had in the hospital (except the procedure part wasn't really fun), and I wasn't even on drugs the last two times.

So I am bandaged up pretty good and compression is the name of the game for the weekend. I don't think the fluid will come back, or at least before I can finish radiation. I have my last three radiation treatments scheduled for Monday, Tuesday, and Wednesday. I see my primary doc on Monday and the surgeon for follow up on Tuesday. I am hoping that will be the end of it and I can start the Tamoxifen on Thursday.

I asked the doctor who did the procedure today his opinion. "Do you think when radiation is over, the abscess pockets and all that is going on in the chest area will heal without surgical intervention?" He is a chicken and said fifty-fifty. How careful is he in his response?

Overall, glad that I had the procedure done and hoping I can finish up radiation. I don't want to be a quitter but at some point, in my head, there is a time when fixing my chest and going on Tamoxifen would be more beneficial than doing the last three radiation treatments. I could be wrong on that but that is what is in my head. I started radiation on September 5 and it was supposed to be about 30 treatments.

Looking forward to seeing Riley perform his tech crew duties this weekend at the the high school musical and a family Thanksgiving dinner with the Browning Family on Sunday.

I hope you all have a good weekend and that I have nothing significant to report until radiation is done.

Take care, Marcy

P.S. I didn't make up the words "abscessogram" and "sclerotherapy," those were written on the board in the interventional radiology room under my name.

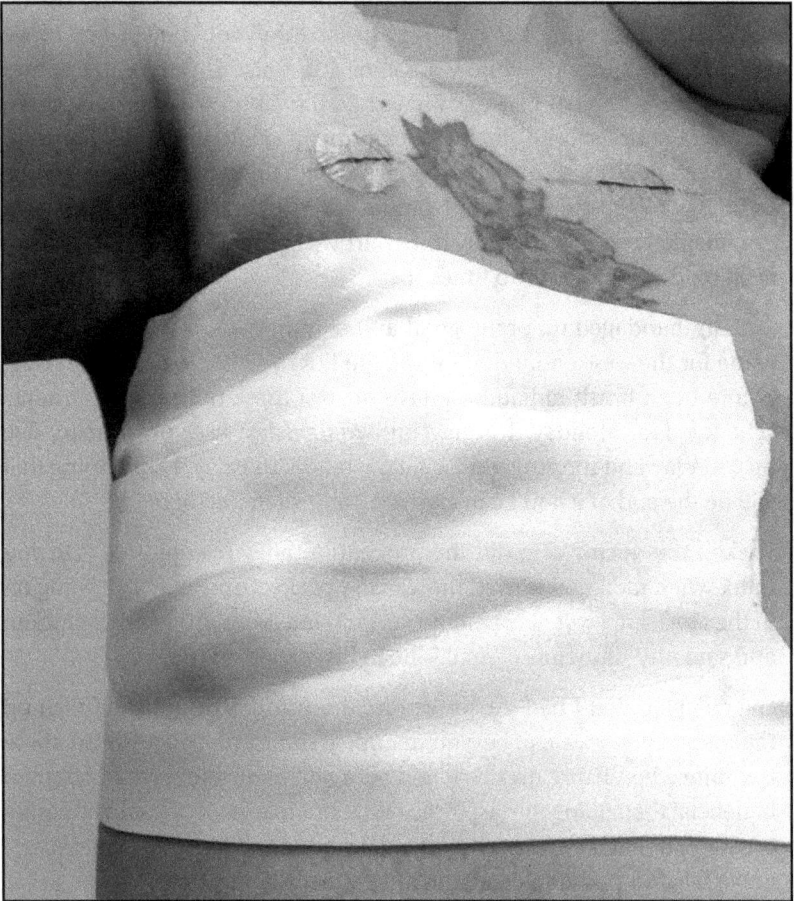

Figure 4-3. Tight dressing after sclerosing procedure

Lucy: Marcy—Sounds like things are progressing and I'm sure that is what you want, so I wish you a good weekend! Regarding the radiation, listen to what your body tells you. This was also an issue for my brother, so it is very real and you will know what is best for you. There appears to be a very fine line there for the patient—enough, but not too much. Love and prayers!

FB: November 17, 2012

Planning on resting all day until Riley's musical. I didn't realize how much the complications were taking out of me. It's almost over... Three more days of radiation and praying my chest will heal without more surgery or having to get skin grafts.

CB: November 17, 2012

Sclerotherapy Didn't Work

Well, I got to see Riley perform his tech crew duties in the musical, and I know he was really happy my mom and I went. I was a bit distracted though because during the musical my chest was leaking again, soaking through gauze and my shirt. I guess it is better that it is leaking out instead of building inside, but I think it is doing a little of that too. I just don't feel good, a little nausea and indigestion and pain from that chest area through to the shoulder blade... Nothing I can do anything about on the weekend.

Our family Thanksgiving is tomorrow and I don't want to go like this. I just want to stay in bed until I can see what the doctors are going to tell me about it...this time.

The other thing is, the D601 nurses are now part of the teacher's union and with an impending strike, they advised us to get medical stuff done and medicines before December 3, which is likely the strike date if negotiations don't improve. Then there would be about two weeks of insurance coverage before COBRA [Consolidated Omnibus Budget Reconciliation Act] would be involved if the strike lasted any length of time. Just what I need to think about, insurance issues.

The good news is that when I wear makeup and big earrings no one calls me "sir."

Really feel like I am hanging on by a thread here.

FB: November 17, 2012

This Irish proverb happened to come up today on the twenty-seventh birthday of my firstborn son. I held him for five months before having the strength to place him for adoption so he could have a better life, one that would be better with two adult parents and not a seventeen-year-old girl. I still think about you Joseph Mason (aka, Steven Douglas, not named after the politician). [In hopes that I would someday see my oldest child again, I taught my children that their older brother's name was Joey, so they learned the name his adoptive parents gave him instead of his birth-name, which was after my brothers.] I hope someday we will meet again but more importantly I hope you are healthy and happy.

"Mothers hold their children's hands for just a little while and their hearts forever." —Author Unknown

EM: November 18, 2012

From: Alan

To: Marcy

You've got family, friends and life. They'll clean it up surgically. It will heal. And the good times will roll. You'll see.

From: Marcy

To: Alan

Yes, thank you. Just anxious to get it done. I know it will all work out just not on my timeline I guess. How are you, Sophie, and the dogs? Very, very concerned about the Bears game tonight. Wear your hat and do whatever else you can. The Packers won yesterday so we really need this to stay on top. Let's worry about what really matters!

From: Alan

To: Marcy

Go Bears!

CB: November 19, 2012

No More Sclerosing, Time for Surgery

I saw my primary care doctor today. With the fluid leaking and some buildup and the red skin, she thinks no more radiation and I should get surgery to fix this. She is extending the antibiotics as well until this is resolved. So far I have had seventeen days of IV Vancomycin and eight days of Levaquin. If I go off them before the problem is fixed and that fluid becomes infected, I could end up really sick again. The skin integrity is not good enough for radiation. I called the radiation oncologist and he is in agreement (I'm glad, I really don't want to be a difficult patient). The hope was the sclerotherapy would hold off the fluid long enough to get the radiation completed. After about thirty-four hours, it built up so much it leaked everywhere.

This happened while I was at Riley's musical, the only thing I could do was wear the big fleece sweater over it to hide the wetness.

I see the surgeon tomorrow. I guess she had already discussed this with my primary care doctor on Thursday, telling her that if the sclerotherapy didn't work that surgery would need to be done and radiation should be on hold. I don't really know any details on the surgery, outpatient vs. inpatient, skin graft or not, what exactly she will do and if she will fix the other side that has a clump of tissue that might have gotten in the way of good-fitting prosthetics. Will she fix that while I am in surgery so I don't have to go back in again? I can't help but think if I had any reconstruction surgery what a mess this would be. Knowing what kinds of complications can occur I am very comfortable with my decision not to have reconstruction. With this being Thanksgiving week, I don't know when surgery will be scheduled. Maybe next Monday? Would have been good to get it done this week, while I was off work but the timing on all of this just hasn't worked out. I just want to get it done and heal before my mom's total hip replacement that is scheduled for December 3. I still want to try to take Riley on vacation to California during winter break... We deserve a vacation, right? I will let you know what the surgeon says tomorrow and when surgery is scheduled.

EM: November 19, 2012

To: Marcy

From: Alan

Hey Marcy,

Just a thought on the surgery and something to ask the surgeon about: the merits of a skin graft versus leaving it somewhat open to close as it heals.

Skin grafts can be fragile and need delicate care. You're a smart lady and an RN [registered nurse] so that shouldn't be a problem.

There's a process of wound healing known as "second intention." Google it. It's when an infected area is left open so healthy tissue can replace the infected stuff. I'm sure you could manage that too.

On another subject: going to my dad's tonight for the game. The Bears hat is being prepped and warming up.

Go Bears! and *go Marcy!* I've got faith in one of you and it ain't the Bears.

From: Marcy

To: Alan

My question is, if the infection is cleared and it is just the pockets or seroma [sack of clear fluid], is secondary intention needed? Which will heal faster, which will allow me to go back to work sooner, which will allow radiation sooner? Will skin grafts hold up to radiation? Lots to consider I guess. I hope it is outpatient, really don't want to stay in the hospital again.

I am hopeful yet worried at the same time about my boys, Da Bears, in San Fran tonight.

From: Alan

To: Marcy

My guess is the infection is long gone but the pocket/capsule and the fluid will be a setup for a recurring infection. Primary closure with or without a graft would be ideal and you'd of course take really good care of the site. I hear the Jell-O at Good Samuel is really good but it should be a twenty-three-hour stay at most I would guess.

My suggestion, turn off the TV, take a deep breath, clear your mind, and get some rest.

From: Marcy

To: Alan

I left my brother's house after third quarter, couldn't take it anymore... Da Bears looked awful. Felt like after your email I had a good excuse to not watch the last tortuous quarter, "Doctor's orders."

I will take good care of the site no matter what she does. Probably could have taken better care of myself before but couldn't prevent the capsules from forming I guess. I do so much better at taking care of other people but I will try to put my A+ personality on my self-care now.

Wednesday I have a shopping date with my sister-in-law, Patti. I don't usually like shopping but we are going to Bass Pro Shop, they have "Browning" bedding in pink and brown reversible fabric on sale. We are also going to the outlet mall.

Talk to you later.

From: Alan

To: Marcy

Speaking of pink and brown Browning items you just might get something from Santa in the mail in the next day or two.

I'm sure you'll take excellent care of the site, which is definitely an advantage you have.

One of the docs I work with is Indian and he's off to India for December, which means I work a lot for the holidays. Oh well.

Enjoy shopping!

FB: November 19, 2012

Should probably go into work tomorrow and do paperwork but I think I am going to do the annual "kidnap your student for lunch day." Don't tell Riley. He has acted all tough with my recent setbacks but he struggled while I was in the hospital this last time, I can tell by the number of missing assignments. He seems to be back on track now, but it made his grades go down.

Marcy: Left a message with the attendance office to have Riley ready at 10:55 a.m. for pick up, he has an appointment but would be returning to school after the appointment. Well, I didn't lie, he does have an appointment, for lunch, with his Mom, he just doesn't know it yet. I remember one time a grade school classmate went out to lunch with her mom, they took me with them...we went to a hot dog place in town. I thought that was so cool! Even during my single parent years, I have always taken them from school for lunch once a year. When they were in grade school I would bring back dessert for the teacher.

FP: Can you call me out of work?

CB: November 20, 2012

Frustrated

Don't even really want to talk about the frustrating doctor appointment that I waited all day for. I don't know any more about the type of surgery, recovery time, when it will be, etc., than I did before the appointment because my surgeon isn't going to do it. She referred me to a plastic surgeon. Hopefully after a phone call from my surgeon, he will be able to fit me in sooner than later, as it was I couldn't get in to see him until Nov. 28. It really isn't long for a specialist, *unless you are leaking or accumulating fluid and on antibiotics until this is corrected.* I need to get this done for so many reasons. I realize he has other patients and is busy but I really don't want to end up in the hospital again, or delay getting the rest of the cancer treatment or end up getting surgery and being in the hospital the same time my mom has her hip replacement. There is so much going on. I spent a lot of time crying on the phone tonight.

You all have been amazing through this entire ordeal. Looking forward to better times.

I'll update when I have more details, unless I am in the psych ward by that time.

Lucy: I'm so sorry for the disappointing visit. Remember, it is all in His time, not ours—hate to say that to you, but I'm always saying it to myself. Take a deep breath and one day at a time or hour at a time. It will all work out. Oh and yes, it is definitely understandable to cry and be totally disappointed. I'll pray harder for you and no psych ward please—don't think you could take that! I'm thankful you are in my life and wish I could do more for you—just don't know what to do besides pray.

I was definitely getting to the point in cancer treatment and complications when I had to use all my "lifelines." My friends and family weren't the only ones feeling trepidatious about the complications and delay in finishing the treatment, although they expressed it rarely. They wanted to stay strong to hold me up as much as I wanted to stay positive so they didn't lose hope. Although I was keeping people updated via Facebook and CaringBridge, I was slowly crumbling and I believe now there were a few people who could see that. While I was in the hospital I was mostly quiet and withdrawn or agitated. I became less withdrawn when I was able to get back to work and on some type of schedule, but the frequent fluid accumulation, procedures, and delays were becoming heavier on my shoulders. I wasn't sure if I wanted to stand up and fight at that point or lay down and wave the white flag. I spoke with Hannah in Arizona, Miriam in Florida, Laurie, Liza, and Alan frequently. I went to counseling to try to process some of these thoughts and feelings. I cried a lot but also called people to hear about their lives, which helped me take the focus off how despondent I felt.

EM: November 21, 2012

From: Marcy

To: Alan

Hey Alan:

Got the Browning shirt, awesome! It was in the mail when I got home from buying supplies to make you (and Sophie—if you share) something. It will keep me occupied for a little while and that may help my mood a bit.

Still waiting to see if they will fit me in today. He is in surgery Fridays so if he can't see me this afternoon, it will still be sometime next week. I am ready to jump in the car and go to Elk Grove right now if they call.

Talk to you soon.

From: Alan

To: Marcy

I really hope you can be seen today. I wish there was more I could do.

I can't imagine all you're going through with the wound, your mom, your kids, your job and the holidays. You're being a lot tougher than you realize. It has to get better at some point right? You gotta keep battling. I figure a small gift might bring a smile for a few minutes.

I'm off to work shortly. I think we'll be busy tonight.

I know that life keeps asking more and more from you. You'll find the strength and the toughness to persevere. Imagine the joy when you cross the finish line.

From: Marcy

To: Alan

I liked the surgeon, Dr. Lovejoy, and he will do surgery at Community Outpatient at 4 p.m. next Tuesday! No skin graft. Will update online journal later but I am encouraged by what he said! I hope you aren't too busy tonight.

From: Alan

To: Marcy

I am so relieved for you. Better days are coming.

It's busy and some people are drunk. Good times. Happy Thanksgiving.

From: Marcy

To: Alan

Vegas story: We were there a brief time to see shows with the kids, Riley saw *The Lion King* and Dani saw a comedian. It was early in the morning and when Riley and I went for breakfast, there were some people in the elevator very drunk but Riley's comment was, "Mom, I think they are a little under-sober." I really didn't enjoy taking care of drunk people when I worked at the immediate care center. I worked 10 p.m. to 6 a.m. so I got more than my share. Usually it was an injury that was stupid and I had to be professional and not say to them what I say to Riley: "Stupid should hurt."

Hang in there,

Marcy

P.S. I am excited to start on my project for you, Dani even offered to help me, but I want to do it myself.

Reflections

This period of time clearly had to be one of the most discouraging. We (the medical team and I) had a plan to treat the cancer. It was supposed to be done by now. I had planned a road trip with Riley and put deposits down on lodging at the Grand Canyon. We talked to friends about visiting. All of those things had to be canceled and plans changed. My mom had been putting off her hip surgery. As if it wasn't lousy enough to be sick myself, watching my mom in pain because she delayed her own care on my account was distressing.

I was trying to avoid more surgeries by not having reconstruction and yet I was relieved that the decision to have surgery was finally made so that the breast area could be debrided and healing could start. My goals and expectations had changed yet again and now I was just hoping to start the new year with the ordeal that myself, family and friends had to endure in 2012 behind us.

— 5 —

Surgery Again

Hot Mess

CB: November 21, 2012

Good News, Surgery Scheduled

Hi and Happy Thanksgiving.

I hope you get to enjoy whatever you decide to eat with people you love. The kids, my mom, Roger, and I have reservations at an upscale restaurant. We went last year, it was yummy.

The good news is that surgery is scheduled for Tuesday, November 27 at 4 p.m., at Community Hospital. I didn't want any more surgeries and wanted to minimize complications, which was why I didn't want breast reconstruction. I am ending up in surgery anyway. I am grateful Dr. Lovejoy was able to fit me in and schedule the surgery. I liked him and his staff. He said I could get it sooner if it didn't matter when or where.

About the surgery: Outpatient surgery—wooohooo! He also thinks I have plenty of skin to not need a graft. He will open the area that has the seroma, remove calcifications, and, if there are capsules that are holding fluid, he will take that out, not really sure about the details of the surgery much more than that. Honestly, for once I don't care. I just want him to fix it. I would sign an open-ended consent right now...just do what you need to do. He will also repair the left side that has too much tissue—it is like having a mini breast close to being under my arm. I didn't ask how long it will take but I don't expect it will be a long surgery. He said to give myself a few days for recovery and I will be able to go back to work December 3 (unless we are on strike). My mom's hip replacement is Dec. 3. Now I want to be on strike for one day only so I can be with her.

I liked the surgeon, not just because he said I was beautiful or because he squeezed me in for an appointment today but because I think he understood my situation, the type of breast cancer I have and my desire to get finished with breast cancer treatment. He asked "Feeling pretty beat up?" I said, "Yeah, a little bit." I am confident we tried everything we could to prevent surgery and get radiation done but now it is time to fix it permanently. I am still dripping fluid from the chest area, even with trying to keep it compressed with a breast binder. Only 6 more days of dripping.

The lymphedema is starting to come back in my hand and fingers; I will wear the Caresia glove and sleeve and try to keep it under control.

Before I end this entry I just want to express my gratitude. You all have contributed to me getting through this horrific year in one way or another. Calls, emails, cards, flowers, gifts. You have let me cry when I needed to let it out and also brought out the laughter too. This last month has been particularly rough and you guys haven't given up on me. I know I am sick of all this medical stuff. I would think you would be sick of hearing about it. Still, you all are so patient and understanding. So thankful for my friends and family and that I am still alive.

Have a happy and healthy Thanksgiving, Marcy

Hannah: Oh, Marcy. I wish you would give yourself a break and stop feeling like you are disappointing all of your fans. (That's right, you have a fan club.) You have been through so much physically and emotionally in just the last six months. You are doing so well fighting the cancer demon. It puts up a big fight to make the triumph that much sweeter.

I am so appreciative of the updates you give as you are always on my mind. Some good advice I rarely follow: Stop worrying so much about everything you can't control. Worrying doesn't help the situation, it just makes you miserable.

Love you much!

Grace: Marcy, you are an amazing person. Thank you for being just who you are. I am so thankful that God brought you into my life. I wish you and your family a wonderful thanksgiving. Have a great time at Jameson's. You are in my thoughts and prayers.

Dad: Good. I am happy you finally caught a break. Enjoy your dinner out. God bless you.

Lola: I was hoping that you'd get at least one overnight stay. I wanted to clean your house and finish the windows without you telling me to stop doing stuff.

CB: November 22, 2012

Growing It Back...

The hair is coming in enough that with some mousse it looks almost like I wanted it that short. I'm still waiting for the eyelashes and eyebrows to come back in more, but at least I have some.

FB: November 24, 2012

Dani said, "You are like a form of entertainment when you go from being okay to having a hot flash." Nice kid, huh? Then she asks, "How often do you post about Riley and I," and I said, "All the time, that is why I can't be friends with you guys on social media." "Oh," she says, "I didn't mean that in a baaaaad way."

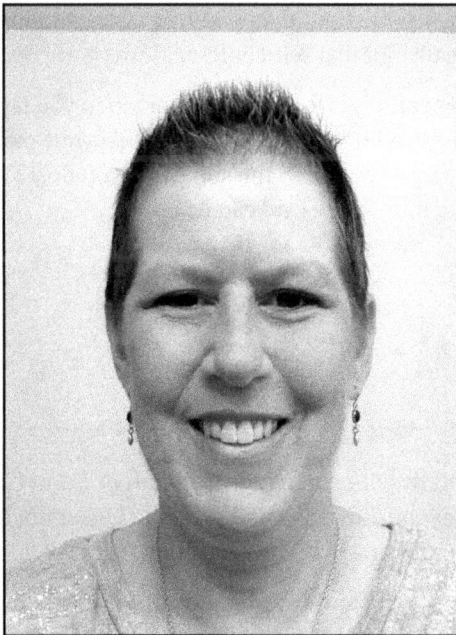

Figure 5-1. My hair growing back

EM: November 24, 2012

From: Alan

To: Marcy

Yesterday we saw a bunch of people from out of town and a bunch of college kids home with coughs. It was really busy.

It's sweet that you're working on something for me. It makes me smile. It's OK if it doesn't work out. It's truly the thought that counts.

Unfortunately, things are not going well for me. My back pain has become intolerable. I will likely stop working soon. I can't do much at all this holiday season. I'm fairly depressed.

Hope you have a nice weekend. Hope things go well on Tuesday.

Be good.

From: Marcy

To: Alan

Hi,

I was going to ask you about that, you had not mentioned your back or therapy. I am really not that self-centered, I was going to ask.

So, stop working entirely? Does it feel better when you lay down? Do any medications help? With the way you described your pain before I have always been amazed you put in the shifts that you do, I know how physically demanding immediate care can be.

Tell me more...

From: Alan

To: Marcy

Good evening,

I don't think you're self-centered at all. Truth is, I don't like to share my troubles with anyone. I'm supposed to be the healer not the patient. And it's kind of embarrassing that I can't help myself.

Sophie keeps me going and your remarkable strength has been a source of strength for me.

I work tomorrow and I'm gonna have to take a lot of Aleve and Tylenol even though it won't help. I have some old Vicodin at home but I won't take it at work.

Thursday I'm getting an injection in the hip joint. Then I'm gonna go back to the ortho guy and maybe a pain specialist. I'd do whatever it takes to even make this tolerable.

I'm bringing the hat to work tomorrow. It probably violates the dress code but I don't care.

Have a pleasant evening.

From: Marcy

To: Alan

Hey there tough guy,

I can't go "all doctor on you" but I can go "all friend on you." One thing that has helped me is when others let me help them, it helps take my mind off my situation for a while. My friend in Arizona calls and we talk about some of what is going on with her and her family and for a moment I feel like I am helping and have purpose. Who are you to deprive me of that purpose and suffer in silence, not allowing me to be there for you? I was going to ask how things were with you and Sophie, even though it is none of my business. I know chronic medical problems can be hard on a marriage. I am glad she is there for you. If you need to vent to someone other than Sophie sometime, I am here for you.

The injection doesn't sound fun but I know what it is like to feel so desperate you will try anything. I pray it works to give you relief and the pain specialist has some ideas. I'm curious, do you have/use a TENS [transcutaneous electrical nerve stimulater] unit? I have one, it isn't a cure but has helped at times when my hip joint flared up and I had the buttock pain. The electrical stimulation really made my muscles relax.

Screw the dress code. We need this win!

The lymphedema is back, quite quickly and my fingers were going numb and tingly. So I try to wear the Caresia when I can, it is just really hot and annoying. Such a noncompliant kid I am sometimes. I did get Riley back into knitting with a loom though and he is working on making a scarf for himself. I like that he is doing something involving creating and not destroying.

Dani has been coming in my room almost every day and laying down with me for a while, we talk and laugh and it means so much to me. Wish I got a bigger bed a long time ago, the moments with her have been priceless. I make her laugh and she says how much she loves me and we giggle and tell stories and reminisce. I am in bed a lot lately; going off the Mobic [the only anti-inflammatory medication that helps my arthritis] makes a big difference in my back and knees and the stairs in my house suck. Didn't realize how much the Mobic helped until the times I had to go off of it for surgery. Next time I move it will be to a one-level home so I don't have to deal with the stairs.

Keep it real. I would never think less of you for having pain or having a hard time with it. Even caregivers need care, as I learned the hard way this year.

Your friend, Marcy

From: Alan

To: Marcy

It does help to talk to friends. It's just a little hard on the pride. I have a TENS unit. I use it at night. I should probably use it more often. Sophie has been supportive about the chronic pain but I feel like I can't be the husband I want to be, which is hard on a relationship. I always wonder when she'll have had enough.

Several people just registered at immediate care. Hopefully it will be quiet during the game.

Enjoy your Sunday!

EM: November 25, 2012

From: Alan

To: Marcy

Screw the dress code!

From: Marcy

To: Alan

Gonna take a shower soon and put my game face on, along with my Bears pajama pants, Bears socks, Bears hat, Bears shirt, and Bears sweatshirt.

Then going to watch the game with my sister-in-law. I hope your shift goes fast. Maybe it will be kind of slow, people lying around tired after a long weekend?

From: Marcy

To: Alan

A friend sells natural cosmetics, nutritional supplements, and such. She is suggesting their "hormone balancing cream"; it has progesterone, any thoughts?

From: Alan

To: Marcy

Well, progesterone isn't supposed to effect breast cancer cells and it's said to be good for the skin. But you never really know the nature of the hormones in these products (if they contain any form of an estrogen).

My feeling is, why take a chance.

I'm a big fan of Aquaphor and the udder creams [heavy-duty moisturizers]. I use an udder cream every night on my hands.

When all this is over and your nutrition is back to normal your skin will get better. You'll see.

From: Marcy

To: Alan

She was claiming a positive effect on hot flashes. I like Aquaphor for skin too.

From: Alan

To: Marcy

Well, if it's good for hot flashes it might contain estrogen. I'd be wary.

Hot flashes must suck. Sorry. Have a good evening.

From: Marcy

To: Alan

You were right, I looked up the ingredients and they contain a lot of phytoestrogens, then I found an article on phytoestrogens, *not* a good idea for me.

I finished the project today! Will try to get it in the mail tomorrow, didn't put a note in the box. It is big enough to share and I made it the way I did so that you can enjoy it more months out of the year...

Take care

FB: November 26, 2012

Dani asked if I was nervous about surgery tomorrow. Not nervous about the surgery itself just very anxious to get it done. This complication has been holding me back since October 22nd. Thank you friends and family for all your prayers and words of encouragement. This really should be

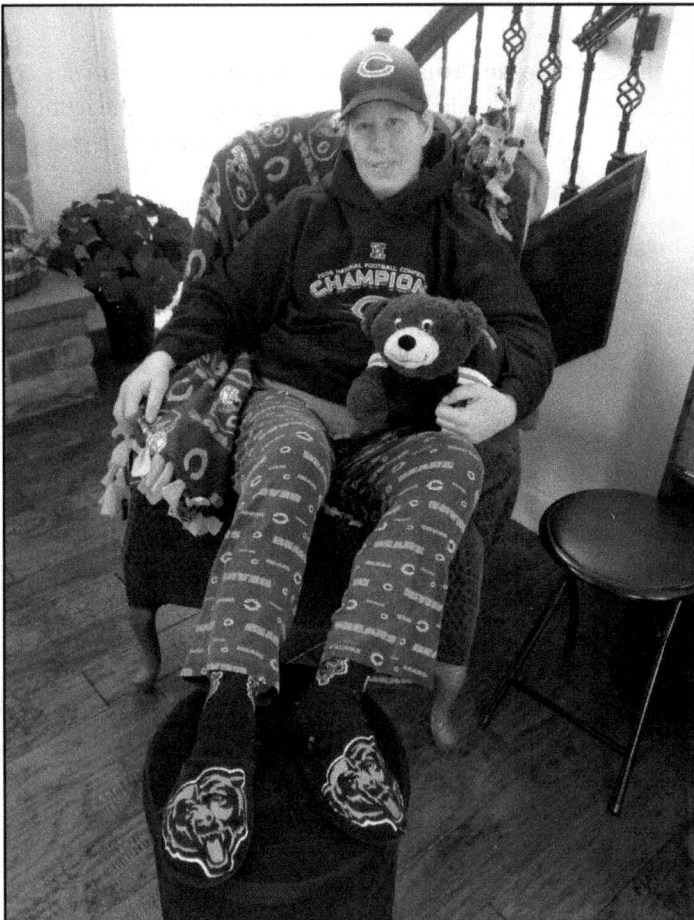

Figure 5-2. My Bears attire

a piece of cake compared to some of the other surgeries I have had, just want to get it all done and put this medical stuff behind me for 2012 so I can bring in the new year healthy.

There is a proverb that says, "It takes a village to raise a child." I think it takes a village to take care of a cancer patient. My surgery was scheduled for the end of the day. Patti was going to take me for the outpatient surgery as the hospital that I was going to was close to her hair salon and she could take me after work. Since I couldn't drive my car, I asked Harrison to drive me to Patti's salon. It was nice to have that alone time with him to just catch up and make small talk.

I started that hospital experience with being misgendered by the volunteer, who immediately apologized and escorted us to the pre-op area. Truth be told, at this point being called "sir" was taking its toll. Not wearing makeup and jewelry made a difference in people seeing me as a female. This whole hospital experience and surgery wasn't the piece of cake I thought it would be.

EM: November 27, 2012

From: Alan

To: Marcy

The blanket is truly awesome! I love it.

It looks like a lot of work. That couldn't have been easy.

I'm guessing you'll be home from the hospital soon. I really hope it went well.

Better days are coming.

Hope you get some rest tonight.

Thank you again

From: Marcy

To: Alan

You got it already? They are super easy to make. I'm drugged and waiting for a wheelchair to go home.

From: Alan

To: Marcy

No stopping for drinks on the way home. Good night.

To: Alan

From: Marcy

I'm taking my drink in the form of Percocet, this wasn't what I expected at all. Will update later. Going to bed now, really. Think about you a lot and wish I could do something to help you.

Good night

FB: November 28, 2012

Dani sent me a quote from Teenager Post #928: "The worst sight in the world is seeing your mother cry." I responded, "That made me want to cry." She pleaded, "Nooooo, don't cry."

CB: November 28, 2012

Surgery Was Not as Expected

On a 1–10 pain scale after surgery, I said it was a 5–6 but I don't think the post-op nurse believed me, as slow tears were making their way down my cheek and dripping into my ears. I would have wiped them away but I didn't want to move my arms causing more pain in my chest. In what must have been a barely audible voice I said, "I am surprised this is more painful than the original mastectomies." She gave me more medicine.

I never saw the surgeon after it was over because he went into another surgery. He talked to my sister-in-law, Patti. I will try to repeat what she relayed to me. If I get it wrong and correct myself later, please forgive me, it could be the anesthesia/medication making me foggy or just emotion itself. He said I looked "pretty ripped up in there." There were several "capsules he needed to remove" and I think he was (we were) expecting one, maybe two that were connected. He told Patti that he took more than he expected he would have to (not sure what that means), but that it is all cleaned out now. I do have another drain...this time a lot of bright red blood. I guess blood is good in a way, dead tissue doesn't bleed but healthy tissue does. I don't know how long I will have the drain in. He also said it will feel tight. He didn't do a skin graft but I think he really pulled it together tight with the remaining tissue after he cut away all the damaged stuff. He will see me in his office on Thursday and then I will get more details on exactly what he did.

You know how patient I am waiting for test results, especially pathology? Well, here we go again.

I usually go to Good Samuel Hospital and missed the people there, but I have only nice things to say about the staff at Community Hospital. It wasn't their fault that it took four tries to get the IV started. The anesthesiologist even took two stabs at it and they usually get it the first time. After my experience in the hospital in October, I was worried that would happen. I guess my veins are sick of this cancer treatment just like the rest of me. The anesthesiologist was great about listening to my past experiences and because she listened to me I haven't had any issues with lightheadedness or low blood pressure. She gave me a fluid bolus and monitored my BP closely. She listened to my history of GERD [gastroesophageal reflux disease] and all the esophagus problems I had during chemo and premedicated me to prevent issues. Not sure why she gave me steroids before surgery (come to think of it, that could be why I am not asleep right now). The nurse said it was because I had them with chemo but that was four months ago. I didn't object though; since I had to go off my anti-inflammatory medication due to blood thinning effects, my arthritis has been bothering me. Steroids usually make the arthritis pain feel better. Any physician friends or nurse friends who know why she would give them to me for surgery because I have had them in the last six months please feel free to educate me on that one.

I thought this was going to be a piece of cake and I would just be taking Tylenol at home but he wrote me a prescription for Percocet (never have used that before). Very grateful he did that. I took two of them at 9 p.m. and although the pain is lessened, it is too painful to sleep right now. I can type and do small movements in my arms but even reaching to my night stand hurts. The left side hurts more than I expected. I thought that would be a simple thing, just cut off they extra tissue to make that side flatter so that prosthetics fit better and so I don't have the clump of tissue off to the side. Really surprised that it hurts as much as it does and of course the right side is worse.

I am glad I am at home in my own bed and will try again to get some sleep now but not before saying thank you again to Harrison for driving me to meet Patti at work so she could take me to the hospital. I love you and Grace so much and have been so blessed to know you and have you in my life consistently since I was a teenager. Patti, what can I say to you? I can never repay you for all you have done for my family and me, but I will try. I really want to be more like you. I respect and admire you.

Tomorrow if I feel good enough I will lay on Patti's couch instead of my bed. My entertainment will be listening to my sisters and Dani in the kitchen baking cookies. I'll let you know what the doctor says after Thursday's visit. If you have any questions you think I should get answered feel free to let me know. I will write them down. I hate going into a visit and then leaving and thinking I wish I would have asked him this or that. I have been better about making lists when I need to. Still have the goal of healing from this soon enough to get my last three radiation treatments and still be able to take Riley to see our wonderful friends in California over winter break. Thank you for the prayers, well wishes, texts, guestbook comments and for being there for my family and me. I couldn't have made it this far without all the love and support from you all. Love, Marcy

FB: November 28, 2012

A most excellent day with my sisters and Dani, making cookies and watching movies. Well, they made cookies, I did nothing today, except laugh, which hurt quite a bit but was worth the pain. Although at one point I thought I could bust my incisions open. They were silly enough to give me the job of unwrapping chocolate for the top of the peanut butter cookies... "Suuuuuurrrre, I can do that. Unwrap one for the cookies, unwrap one for me and so on."

EM: November 28, 2012

From: Alan

To: Marcy

In no particular order.

You were likely given a "stress dose" of cortisones (steroids). Surgery is a "stress" on the cardiovascular system. During surgery and couple days after the adrenal glands produce extra cortisol that helps maintain the vascular system and the cardiac pump.

At this point, four months after chemo, your adrenal glands are *probably* functioning fine and you're right, you may not have needed the bolus dose. That said, there is no harm in a single bolus dose unless you have bad diabetes, which you don't. In the long run vitamin D is a good idea and a bone density scan down the road. To an anesthesiologist, "cancer patient" + surgery = stress-dose cortisone, which is very reasonable. The benefits clearly favor giving them.

Over the years I've pulled some sebaceous cysts [sacs of fluid from the sebaceous glands] out of the backs of old men. They always come out with one large capsule and one or two adjacent capsules. Often times they look like the Mickey Mouse head silhouette. The skin is rather thick and complex. The epithelial layer is the one that "sheds" but the deeper dermal layer is fibrous and doesn't change much over the years—it's where tattoos are placed so they remain forever. These epidermis, stratum corneum and dermis should always remain opposed to each other with no space between. When a cleavage layer forms (as the result of surgery or infection) a capsule or two forms between the layers and becomes a problem (as you know). Now you're all good with the capsules out.

The skin can be stretched very tight and will loosen to an appropriate tension over a few weeks. Children who get plastic surgery for skin defects sometimes have "skin expanders" placed and they are tolerated very well. You don't need a skin expander—the message is your skin will adjust and won't remain tight.

Take the pain meds for a few days. My doc says you don't get any points for suffering.

Hope the healing begins today.

From: Marcy

To: Alan

Awesome explanations, thanks for taking the time to do that. I had no problems with her giving me the steroids because I knew it would help the pain in my back and knees and it did. I just wanted to understand why. Thank you.

I figured the skin will stretch, it is just really tight right now. I know they use expanders before reconstruction and then replace them with the implants. Still have no interest in reconstruction. Percocet does make me feel a little zoned. In a way, a little pain is good because it is a reminder of what not to do; pouring coffee was too much this morning, too heavy on the right side, I could feel it. I was low on vitamin D a few years ago when I was tested so I take calcium and D. Had a DEXA [to measure bone density] years ago but will get another one at some point. It's a lower priority. I have a colonoscopy scheduled in December, moved it from November because of the hospital stay and complications. Yay me, love those things—*not*. I do want to start 2013 healthy!

I am going to take the meds today and let my sisters entertain me.

Will also be thinking about your injection tomorrow and praying for relief for you.

Keep me posted, OK?

From: Marcy

To: Alan

Hi, I just wanted you to know I was thinking about you today and hoping your injection will provide you with some relief. When you are up for it, let me know how you are doing.

From: Alan

To: Marcy

Thank you. As fate would have it I also have a cold but I'm staying warm under my Bears/Sox blanket. How's your arm? Less painful I hope. When does the drain come out?

Talk to you later.

From: Marcy

To: Alan

Hey, the drain comes out when there is less than 25 cc in a twenty-four-hour period of time. I am to call them on Monday and give them an update. There was 25 cc in the past twelve hours. There was 75 cc in the twenty-four hours before that. It is slowing down some.

The surgeon was concerned about the size and thickness of the capsule. Then I reminded him of the sclerotherapy and he said he felt better, that could be part of why it looked the way it did. I told him I was glad I could make him feel better. We are both anxiously waiting for the pathology. He said he would call as soon as he had the report.

Apparently the capsule went from the center of my chest up into the armpit. He said it was a challenging surgery and he did a lot of debridement [removal of damaged, infected, and dead tissue]. He also said he was very aggressive with getting to healthy tissue and that is why he prescribed 50 Percocet, because it may take a while to feel better. He had to work around the major artery in my axilla [armpit] and the veins to get the capsule out. Honestly, it hurts, I can't lift my arm to get to the second shelf in the cabinet and a full pot of coffee is too heavy. The left side is much better. In my case I think a little pain is good, it will prevent me from doing things I am not supposed to. I won't be able to drive for a while and I won't be able to go back to work for a while. This was more extensive than the original mastectomy. I would be interested in getting the operative report when it is ready.

Dani is going to do the grocery shopping tomorrow and I am going to ask my sister to drive Riley and me to his dermatology appointment on Saturday. I am at the point when I can acknowledge I need help and accept when it is offered. That is huge for me.

Yesterday my sisters and Dani and I hung out. They made cookies and we watched a couple movies. Even with all the pain it was a great day. The pain that the laughter caused was worth it. It was good for all of us. Take care.

From: Alan

To: Marcy

I'm glad the drainage is slowing. From what I understand we need our blood to stay in our blood vessels.

To be honest, I wondered why they didn't do surgery when you were in the hospital, but I guess they did a step-wise thing (taking the treatment plan in steps, less aggressive steps first and more aggressive steps only if the initial steps weren't effective).

Hopefully every day it's a little bit better. Spending all your time waiting for a better day gets old, but I do think it's not far off now.

I understand your anxiety over the pathology. It's rough. I still think this abscess was a surgical issue, not a cancer issue. I'm hoping and praying with you.

Acknowledging the need for help is a skill I need to learn. I'm working on it.

The injection went well today. The whole thing took 10 minutes. But now I have a full-blown cold. A very adorable 4-year-old girl coughed in my face last Sunday—my fault. I know better. I'm gonna watch a little Thursday night football and go to sleep.

Have a good evening.

Be good.

From: Marcy

To: Alan

You're right, I know you're right about the pathology.

Most four-year-olds don't know how to share, apparently that one did.

Sweet Dreams

Text: November 29, 2012

Dani: I think I might start working out after class on Tuesday and Thursdays.

Marcy: That would be awesome. I can't wait to start working out again. I'm gonna be smokin' hot by my forty-fifth birthday.

Dani: You're already smokin' hot.

Marcy: Yea, from menopause.

Dani: LOL I love you.

FB: November 29, 2012

Posted on my wall

Miriam: Hope you are feeling better soon!

Marcy: You're the best. Today wasn't that great but thankfully I have a comfy bed and I was in it all day.

Miriam: Aww, Did Dani crawl in with you and keep you company? You should tell her some funny stories about when you were a kid.

Marcy: She has been doing that a lot lately, the past two nights though I have had to have her get in slow and be careful not to bump me. We usually watch funny stuff online or tell stories.

Percocet doesn't take the pain away completely but I guess a little pain reminds me about the surgery and keeps me from doing the things I am not supposed to do. It does make me a little lightheaded though, good night everyone.

Lola: What do you possibly need to do besides wash yourself and brush your teeth??!! Healing takes time stop rushing things.

Marcy: LOL you know me well! Actually though, I'm *not* doing a thing. I promise, been in bed all day. Riley got my ice water for me and Dani is doing the shopping for me. Relax I'm behaving!

CB: November 30, 2012

Stagecoach

Happy Friday to you all. Sorry I didn't get the follow-up visit information posted yesterday; I felt fairly lightheaded (still do) but I try not to let the Percocet wear off too much or the pain on the right gets bad. As a very intelligent friend told me, "You don't get any points for suffering."

Haven't had my blood count done since I was in the hospital and with the blood from the drainage tube…I wonder what those counts would be. Maybe best for me not to know right now. The drainage has to be less than 25 ml in a twenty-four-hour period of time in order for it to come out. He said maybe a week or two. But I think I may be ahead of schedule, the first twenty-four hours I was home it was 75 ml and thicker red blood, the next twenty-four hours it was 50 ml and thinner, lighter blood. That is decent improvement! That same friend from earlier also said, "From what I understand we need our blood to stay in our blood vessels." That totally cracked me up. It hurts to laugh but so worth it!

My niece, Clara, introduced me to this quote: "There is certain relief in change, even though it be from bad to worse! As I have often found in traveling in a stagecoach, that it is often a comfort to shift one's position, and be bruised in a new place." From *Tales of a Traveler* by Washington Irving. This is how I feel when I roll from my left side to my right side. My biggest "bruise" was this seroma that I had been dealing with since the end of October. Surgery is not my favorite option but after more than a month of antibiotics and three sclerotherapy procedures with minimal positive results, it was overdue by the time it was done. I went from the presurgical seroma "bruise" to the postsurgical pain "bruise." The way I am looking at it is: The stagecoach, although bumpy and causing bruises, is getting me where I need to go...to a place where I am cancer free again... Stagecoaches move fairly slow though!

Now for the follow-up appointment information: When Dr. Lovejoy came in, I told him I needed more details on the surgery and what he found because whatever he told Patti, my sister-in-law, seemed to make her worry, to the point she didn't tell me all of it until the next morning.

He said it was a challenging surgery and more extensive than he thought it would be. There was only one capsule (correction from previous post) but it extended from the middle of my chest up into my armpit. To release it from my muscles he had to score the muscles and scrape a lot, he had to work carefully around the major artery in the armpit and the veins in there. He took a lot of tissue out to get to healthy tissue and that is why the drain that I didn't expect is there. He said he was concerned about the way the capsule looked: it was very thick and he made a gesture with his fingers to indicate between a half inch and an inch in thickness. He sent it all to pathology, maybe even a few more lymph nodes with it, not sure on that. I asked him if he was suspicious if those changes were from the cancer, and he said he is always suspicious and that is why he was aggressive with the surgery. We discussed the definition of the inflamma-tory breast cancer and how it can cause tissue thickening and lymphatic vessel damage, which can cause the fluid, *but* he reminded me the cytology from the fluid in the hospital was negative for cancer cells and I reminded him that I had sclerotherapy three times. He instantly looked at ease and said he felt so much better about the way the capsule looked because sclerotherapy can cause the scarring and tissue damage that he saw. I was so glad we could spend the time to discuss it and to make each other feel more at ease. He said he was still anxiously waiting for the pathology results and so am I. He would call me when he got them. Most likely on Monday. I told him I wasn't good at waiting for those...he isn't either. We laughed a little about nurses as patients (I think I have improved a lot) and by the time I left his office I was more at ease. The incisions are healing well. I am very happy not to have the clump of tissue on the left side. He did a beautiful job. On the right...the skin looks better, the incision is good but when I put my hands on my hips and look at myself in the mirror now...it is the first time I really notice a chunk of me is gone. Before I was flat, now I have a big divot... Damn stagecoach!

As far as recovery goes... I think it is going to be slow. It is difficult to lift my arm beyond a certain point. I can't drive on Percocet and I won't drive until I have better arm mobility. I think cancer has brought me down enough now that I am at the point I will acknowledge I need help and can sometimes ask for and accept it. That is big for me, especially now that my mom will be in the hospital and rehab for the next few weeks recovering from her hip replacement that is scheduled for Monday.

Although this totally stinks, I am happy to have had the surgery and know that it is fixed. After some healing I can resume the last three radiation treatments and go on Tamoxifen the day after radiation is done. I want all this to be done by Christmas. I do have an appointment to see Dr. Jacoby on Dec. 7, not for radiation but to check in on how I am healing and when to restart radiation. I miss them at the office, they are so kind.

Have a good weekend,

Love, Marcy

P.S. I am sure the pathology will be fine but a few extra prayers, good vibes, happy thoughts, or whatever you all have been doing to get me through this wouldn't hurt. Thanks

FB: November 30, 2012

Comment on an anticancer meme I posted

Jade: I know this is incredibly difficult and that is putting it mildly. I want you to know you are in my thoughts and prayers daily. In March it will be twenty years for me. I want you to be able to say that to someone else one day. You can do this. I know you and you have what it takes, you are tough. I remember I used a lot of visual imagery...have you tried that? I know it sounds silly but I used to sit quietly and alone in a room a visualize little soldiers marching through my blood vessels blasting all the cancer cells. You can use any image you like. I also used essential oils. When you join me we will do a walk together! Just tell me when you are ready.

Marcy: I love visual imagery. I have used Pac-Man eating the cancer cells when I got chemo and also Da Bears defensive line killing the cancer so we could get the offense on the field and I can run it in for a touchdown—touchdown being cancer free.

Jade: That's great. Do you have a wellness center anywhere near you?

Marcy: Yeah, in Palatine but I haven't gone to it yet.

Another day in bed. See Lola, I am capable of doing nothing except "washing myself and brushing my teeth."

Sending Dani and Riley to the grocery store with my debit card because I can't do it and yes, Lola, I am asking for help from them and they are doing it...but what could possibly go wrong with them doing the grocery shopping?

Miriam: Did you send a list or do you want to be surprised?

Marcy: There is a list but Dani said, "There are sure to be some surprises."

Miriam: She's spot on!

Marcy: I have a craving for the Beelow's Steakhouse's beef stroganoff, and carrot cake [which I hadn't had since the kids and I went there on Mother's Day]. After they put groceries away, they are going out to eat *together* and bring back food for me. Dani called it a brother-sister bonding moment. I call it a quiet house and no dishes!

Miriam: They will have fun and you can relax.

Marcy: I already got a call from her while at the grocery store to clarify the list, LOL. I was just telling her about how when I did the shopping for my grandma at the bottom of every list was "and anything else you see that you want" but I didn't have a cell phone to call and clarify the list.

Marcy: They are back, unloaded and put groceries away and are off to dinner. I am trying to work up the courage to go see what they bought.

Miriam: Take a deep breath and remember that your reaction will determine whether or not they ever help you with this again.

Lola: It's groceries...how bad could it really be? I am happy to hear that you are taking it easy and being a good girl... I was going to ask you what kind of things you like so I can prepare some meals to bring you. I can only make stuffed shells so much. I can't wait to hear what jumped on the list.

Marcy: Snack cakes and spray cheese but she also got grapefruit which wasn't on the list either.

Lola: Spray cheese? LOL love it.

I am not sure what I did to deserve the confidence other people have in me but it brings tears to my eyes that people express it and it makes me stronger because I don't want to disappoint anyone. With that said, time to go to sleep because I am getting a bit mushy.

GC: You can do this, Bad Ass—I know you can! Love you.

Marcy: See, it is comments like that, that make my pillow wet, mushy and snotty, stop already and thank you.

GC: Mush all you want. Sleep well.

PO: We know your love from friends and family will hold you up when you are weak.

Marcy: It was your comment on the tattoo photo, "I am sure you will," about dealing with the change in body shape that made me think of this status and cry a bit. Thank you for having confidence in my ability to deal with it all.

I had posted a photo that was going around Facebook of a woman with a peacock tattoo over her mastectomy scar. At that time I said I didn't really think I wanted to get a tattoo over my scars as I was afraid it would obscure any sign of the cancer returning, but I thought it was cool that she did that. I shared that it was difficult to look at myself at that time but I knew I would have to figure out a way to deal with the body changes. PO expressed her confidence in my by saying, "I am sure you will." That comment was what prompted my post. It made me cry to know my friends had confidence in me when I did not. That carried me through often.

FB: December 1, 2012

"Patience is not the ability to wait but how you act while you're waiting." By Joyce Meyer. I am not doing well at this, just want Monday or Tuesday to come and hear that the pathology was negative.

In the words of Cindy Lou Who, "I just wanted everyone to be together for Christmas."

In a family with six kids and a sixteen-year age gap from eldest to youngest, it is quite a challenge to get us all together at the holidays. The younger generations' age groups spanned even more years. You can't have a family as large as ours without some communication and scheduling issues. During my illness and treatment I had proven that I was calmer and more patient with the Browning shenanigans in smaller groups. My heart's deep desire, though, was to have the family all together. I was still wishing for the perfect family holiday reunion, even knowing it was unrealistic. If having cancer was teaching me anything, it was the value of family and friends and time spent with them. Although I had been joking about wanting foobs and a vacation for Christmas, I really cared most about time and health so I could be with my family, all of them.

FB: December 2, 2012

Big day tomorrow. Mom's hip surgery, find out about the pathology from the surgery (and it better be ready), and also find out whether or not the teachers union goes on strike. My concern is in that order.

FB: December 3, 2012

This is the look that says, "I talked myself into being strong to be there for my mom's hip surgery, follow up and get my pathology reports, and accept whatever the union decides about a strike." It is because of all the love and strength you give me that I can smile on a day like this and be happy to be alive!

Marcy: Great news! Pathology report showed no cancer in all the stuff he took out. Mom is out of her hip replacement and all is well. Now for the 3rd issue… Still waiting to find out how the board/union negotiations are going. All in all, as long as we are healthy we can get through a possible strike.

CB: December 3, 2012

GREAT NEWS!

Pathology report just in—*no cancer* in all the stuff he took out on Tuesday! Now it's time to heal and finish radiation to be done with this!

Dr. Douglass: That's great Marcy! You're almost done. Keep up the great attitude.

Dad: Fantastic.

DA: Thank God! This news made me cry. This made my day!!!!

There was a collection of over thirty celebratory comments via Facebook and CaringBridge in what seemed like minutes after I shared this news. Feeling responsible for being the cause of loads of concern for my family and friends over the last months, I was internally doing my end-zone dance as I absorbed the cheerful words written.

FB: December 3, 2012

Post tagging me

Lola's post: I am overjoyed with the good news my friend Marcy, has received today. The prayers are working!!! I went from feeling like I just want to take all the bad away for all my friends to rejoicing the work of the Lord.

The third issue of the day didn't go as well. D601 is on strike. I am going to celebrate good health and my mom's successful surgery and pray the strike doesn't last long.

Maria: Marcy, I love your unbeatable spirit! I'm so glad for your positive news today and appreciate your support as we all head into unknown territory.

Marcy: I love you guys...such a fantastic group of people who care about others, coworkers, students, parents, and the community. I am going to have to stop reading social media trash talk about the strike though because it is probably getting my blood pressure up and I do need some rest. Hopefully I will get the drain out of my side on Thursday and will see the radiation oncologist on Friday. No one likes a strike but I wish I could be there, right next to all of you physically to show my support. Hang in there, the kids deserve smaller classes where they can get the education they need and the teachers and nurses deserve professional pay, especially after all the sacrifices they have made over the years to keep D601 running. I hope the parents can see that and more importantly

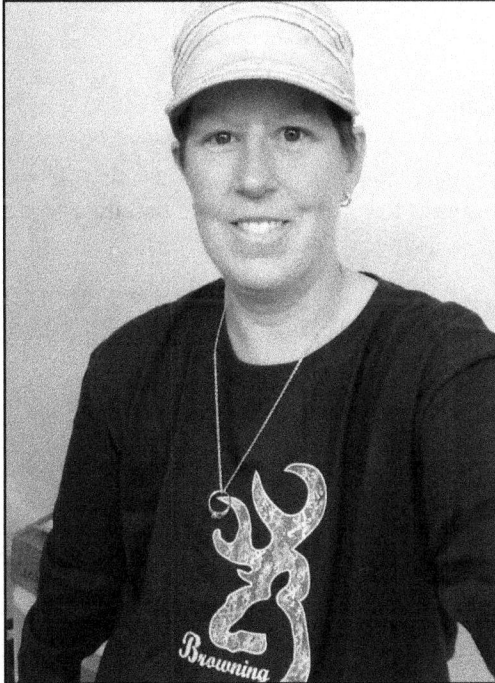

Figure 5-3. My "let's do this" face on while wearing the Browning shirt Alan sent

I hope the board sees it and the strike doesn't last long. The two days before school started all I heard on the walkie-talkie radios were teachers trying to prepare their classes...they were having to call maintenance for more desks...it went on all day long. It was a challenge to even fit enough desks into their classrooms. How can they give the kids the attention they need to help them *learn* the material with those ratios?

Maria: Get some rest...That is an order!

Marcy: In bed now, light will be off in fifteen minutes, didn't realize how tired I was until I got in bed. I am going to let myself heal this time for sure. No more complications!

FB: December 4, 2012

Overheard from Riley while he was playing a video game: "I would rather not die." I can relate, thought that way a lot this year.

Post by LEAD 601 [the teachers union that the school nurses also belong to]

We have a tentative agreement. Stay tuned.

Gaining All I Can

FB: December 5, 2012

My blood pressure is low again today. Too bad the Bears aren't playing, that always raises it a bit.

CB: December 6, 2012

Thoughts and Update

Hi there. When discussing the D601 strike, Christmas, taxes, and a bunch of other stuff, a coworker said...to paraphrase, "I don't want to make you feel bad but for months I have been telling myself when faced with tough stuff, 'At least it's not cancer.'" She said her mom used to tell her, "It's just money, you can get it back again, it isn't like they are taking an arm or a leg." Her father used to say, "Give when you don't think you can—it is the most important time to give." She made a donation in my name to Hurricane Sandy victims...makes me tear up. Her saying that doesn't make me feel bad at all. It is why I talk about my experience; it's why I write about it on this site. If going through this helps no one else how will I get through it? What meaning would it have? If it helps make your faith stronger or makes someone feel more gratitude or giving, it is worth it to share my experience, even if my experience is painful. It is my hope that sharing my experience will help someone now or down the road if they go through something similar. That is why I share and sometimes share a bit too much. It has also given me strength. You have given me strength. When she said the part about taking the arm or leg, I said, "I'm at the point where they can take that too as long as I am alive." I have given up a lot physically but still have my life and a better one for it all. I've gained much more than cancer took away.

Many people ask when I am getting my breast cancer survivor tattoo and I decided on March 29, that will be one year from the time I got the call from my doctor and heard, "You have an invasive and aggressive type of breast cancer." Many times since then, I confess, I didn't think I would make it to 03/29/13. One of those times fairly recently during the end of October. During those times I hung on to your words of hope, your calls, texts, emails, visits, and guestbook comments—it all helped. I needed every one of them to get here. I read them over and over until I started to believe what you told me, that I was strong and would survive. So those who expressed interest in going to get a tattoo, save the date.

Now a medical update: I thought I would have the drain out by now, but I still have 25-40 ml of fluid every twenty-four hours. Pain is there when I try to move my arm, shoulder, or chest like a normal person. I am becoming better at being left-handed for some things. I have physical therapy scheduled for December 13. I should have the drain out by then.

I'm scheduled to see the radiation oncologist tomorrow and wonder if they will have to make some adjustments to the radiation beam due to the new shape (divot) of my chest/underarm area. It isn't terrible, could be worse but will definitely take some getting used to and is a little hard to look at in the mirror and feel it. Many of you have already seen it but I am not sure if I should put the picture on here. Any thoughts? Are you curious? Would it bother you?

I have been pretty lightheaded and can't take my heart rate medicine because even without it my blood pressure is low. Pain medication makes it worse so I am only taking Tylenol for now. When my heart rate goes up I am also short of breath and with my blood pressure low I feel kind of weak. This morning the BP [blood pressure] cuff wouldn't read while

I was sitting up, but when I was on my back for a while it read 94/64. This makes me think when I am sitting or standing my blood pressure is even lower. I guess I will have to manage with Tylenol only and a higher heart rate to keep my BP high enough, so that I am not lightheaded. Don't really want to pass out. Before you ask, yes, I am eating and drinking what I can. Trying to stay well hydrated.

My mom is doing fabulous. Her hip replacement went well and she is walking with a cane and doing some stairs with physical therapy with a cane, she started doing that yesterday and she only had her hip replacement on Monday. They had her up with a walker a few hours after surgery was over. They are transferring her from the hospital to a rehabilitation facility right now (just got the call), so I have to go. Glad it is only five miles from here. I am so proud of her.

That is all I have for now, Take care, Marcy

I had very mixed thoughts and emotions on the appearance of my chest after the debridement surgery. I was pleased to see that the extra tissue on both sides was gone. That extra skin felt odd to me, like I was *supposed* to have something (a breast) there but didn't. I always thought that I would be okay with a flat chest. After the second surgery I was finally flat on the left side but on the right side I was now *concave*. While I felt relief that the unhealthy tissue and skin were gone, I also felt anger that if my team had done what Alan had thought and I mentioned in October and taken care of the seroma and infection, I would not have had the sclerosing procedures or the damaged tissue, and the delay in radiation would have been shorter. I would not have had the scare that the torn-up tissue that was removed was more cancer.

At times I had disassociating spells in front of the mirror that I didn't share with anyone. It was if I was in a trance looking at the shape of my chest as if my chest was not really *my* chest.

Before posting pictures of my debrided chest, I sent the pictures to Kady. With pep in her voice she said that it looked great, so much healthier. When I posted the photos not one person acknowledged the concave appearance; they all could see healthy tissue and clean incisions. I tried to take courage from that. Although I knew it was what had to happen to get back to healthy and my goal was life not appearance, I still had to move beyond the changes. Looking back this is one of the times that my physical brokenness started twisting my thoughts and emotions until I also felt broken in my heart and mind. I continued to "fake it" hoping I'd "make it"

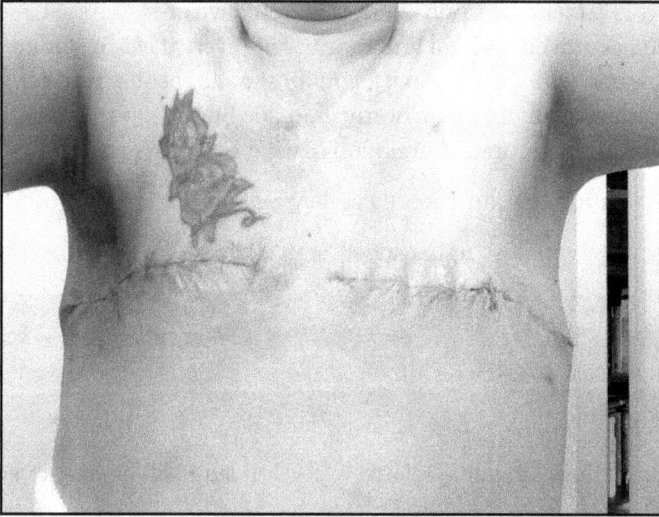

Figure 5-4. My chest after the debridement surgery

before my inconsistent thoughts and feelings on my brokenness leaked out to the point of being obvious to those around me. Maybe it was obvious and they were holding back talking to me about it as I held back sharing it with them. It was one of those times where I yearned to connect yet intentionally withdrew.

CB: December 6, 2012

Better Person

This year I have gained so much more in my life than cancer tried to take from me. Most importantly the time in person, on the phone, and in writing that I have spent with family and friends. I am a better person because of cancer (although physically I still have some treatments and recovery to do and am missing some parts, LOL).

FB: December 6, 2012

Posted on my wall

PO: Marcy, you are the bravest woman I've ever known. Sometimes I think my life is hard and then I look at you and your pictures and I think I have nothing that I can't manage to get through. Thank you for being such an inspiration for me.

Marcy: PO, I feel the same about you. You have been through a lot and all you have given and still give to your kids every day is inspiring to me. You are my hero! I really wasn't sure if I should post the pictures. I tried to describe it without being overly dramatic but wasn't sure if my words were giving an accurate description of what was going on.

PO: I am humbled and honored to be your friend.

Marcy: Now I am just embarrassed, stop it already.

EM: December 6, 2012

From: Alan

To: Marcy

I'm glad things are going relatively good. It sure will be nice to get that drain out.

I'd stop the atenolol [beta blocker prescribed for a fast heart rate but also lowers blood pressure] and stay well hydrated. Maybe add a little extra salt to your meals and extra fluids. I had an MRI and bone scan today— good times.

Gonna try to enjoy some holiday stuff this weekend. I hope you do the same.

I asked Santa for a new lumbar spine but I've been a bit naughty so I'll probably get a sweater—same as last year and the year before that.

Be good.

From: Marcy

To: Alan

Hey Alan,

I hope you get some answers from your tests and it is something they can fix.

I did stop the atenolol. I will call my primary tomorrow and let her know I will be off it for a while and will track my BP for her.

What did you do that was naughty, tell me tell me... LOL on the sweater... He could do better than that!

I will try to be good but only because Christmas is coming soon. I want my kids to get me a Chicago Bears Onesie for Christmas; they are open at the feet, which I like. I'll probably end up buying it for myself "from the kids" since neither of them have jobs right now.

CB: December 7, 2012

Moving Forward

Hi,

Today I saw Dr. Jacoby, my radiation oncologist, whom I haven't seen in a while since radiation was on hold. I am happy the chest looks healthier now but I was expressing to him that in hindsight I really wish they would have done the surgery at the end of October or early November because I could be completely done by now. He told me, "Don't look back, it's time to move forward." I instantly knew he was right and told him so. So what does moving forward look like for me? Here is the schedule so far:

Tuesday, Dec. 11: See Dr. Lovejoy's nurse practitioner and get the drain out.

Thursday, Dec. 13: Physical therapy and then rescan my chest. The contour of the chest has changed and the radiation dose has to be precise, so new scans are needed.

Monday, Dec. 17-Wednesday, Dec. 19: Radiation treatments. (hopefully the nineteenth will be my last)

The day after last radiation start Tamoxifen.

Thursday, Dec. 20: Colonoscopy for screening (colon cancer and polyp family history)

Then focus on family and holidays and celebrating being done with cancer treatment.

This is what "moving forward" through the end of the cancer treatment looks like and then in 2013 it will be "moving on" to being cancer free and becoming healthy and physically fit.

What are your plans for the holidays and new year?

Have a great weekend, Marcy

Dad: It sounds like you are finally making good progress. Good for you.

Alan: Have no fear, they're running out of places they can stick needles, catheters and scopes. They should issue merit badges like the scouts do for everything you've gone through. Your uniform would be covered. You'd be an Eagle Patient. The finish line is in sight!

Dr. Jacoby's simple words snapped me out of my funk. Simply looking me in the eyes and commanding me in an urgent tone, "Don't look back, it's time to move forward," was the coaching I needed to get back in the game I had felt like I was losing over the last couple months. It now seemed possible to come from behind and end victoriously. I think he knew there would be time to look back and process later but now was not the time. Back to survival mode.

FB: December 7, 2012

Happy Friday to those who actually get to go to work, from someone who has been on medical leave and misses her job and who also has a teenager who needs a job!

FB: December 9, 2012

I'm glad the Bears play today because my blood pressure is too low and they always fix that.

Lola: Eat something salty!

Marcy: That is the second time I have heard that. Margarita with a salt rim? My last BP was 90/68 with a pulse of 96. Can't take the beta blocker for the high pulse when the BP is low [or the BP will go lower and make me lightheaded]. Salt it is. Da Bears will get my BP up but will probably also cause palpitations!

Riley is really trying to take care of his mama. I'm up in bed on my computer and he is down in the kitchen, asking if he could bring me something to eat or drink. Either he loves me or he is trying to butter me up for spending money for our California trip.

Bailey: I'm glad to hear you're are taking it easy! Hope all is well.

BP before the Bears' game 90/68, after 118/82. Thank you Bears, my blood pressure is back up to normal. My pulse is over 100 now though.

From: Marcy

To: Alan

I usually always watch the Bears game until the end but stopped watching at the two-minute warning. [Although they were behind the whole game at least it was a little closer in the end, with Bears 14 and Vikings 21.] They did effectively increase my BP back into the normal range. Wouldn't have to worry about low blood pressure if the Bears played every day.

Hoping to get the drain out tomorrow, two weeks since surgery and the output is still borderline 25–30 cc/24 hours... We shall see. I don't know how long they can keep it in, I want it out but don't want to have the fluid accumulate.

What did the doc say about your tests, any ideas on how they can manage your pain better?

From: Alan

To: Marcy

I'm guessing that having that drain is beginning to suck—no pun intended. However, removing too soon would suck more. Is the site clean?

Today they decided I have pain from the L5-S1 disc that is nearly gone. He referred for an injection into it. The first guy doesn't do that procedure and the second guy doesn't take our insurance. I'll try again in the morning.

Be good!

To: Alan

From: Marcy

The drain site is still good. How long can it stay in? If it doesn't stop soon does it indicate there is still some kind of problem in there? Grrrr.

I went to two different Wal-Marts to find those Bears onesies and they are gone. I may go to the original Wal-Mart that I saw them in tomorrow. Wish I would have given myself permission to buy them when I first saw them.

So are you back to work. What do you mean "they decided" about your pain? What have you decided?

I'm trying to be good.

From: Alan

To: Marcy

It could probably stay for weeks as long as it stays clean. Of course, any indwelling catheter is always a risk for the infection but this sounds clean so no worries.

The whole pain treatment thing has become frustrating. Sophie is sick so we're gonna take the dogs out and go to sleep. I'm hoping for more clarity in the morning.

Sleep tight.

FB: December 10, 2012

I have to get some Christmas shopping done. Thanks to my sister-in-law Patti, I won't have to do the driving or think much. Hopefully not too crowded on Monday and I can get it done.

I am scheduled to get the drain out tomorrow afternoon but the fluid output was supposed to be less than 25cc/24 hours and the last three days it has been just under 30 cc. I really want this out but if it comes out too soon, there could be problems with fluid accumulation again. I guess I will just have to call and see if they want me to reschedule.

EM: December 11, 2012

To: Alan

From: Marcy

They are going to take the drain out...a bit nervous about that.

From: Alan

To: Marcy

Just keep it clean. It's time to get it removed. It's clean and healthy inside. That's what counts.

CB: December 12, 2012

Change in Plan...Again

Howdeeeee,

Change in plans and some things up in the air. Went to get the drain out yesterday. I was told they are leaving it in. Still too much drainage to pull the drain out. It is lighter and clear and the site looks good. I can still get the scan for radiation to recalculate the treatment but he will have to see where the drain tubing is and if we can still do treatments while it is in place. Maybe it can be pulled Friday or Monday. Physical therapy cancelled my appointment too, they won't see me with a drain in and with the holidays. Riley and I ARE going on vacation. Physical therapy will have to wait until the new year. I also have a call out to the gastroenterologist to find out if he is still going to do my colonoscopy. Not sure if there is any concern about blood counts if I have radiation the three consecutive days before the procedure, would my blood counts be okay? That is another thing that may need to wait.

I made an appointment with my neurologist (12/24) to see if he can shed some light on the right hand and arm numbness, tingling, and weakness that is much worse since the last surgery. Some of it could be inflammation I suppose but I am a little concerned. They told me in the hospital to report those symptoms but when I tell the surgeons about it, they don't say much. The lymphedema is back but not terrible and I am wearing the big blue Caresia again. It helps with the swelling but also reminds me not to reach and stretch that right arm too far.

My blood pressure is still too low to take the medication for the heart rate, so the primary care doctor said use more salt and drink more fluids and send her the readings in five days.

It may not have been the most rational decision, financially and timing wise but I booked plane tickets for Riley and I to go to California from Dec. 27-Jan. 4. A *real* vacation, and seeing some of our favorite people. I am so looking forward to that. So whatever needs to be done medically will have to wait if it can't be done before then.

Also looking forward to Christmas at home with the family and seeing some of the younger generation coming in from out of state.

My mom will probably be home on Dec. 22 or sooner depending on how she progresses with OT and PT [occupational therapy and physical therapy] and pain. She will have home care for a little while and then outpatient PT. We have a home assessment tomorrow to see what equipment or safety things we need to get. She is doing very well.

So that is my story for now...until it changes yet again. Trying to go with the flow.

TTFN ("Ta Ta For Now" as Tigger would say), Marcy

FB: December 12, 2012

"When you can tell your story and it doesn't make you cry, you know you have healed." —Author Unknown

FB: December 13, 2012

Today I had to put my arm above my head to be rescanned for radiation treatments to start next Monday. I can't reach my arm above my head like that since the last surgery. Now I am in pain, my hand is swollen and I have more fluid coming from the drain. I had to cancel the appointment to get the drain out. The good news is, since I am not going to drive tomorrow, I can take the Percocet!

Willow: Thank God for Percocet right?!

Marcy: Yeah, helps with the pain but makes me feel lightheaded. I haven't taken it in a while because I wanted to drive.

Sorry I am not going to do Christmas cards this year. My hand is swollen and numb and I can't write that much. Please know that I am thinking of you though and wishing you a very Merry Christmas and a Happy New Year.

Hannah: What's my excuse?

Marcy: You have been busy being an exceptional mom and student?

FP: Ho Ho Ho! No cards needed. That's one of the good things about Facebook, by posting this you did send us all a holiday "card."

FB: December 14, 2012

This was posted by a friend and one of the teachers who taught in my son's 4th grade classroom. Teachers, God bless them as well as the little ones and families at Sandy Hook Elementary. Thank you Dakota.

"When I was a boy and I would see scary things in the news, my mother would say to me, 'Look for the helpers. You will always find people who are helping.' To this day, especially in times of disaster, I remember my mother's words and I am always comforted by realizing that there are still so many helpers—so many caring people in this world." —Mr. Rogers

CB: December 14, 2012

Blah Blah Blah

Blah blah blah, that's how I feel right now. Tylenol doesn't help the pain much and Percocet does but gives me a headache.

The pain in my shoulder, chest, and arm is limiting my abilities. It became much worse after putting my arm above my head to be rescanned for radiation. It didn't take long to be scanned, just long enough for some silent tears to slowly escape. I still get the numbness and tingling down into my fingers. My hand and fingers are swollen.

My blood pressure is still low enough not to take the beta blocker but my pulse was 112 this morning and when it gets like that I am short of breath.

The drain is still in and having outputs of 25–30 cc. I didn't get the drain out today but will call with a report of output on Monday.

The gastroenterologist still wants to do the colonoscopy on Thursday but I may cancel. If my BP is still low and then I have to do the colonoscopy prep, I just can't see that going well with radiation next week too. [Prepping for a colonoscopy often dehydrates people, and if I had become dehydrated, my blood pressure would have been low, and the sedation meds would have made it even worse. I was worried it would make me feel weak, especially with radiation the next week.] I have become a pretty difficult IV stick and I think maybe when I am healthier it would be better. I am not having problems, it is just screening and family history. So have I convinced myself to cancel? Probably.

My mom had her home visit with the physical therapist. We got some good suggestions. It wore her out though and now she is in more pain. She should be home by the twenty-second still.

Have a good weekend. Go Bears!

FB: December 14, 2012

My bed is feeling very friendly right now. Riley got an ice pack for me and tucked me in.

FB: December 15, 2012

Lazy morning. My sweet boy, Riley, brought me coffee in bed. I guess I will have to get in the shower after him, hope he leaves some hot water for me or I will have to stay in bed longer while it warms up. Staying in bed longer would be a darn shame. *dripping with sarcasm*

EM: December 15, 2012

From: Marcy

To: Alan

Hey there, how are you today?

Got your package and thank you. I put the present under the tree, although I am not good at waiting. Again, thank you so much.

I really don't know how you do this chronic pain shit. How do you do it? I know it is a struggle. My arm is getting so bad; it started with the numbness and tingling, worse at night, now the swelling is worse and the pain is getting bad. It's the shoulder, shoulder blade, and chest but this morning even my elbow was screaming. I wake up and the thumb and second and third fingers are numb, that gets a little better, and then the fourth and fifth finger goes numb.

Bright spots: They always involve people for me... My friend who drove me to the hospital and was one of the ones there when Riley was born is coming over. Haven't seen her in years. My nephew is home from the marines for Christmas (he leaves for Afghanistan in February). I am very much looking forward to seeing both of them.

I'm done with Christmas shopping and as soon as my arm is a little better I will wrap. Typing isn't easy. I paid a friend and her friend to clean my house so that is done. I think I did too much getting the clutter taken care of, maybe I made it worse for myself. I have the kids doing dishes and garbage, dusting and vacuuming but I don't ask them to clean my bathroom, bedroom, or to do my laundry. Have a good weekend.

From: Alan

To: Marcy

Hi Marcy, sorry to hear about your arm. I hope it turns for the good really soon.

I haven't been very communicative lately because things are not going well. I took time off work and saw a physiatrist. He advised no more injections (which was good) and had me start with his PT guy. The problem is he also started me on Cymbalta for chronic pain. I finally stopped it this morning. I've been so sick for the last several days. I'm nauseous, I can't eat and I'm exhausted but can't sleep. I've been on the couch for days.

We have tickets tonight to a show in Arlington Hts. I'm gonna try coffee, Tylenol and Naproxen and see if I can go.

I'm sorry about your arm. It seems like one thing after the other. Are you seeing the surgeon next week?

Hang in there. Always believe that better days are coming.

From: Marcy

To: Alan

Hi Alan,

That is the thing...I do believe better days are coming... Do you? Don't worry about times when you don't feel like communicating. 1) Sometimes I feel like I am bothering you but if you don't respond I won't take it personally. 2) It is probably in the times you feel less communicative that you need to communicate the most.

I am glad you saw your physiatrist. I was on Cymbalta once, didn't tolerate well and also Lyrica...made me so sleepy.

Fairly certain the arm will get better. I had surgery for cubital tunnel on the left and tarsal tunnel on the right, so I obviously worry about all my "tunnels."

I really hope you feel well enough for the show. Sometimes getting out is the best thing, even for a short while. For me, I think I am going to have to take the Percocet again, so I am going to have to ask Dani to take my mom's mail to her and go to the grocery store for me.

I won't think any less of you if you have pain, are depressed or not working. You rock and I love you for being the caring person you are, sticking by me when my world was crumbling. I want to do the same for you if I can.

Take care, Marcy

From: Alan

To: Marcy

Thank you, your words mean a lot to me.

I'd certainly ask the surgeon about the persistent fluid production.

Hope the Percocet works tonight.

Take care, Alan

FB: December 16, 2012

Riley and I have an early flight the day after Christmas, so my Christmas present from my mom is a limo to the airport, win/win. She doesn't have to get up and do it and I can relax about getting there. Thanks Mom.

Reflections

Hindsight has me thinking I could have handled this last period of time much better. There have been a few times in my life I was consumed by emotions and trying to process what I was going through—such as placing my child up for adoption—and craved to have the support that was offered for my battle with cancer. Why would I use the support I had less during the time I needed it the most?

And then there was the physical gauntlet I had to run. Looking back now I wonder if I felt like I was becoming too whiny about my physical health during the treatment. I worried my friends and family were tired of hearing about it. I was just tired of dealing with it all and thought they may be also. In all likelihood it was moreso me than them. Sometimes I think it really comes down to society's chants of "keep fighting" and "stay positive." As much as we want for it to be helpful to a cancer patient at times it can have the opposite effect of making people think they are not handling themselves well if they have a weak period or get scared. I think sometimes it instead encourages people to put on a happy face and keep their feelings bottled up. I want to be the kind of friend that I often had, the ones who not only are the energetic, happy cheerleaders but also the ones who say, "It's okay to have a bad day, to cry and to want to hide." Those are the ones who met me where I was and would just lay on my couch and fall asleep with me while watching a movie. Sometimes fewer words have more impact when it comes to supporting someone.

One thing was certain, I still just wanted to get treatment done and get out of town. I wanted to take Riley away from it all. I would have loved to have had Dani with me also but her work schedule wouldn't allow it. I was doing my best to try to get through this last week of being a cancer patient and moving on to being a cancer survivor.

— 6 —

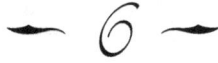

Finishing Radiation

Mourning All I Lost

Pain and Frustration

I was in my bed crying a couple hours ago, Dani came in and gently rubbed my leg while I tried to explain how frustrated I am. I hate that she had to see me like that. I think I was able to hide it from Riley today. He already has seen too much of my pain.

Four medical contacts today...

First, I called the plastic surgeon, drainage is finally subsiding to 20 cc/24 hours. Appointment to get the drain out tomorrow afternoon was made.

Second, a new medicine for neuropathy by phone, will try it and see Dr. Douglass, the neurologist, in person on 12/24.

Third, the radiation doctor listened, gave me a tissue, and asked how he could soothe me, then I went into the radiation machine for a simulation. Raising my arm hurt me to tears, they had to adjust the treatment plan to accommodate the fact I can't raise my arm without pain. By the time it was done, half my hand felt dead and the pain in the arm and shoulder was ridiculous.

Fourth, I called in my blood pressure and pulse readings that I have been monitoring twice a day to the nurse at my primary care physician's office. I let the return call go to voice mail. The nurse said the doctor has instructions for me and to call tomorrow. Just after I let that call go to voice mail was when Dani came in my room. Even typing this is frustrating with fat, numb and tingling fingers. Don't want to talk to anybody about anything, for a while.

Hannah: ((hug)) But gently, so I don't squeeze your arm or shoulder.

CP: My prayers go out for God to be with you and ease your pain. Love ya!

FB: December 18, 2012

Think I am going to take myself out to lunch before going to radiation, then the surgeon's office, and then for lab work. Hell, I may even have dessert first.

CB: December 18, 2012

Sweeping It under the Rug

This is my third attempt at this journal entry. The application I typed it in wouldn't save, and then I redid it in another application and it wouldn't save. Each time I have to stop several times because of my hand and arm pain and numbness. So I am trying to type it directly in here instead of trying to copy and paste it. Here it goes:

I have lived long enough and seen what happens when, in an effort to preserve the look of being positive, people do all the dusting and polish the things on the shelf yet sweep the dirt and dust under the rug.

I think that is what I have been doing. Although I have acknowledged and wrote about the dust and dirt, I never accepted it or the work it takes to get rid of it. So it is coming out from under the rug again causing a mess and being tracked around. It is much easier to go back to polishing the shiny stuff that everyone sees and compliments me on than to admit that I have dirt on the floor and I may need help getting it out of my house.

So what brought me to this line of thinking? My friend responded to the question I posted: "What the hell is wrong with me?" I had extreme sadness and tears all day yesterday. She said, "Nothing is wrong with you. You have put off your mourning. I think this is normal and you should let it out. It's not normal if it goes on for a long period of time" (I don't know what "a long time" is).

Yep, I've swept it under the rug and put off the mourning. While actively getting treatments and dealing with the complications of the treatments, I have put off mourning to be a stronger fighter. Treatment is going to be done this week, I hope. I am very grateful for that, glad to still be alive. In my mind, we have all been looking forward to the last treatment day and I attached a lot of meaning to it, the "light at the end of the tunnel," the moment I can put this all behind me. The fact is while I was polishing my shiny stuff and celebrating treatments soon to be over, I was sweeping what cancer took from me under the rug and not dealing with the uncertainty of how long the pain, neuropathy, and lymphedema may last. How it will affect my future career worries me. It makes me sad and angry that to write this (for the third time) I have to keep stopping because it is difficult to use my fingers and my arm hurts. Will that get better? It has been getting worse the past two weeks. How long will it last? Will I get the fine motor skills back and will I be able to get the full range of motion back in my shoulder? Holding the phone to my ear makes my hand go numb after five minutes. I can't put a cup of coffee in the microwave with my right hand, it is too high and causes pain. These are the things that I have a tendency to sweep under the rug in order to focus on the positive. The treatments are almost over...yet the effects will be with me for a while. How long? The doctors say give it time. They can't know for sure. I guess I can't expect them to know, they don't have a crystal ball.

It's difficult to accept that even though I can see that light at the end of the tunnel, I may still be in the tunnel for a while. I know I am not going to die of cancer but I also realize that I will have the effects of what cancer took from me and the consequences of the treatment, some forever (mastectomies) and some may get better. I also now understand that there are people in my life who are really good at polishing the things in view on the shelf and I need those people to remind me sometimes of the joys and celebrate with me. There are also the people who are comfortable seeing the dirt and helping me to get it out from under the rug and out of my house so it doesn't resurface later. I need those people in my life too. There are also the people who are good at both and that is the person I would like to be.

So I want to say sorry for yesterday. I'm sorry for shutting some people out, while I was overwhelmed with the dirt from under my rug. I'm learning that in fighting cancer physically, there is also an internal fight, both emotionally and mentally that sometimes becomes externally visible for all to see.

So I guess the bottom line is: There is a light at the end of the tunnel, I can see it but it seems farther away than I thought and the tunnel can get dirty sometimes. I need all kinds of people in my life to get through this and

I appreciate all of them and the variety of support I get, especially from the ones in the tunnel with me. Thanks for continuing to be there for me, even though the tunnel is longer than I expected.

Love, Marcy

Forward Movement

Hi, today was a little better. I am not magically healed but I am not as emotional. It helps that there was more sleep last night and forward movement today.

The drain came out today. I did not realize how long the tubing was inside me, it seemed like she was pulling it out for a long time. Like the magician who pulls out the never-ending handkerchief. Maybe now that it is out some symptoms will settle down. As I type my fingers are getting numb though. It will probably take time and I need to learn to be patient.

I had radiation today, only two more left... Woohooo!

I did get lab work done, to see if my B12 is low. I will also see the neurologist next week. Maybe after vacation, after I get back into physical therapy things will get better. It isn't like I am completely helpless. I will learn to manage with the symptoms I have and pray that they get better over time.

My other therapy today was talking to friends (I could actually have a conversation without crying), listening to good music, and eating whiskey cake from TGI Fridays. Boy, was that goooood!

Thanks for hanging in there with me and keeping up with my posts. I know I can be really honest and open about the good and bad and that makes me a little vulnerable but it helps me deal with it and maybe helps others deal with their stuff too, whatever that stuff may be. I also get a lot of support with the comments, emails and phone calls. I appreciate it, knowing you are there. Take care of you, Marcy

Lucy: Marcy—I always appreciate your honesty! Of course you are going to go through a mourning period of what you have been dealing with and what you have lost as a woman. I hope you will let the gates open and cry to your heart's content—you are entitled to do that and need to do that. We all need our days when we are on the "pity pot," but you actually deserve some of those days!

Hopefully once the treatments are over and you can get some of those toxins out of your body and give your body the good nourishment it needs—your body will regenerate its strength. A doctor once told me that if you give the body what it needs, it can perform miracles, and I believe that!!! You are doing so well and the fact that you realize all this is such a blessing. Love you dear friend!

I'm always more emotional when I'm tired, so I can certainly understand that! Get your rest young lady and take your vitamins, eat fruits and veggies and be patient with yourself. You are doing great! Love you!

SS: Marcy, I am so glad that you are moving ahead. I miss seeing you and tomorrow is my last day at Hamilton before the new year begins. So I will be seeing you and wishing you a happy new year. Wow...things are really moving on. Love you and have a great Christmas.

EM: December 18, 2012

From: Alan

To: Marcy

Your honesty in your posts is a good thing. All that you've been through just sucks.

Feelings I've had over the past few years related to my back pain (some in the past few days):

I hate everybody.

Leave me alone.

This isn't fair.

Everyone else is fine but me.

I deserve better than this.

There's no such thing as God.

I wish I was dead.

I've hated some doctors. I pretend to be OK at work. It pisses me off to lie to myself.

People ask me how I'm doing, I say fine. It's not true, but who wants to hear the truth? And what can they do?

I have a close friend from college (whose house I was at Sunday for the Bears game). Sometimes I email him if I'm going through a bad time. He emails back and says, "That sucks man."

That helps more than anything—just expressing an understanding that it does in fact suck.

It seems like despite being a good patient so much has gone wrong for you.

Wondering when, if ever, the pain, neuropathy, and lymphedema will improve is the worst. I know that feeling. It's scary, frustrating and depressing. This cannot be understated.

I can't imagine what the loss of your breasts feels like emotionally. I just guess the sadness will lessen as the years go by.

I had physical therapy today. I'm doing all I can to not take a Vicodin. I'm tired of this.

Like every day I still hold the belief that better days are coming. I go to bed and hope to wake up feeling better.

I can't think of a reason why your arm wouldn't get better. Maybe tomorrow.

I hope the good times outweigh the bad. I really hope your arm improves soon—wish there were something I could do for you. Hang in there, always hang in there.

From: Marcy

To: Alan

Thank you. I knew you would understand and I pray things get better for you too. The acute stuff was intense but the chronic stuff (including the back pain and arthritis) can be really hard to deal with. You don't deserve this is right!

The drain is out and part of me hopes that it was irritating things and the numbness, tingling, and pain will settle down. I am sure it will get better, it just will take time. I am afraid it will affect changing jobs and getting back into home care. The mobility in my chest, arm, and shoulder is part of the issue, but it should get better in time, especially when I get back into physical therapy after the new year.

Today was a better day, there was movement forward. Got a radiation treatment, got lab work, got the drain out. It is when there are many days of no movement or progress or even back stepping that I get like I was. Especially when the pain interferes with sleep, waking up every couple hours numb and with a dead hand. When I don't sleep I get out of control emotionally.

I don't hate any of the doctors now. I have hated some of the ones who treated me like a drug seeker in the emergency room, when my back flared up, before I had a "real diagnosis" and a rheumatologist.

Thank you for being honest with me. You never have to lie and tell me you're okay when you aren't okay.

Thanks also for understanding me not coming out yesterday. I want to see you. Maybe after we get back from California.

Take care. Marcy

P.S. The good does outweigh the bad, wish the bad wasn't so intense though. If it wasn't for my kids, there are times this year and during my marriage with Jack that I would wish to be dead. Fingers are getting numb so I will go, but thanks again. I'll hang in there if you do.

From: Alan

To: Marcy

I shall.

FB: December 19, 2012

My last radiation treatment will be tomorrow! Trying to get comfortable in bed, so I could watch a DVD on my laptop. Adjusting pillows, bedding, etc. I realized that if I were a dog, I would be one of the ones that circled around on the bed twenty times before settling down. Sheesh!

EM: December 19, 2012

From: Lucy

To: Marcy

Hi lady—I've been trying to keep up with you on CaringBridge, so I think I'm up to date. I think I understand all your feelings—the being positive, staying strong, but occasionally being emotional, feeling the impact of what your cancer has done to you and your body, and so many more feelings—just wanting life to get back to some sense of normal. I think all of those feelings are absolutely normal and important to go through in this whole process of being sick, getting treatments, and then finally getting well. You have done an amazing job and I just wish I was there to give you a big hug, because that's what I'm feeling—so darn proud of you for fighting so hard and doing what you had to do. I pray for you every day—that He gives you the strength to get through another day.

I'm so happy you and Riley get to go on a vacation and get away for a short time. I sent you a package today, so hoping you get it before you leave. I think you should get it maybe Saturday or Monday. I hope your mother is continuing to do well with her hip replacement.

Wishing you a very merry Christmas and best wishes for a healthy, happy New Year!!!

Love you, Lucy

From: Marcy

To: Lucy

Hi, it was great talking to you. I have read this email several times tonight. It means a lot to me. Yes, it sounds like you understand. Thank you for your consistent prayers.

California Dreamin'

CB and FB: December 20, 2012

From Fighter to Survivor

Hello,

So I don't know what my doctors think about this but in my mind, the moment I walked out of my last radiation today, I went from a cancer fighter to a survivor.

The radiation machine was in need of repair when I arrived. I told the tech that I wasn't leaving until I got my last treatment. He would have to find me a pillow and a blanket for the night. The repair guy came in twenty-five minutes and a little over an hour later I got my last treatment.

I will still have many medical appointments in the month of January, physical therapy and some screening tests to do, but the actual active treatments are done. I start Tamoxifen tomorrow. I will do what I can about the things that I can change and try to accept the things that will never be the same again. The trick is knowing the difference and being patient.

So to cancer I say, "Adios Mother F***er! With the help of my medical team, my family and friends, WE beat you. Even if there is a cancer cell or two hanging around, the Tamoxifen will catch up to you and keep you away. So na nee na nee boo boo, we beat you."

Okay, so I know that wasn't very mature but really, that is how I feel about it!

Be safe, Love, Marcy

CB: *Love!*

CP: Way to go Marcy!!!!

FP: *Awesome.*

DA: Wonderful!!! Enjoy your trip to the best you can!!!

Liza: *You are my hero!!*

Marcy: Aw Liza, I could not have done it without you. You were there at my hardest moments. Thank you, thank you, thank you.

Willow: *Woohoo!!* I am so proud of you!! You are the strongest woman I know!!

Laurie: Strong, sassy, beautiful survivor!

Jade: Now we are in the same club! I am so happy for you, Riley, and all whose lives you have touched, including mine.

Marcy: Yes, Jade, we are in the same club, now it is going to be focusing on recovering and getting healthy and fit in 2013!

Jade: Any of your docs talk to you about taking vitamins? My oncology doctor had me start taking quite a few when I was finally finished with treatment.

Marcy: I took some before and there are some I am taking specifically for the neuropathy. I just had my B12 level checked too, was deficient years ago and already supplemented that. Waiting for the results. Before this I was Vitamin D deficient and take that and calcium. So right now I take a multivitamin, calcium with D, B12 and B6.

Jade: No antioxidants?

Marcy: Relax Jade, LOL, one thing at a time. I'll talk to the medical oncologist about that at my follow up in January.

Jade: Okay, I will behave.

Melanie: Way to go Marcy. You kicked butt!!!

GG: Who says we have to act mature anyhow. I love the naneenaneebooboo. So happy for you that the radiation is over!

Alan: I'm proud to call you my friend. You did it!

PH: Yay!!!!!!!! Yeah!!!!!!!!

JY: So glad you got that last treatment in... that was *determination*!!! Merry Christmas Marcy... I hope your mom is hanging in there too!

Lucy: Congrats and amen!! You are one tough cookie!

EM: December 20, 2012

From: Marcy

To: Alan

Hi friend, Thanks for what you said on online journal. I am so grateful we are friends and I hope someday I can help you like you have helped me.

You were one of the most significant people in my fight. I really could not have made it without you. You always seemed to know exactly what to say and when. Funny, you didn't need to do anything physically to make such a difference in my life. The contact we had was mostly, mail, phone, email, etc. Hmmmm, I guess that means that even if you don't work as a doctor in a medical facility you still can save lives.

Thank you!

From: Alan

To: Marcy

Thank you. That means a lot to me. You have no idea how much you've helped me.

Have a great day!

Reflections

I clearly remember getting ready to pull out of the parking lot of the radiation oncologist's office and posting to CaringBridge and Facebook that I finally made it through the last treatment. The panic I felt when the radiation machine needed repair was intense. I wasn't sure I would ever return if I left without my last treatment. It *had* to be done and over with that day! I was not sure if everyone in the office knew what had happened to me in the previous months. They were so sympathetic but may not have truly understood how done I was with radiation. Telling them I was not leaving until it was done sent them the shockwave they needed to empathize with me. I like to believe it was their "aha moment" to understand how done I was with this treatment. The elation to finally be done with cancer treatments was spectacular. I knew I would have pain and fatigue. I would need to have physical and occupational therapy when I returned from California. I expected that when I started to improve I wouldn't have to back step again. I celebrated with my family and friends. I felt like a survivor.

I often think about Alan. Cancer is a terrible disease and the treatments can be horrific but I looked forward to the last chemo, the last surgery, the last radiation. I knew after the last radiation when I started to feel better I wouldn't have to feel beat up like that again. Alan lives with chronic pain, pain that impacts his daily life. I planned my life around treatments, he plans his life around pain. Learning from him how he managed and knowing he understood was one of my lifelines. I think our need to feel productive, useful and not a burden to anyone are commonalities we share. My friends, family, and even strangers embraced me and held me up often because of the cancer, but people with chronic pain do they get the same support? I don't think they do. I think they get judgments and criticism. They are treated like they are lazy or seeking drugs.

I know from experience as a nurse and a patient with chronic arthritis that chronic pain sufferers are not treated with as much compassion as a cancer patients, but why shouldn't they be? I have had chronic arthritis that has left me unable to walk during a flare up. Often I believed I was not being understood by emergency department staff. I am hoping someday this will change, someday society will see pain as pain regardless of cause and will try to ease suffering in whatever way possible instead of placing blame and making accusations.

— 7 —

Recovery

What Do You Live For?

FB: December 21, 2012

For those who have suggested a specific vitamin, mineral, antioxidant, supplement: I will evaluate all suggestions and talk to my doctors about them... as it is I am taking thirteen and a half capsules/pills per day that are doctor-recommended—some are vitamins, but still, three times a day, 13.5 pills! I want to be sure it will be beneficial before I spend more money and swallow more pills. With that said, if you have a specific recommendation, please post what it is and why you think I should take it and I will bring this info to my doctor in January when I go for follow-up. Just because it is "natural" doesn't mean it is safe or won't interact with what I am already taking. Thanks for caring enough to make suggestions.

FP: How do you have an appetite for food after all those pills?

CC: I would recommend that you {{HUG}} those you love. Because it makes everyone feel great, doesn't cost a cent and will not interact with any of your current meds.

Marcy: Half of them are vitamins and calcium because those levels were low. Unfortunately, one of them increases appetite and the other one decreases metabolism. I've got some work to do with diet and exercise in 2013.

CB: December 22, 2012

What Do You Live For?

Fingers are really too numb to type what has been on my mind. I will at some later point but I wanted to share this quote:

"The mystery of human existence lies not in just staying alive, but in finding something to live for." —Fyodor Dostoyevsky, *The Brothers Karamazov*

If you have read my journal you probably know that for me, it is my kids and helping other people when I can. What about you? What do you live for? Even with this amount of typing my fingers are now on fire. Good night.

Alan: I've always thought the following: 1. You do what you need to do to keep a roof over your head and take care of those who depend on you. 2. You live by the golden rule and then some extra when people need you. 3. You have as many good times with friends and family as possible, and make good memories. Life always has value.

JS: [...] St. Paul's answer to your question was "For me, to live is Christ; to die is gain." I don't think I can top that.

CB: December 25, 2012

Merry Christmas! And a Very Happy and Healthy New Year!

Quick update from the visit with the neurologist. After the physical exam and getting the history of what has been going on with the numbness, tingling, and pain from my shoulder to my fingers we have decided that it is bilateral carpal tunnel [wrist] and right cubital [elbow] tunnel. These things existed before the chemo, radiation, and surgery but all those things made the symptoms worse. I figured I had these as I have already had surgery for left cubital tunnel and tarsal tunnel [ankle]. The symptoms being worse with certain activities or positions gave me some clues. The symptoms were there but tolerable so I had not seen a doctor about it before all the cancer treatments started. Neurontin [an anticonvulsant medication that is also used to treat neuropathic pain] doesn't do much for compression neuropathy so I am going off it. I have bilateral wrist braces for night time when the symptoms are the worst. When I get back from vacation I will do physical and occupational therapy for a while and hopefully that will help; if not, we will do some tests to determine if surgery is needed and where to start. I am in total agreement with this assessment and plan.

Now I am just going to manage the symptoms the best I can to enjoy the holiday and a vacation with Riley.

I will be going back to work when the kids return to school on January 7.

Love, Marcy

P.S. At least with the numbness and tingling I don't ramble on as much when typing.

Alan: Merry Christmas! And wear those splints every night. Be good!

GG: Merry Christmas to you Dani and Riley! Have a wonderful vacation. You deserve it.

Lucy: Wishing you a wonderful, well deserved vacation! Enjoy!!

FB: December 25, 2012

Last post until the day after Christmas celebrations with my family are over. I want to give them my full attention by staying off social media, I can do that for twenty-five hours, right?

Lola: Yes...yes. You can!! I was just signing off myself...patiently waiting for the boy's eyes to close. Have a Merry Christmas... Love you!

FB: December 26, 2012

At the family Christmas get together my precious 10-year-old nephew Terry asked me, "Is the cancer all out of your body now?" I said, "Yep." He smiled and said, "That makes this the best Christmas eeeevverrrr!" What a sweetie pie.

CB: December 29, 2012

California with Riley

We had a very merry Christmas with family and now Riley and I are in California with friends. Very relaxed yet getting some exercise and building up some endurance, walking in the hills and on the beach paths.

We plan to go to San Diego Zoo tomorrow, some other beaches, maybe a vineyard, and I made reservations for the boys and me to do a Segway tour of the Hollywood sign and reservoir. After that we will go to the Griffith Observatory.

Feeling pretty good, the neuropathy is still bothering me. I consistently wear the wrist braces at night and it helps tremendously with the night-time pain, although I still have the tingling. Wish I had a brace to keep the cubital tunnel (similar to carpal tunnel but in the elbow) in check; the wrist braces don't help the elbow. I think if they made a brace to keep my elbows in a good position at night, that would help. During the day, certain movements of the wrist cause the shooting pain, andbending my elbow and holding things like the little chihuahua causes the ulnar neuropathy symptoms. Although it is worse during the day I am grateful not to be waking up in the middle of the night in such pain. May need to wear the right wrist brace during the day too if this keeps up.

I'm really *loving* our time in California and with the Rizzo family. I am so glad my health didn't prevent me from getting us out here. It is soooo heartwarming to see Riley with his close friend. I love spending time with these boys. Okay, their parents and grandma are cool too. hahaha.

Have a Happy New Year! Here's to a healthy 2013.

Love, Marcy

FB: December 31, 2012

I wish you all a happy and healthy new year! Goodbye 2012, so much happened in this year that changed our lives and outlooks forever. *Welcome* 2013!

Pinch me, can't believe I'm enjoying live music outside in front of palm trees!

FB: January 3, 2013

Well worth the fatigue I feel right now to have had such a special day with the boys, the laughter was frequent and the memories will last!

The only thing that could have been better about going to California with Riley would have been if Dani were able to go with us. On April 15, after Brayden and Mia visited us from California, I wrote in CaringBridge the feeling that they were worried they wouldn't see me again. Therefore it was so exhilarating to be able to go to California and visit the Rizzo family in December. I wanted to do everything I could with them. We did a Segway tour to the Hollywood sign, visited Griffith Observatory and San Diego Zoo. We walked along beaches and kayaked. We hiked and played.

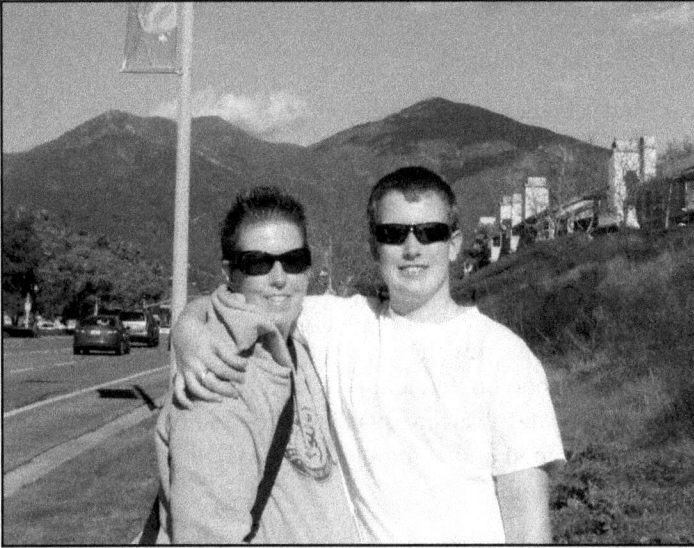

Figure 7-1. Riley and me in California

My heart felt full being with them. The trip itself posed some physical challenges as I was heavier than I had been in a long time, the neuropathy pain in my hands and arms was barely controlled with use of splints at night, and I tired easily. The Rizzos were another family that understood where I was at physically and were able to make me feel comfortable and accepted regardless of my energy level, that in itself gave me motivation to push myself a little more each day.

FB: January 6, 2013

Clothes set out, coffee pot programmed, lunch made, car fueled up, alarm clock set. I'm going back to work full time tomorrow after a long time on medical leave. Excited and nervous. I very much need to be back at HHS!

FB: January 7, 2013

Went to warm up car and take out trash, found thank-you card from Dani on my steering wheel. Thanking me for being her and Riley's mom. She wouldn't trade the moments I sing and dance in the car for the world. Not sure if it offsets the guilt of going back to work when Riley's home sick but it helps! Got to pay the bills. So away I go! Have a good Monday everyone.

Was told by a student that my hair has better spikes than one of the male PE teachers...go me!

CB: January 8, 2013

Motivated and Encouraged

I am feeling very motivated and encouraged so far in this new year.

This week I went back to work full time. I can't think of any other time I was happier to wake up on Monday and drive to work very early in the morning, watching the sunrise on my commute. Everyone at work was welcoming and it felt so good. Made it through the first two days and the rest of the week is looking good too.

Monday after work I saw the medical oncologist's nurse practitioner. Everything was good on that follow up and I don't have to see them for three months. Today I saw the plastic surgeon's nurse practitioner and everything was good at that appointment also, and I don't have to see them for three months.

I started occupational therapy for my carpal tunnel and cubital tunnel symptoms. She was also very encouraging. After her evaluation she said she didn't think I lost a lot of strength and my sensation was better than I thought it was. I am starting to believe that I will be able to control these symptoms without more surgeries. The wrist braces at night are a tremendous help. With some therapy—nerve elongating exercises, mobilization stuff and other mumbo jumbo—I will see much improvement, I am sure. I will start physical therapy next week for my shoulder pain and range of motion. I can do them both on the same day after work.

I also went back to my Weight Watchers meeting. I felt encouraged and motivated there too. Things seem to be falling into place. Planning and preparing is paying off.

I just realized how tired I was when I sat down to write this; it is a good tired. The kind of tired I feel from purposefully living my life and moving my body. Not the kind of tired I feel from being sick and depressed.

The things that bother me now are the things that are manageable— manageable with effort but manageable. Most importantly, the things that bother me don't have the potential to kill me. The neuropathy, the lymphedema (which isn't bad at all right now), my weight gain, hot flashes...those are all manageable.

So onward we go. Thanks for sticking around to read how things are going.

Have a good week, Marcy

PH: Marcy I am so *happy* for you. You have been through so much that it is about time you got some relief and happiness! Looks like some of that rest and vacation did some good too. Love and hugs to you!

JY: Marcy, so happy to read your positive update! Welcome back to school. :)

Alan: Cool. Up until this point in my day (11 p.m.) nothing was going right. Reading your journal just now made everything OK. I feel better now. Glad things are going well.

CP: Hello Marcy, I am glad to hear this good news from you and I also like the word you used, "manageable." I think that is a good word. Take care and I look forward to seeing you in the near future. Love you.

CB: January 10, 2013

The Week

It may not seem like a lot to most and I know I am patting myself on the back for what people do all the time but...tomorrow is Friday, after I get out of work I will have made it through my first week back at work full time, plus three doctors' visits, and two occupational therapy visits this week. It could be why I am tired by 6:30 p.m. I am just happy I am capable of doing it. Wouldn't have been able to last through all of that a month ago. When I saw the radiation oncologist, I thought he was going to say, "See you in three months," like the surgeon and medical oncologist said, but I was wrong. He wants to see me in six weeks. I guess I thought when I was done, I wouldn't have to worry about risks anymore, but for the first six months after radiation there are things that he needs to watch for. I think related to the lung mostly. It got radiated in certain areas with the chest wall. Even with all the precise scans, positioning and angles, you still can't send radiation beams on a curve. So we will watch for signs of pneumonitis but I feel good now and that is what counts. So...I have to say.... Happy Friday (almost).

Looking forward to the weekend. Marcy

Alan: We see others all day long and we assume everyone else feels great, but we don't see what they struggle with on a daily basis. But I've come to learn that some people make extraordinary efforts just to get through a day. It's a big deal to get through a week of work and all those other appointments. Very satisfying. Congratulations!

FB: January 11, 2013

I feel like I *earned* my weekend for the first time in months. What will I do with it you ask? Laundry, shopping, run Riley around and lay on the couch or in bed watching TV.

FB: January 19, 2013

I have an appointment to be fitted for prosthetics on Monday. I wonder if they will have my breasts in stock or if I will have to order them. I wonder if insurance pays for more than one pair, one pair for daily wear and one for going out on the town?

SV: If it makes you feel better I need those panties with the butt implants.

Marcy: I got plenty of that!

SV: I'll take some and trade my muffin top.

Marcy: No thanks, I have a muffin of my own.

SV: LOL! More cushion for the pushin'? *Haaaa!* I'm talking about me.

Marcy: Nobody's pushin' anything around here.

Kady: Well duh...you *have* to have a sexy set for the weekends! How would insurance *not* understand this?

FB: January 21, 2013

Trying to pick up where I left off before the cancer diagnosis. Not many people get a second chance. I was in the process of interviewing on the day I had the mammogram almost a year ago that derailed my efforts to change jobs.

I was super excited that the hospital-based home care company was willing to interview me again. I felt an even deeper financial pressure to change jobs from school nursing to a higher paid nursing job with more consistent hours and not as much unpaid time off. Looking back now, it was so very soon after a year of incredible stress and change. It was a lot to take on. I met with Brooke again and also had a peer interview. I was appreciative that Brooke not only encouraged me from a nursing perspective but also that as a breast cancer survivor she understood more than most how much I needed to pick up where I left off in my life. She gave me the chance to do so and became a mentor in nursing and in cancer survivorship.

Dani is going with me to pick out my new foobs, never thought we would be doing this together.

The prosthetic-buying experience was nothing like I had envisioned it. There was not a lot of teaching in the hospital about what to expect and with all the complications that occurred I had never discussed it in any detail with the surgeon. I thought it would be a bigger deal and wasn't quite sure why I couldn't have done it sooner.

I had an appointment at Benchmark Atlantic, a company that specializes in the fitting of mastectomy forms and compression garments. I didn't know this was something that people could be board certified in. I was impressed by Kathy, the president and owner of this company. Our appointment was actually fun! Walking in, it appeared to be more of a boutique than anything. Dani was welcomed with me. We met in a private room and Kathy spoke about the process and my options for types of prosthesis, also called a breast form.

The remaining time there was spent holding, examining, and trying on different breast forms and pocketed bras. Our laughter and lighthearted banter made the process so easy. At one point Kathy asked if I needed a pocketed sports bra. Dani's eyes widened and my eyebrow furrowed as I declined. I could not comprehend why anyone would want to wear breast prosthetics while working out. I have always been the type not to care what I look like when I go to the gym. You would never find me putting makeup on to go work out.

Before leaving, Kathy gave Dani a fun, colorful knitted hat that she was admiring. She wore it as we drove home laughing about how oddly fun it was to do this together. Wearing prosthetics was something I would have to get used to. I felt like I was just starting to get used to not having anything on my chest. I had gotten used to not buying clothes with v-necks, low crew necks, or tops that were tapered in the breast area. I would have to remember to wear or take my prosthetics with me when trying on clothes now. Thankfully nursing scrubs are pretty basic and I could always wear a thin long-sleeved shirt under a scrub top or a nursing jacket.

Learning to Trust My Body Again

Super excited to start my new job in home health and super sad leaving the people at HHS.

CB: January 27, 2013

Pre-cancer Normal?

Hello all,

So as I try to "get back to pre-cancer 'normal'" my updates will be less often.

The OT/PT is helping my arm, hand, and shoulder symptoms. The biggest help is wearing the splints at night. I occasionally have issues with the swelling in the hand but not as bad as when I first had the lymph nodes removed and had the damage from radiation. I have a sleeve and glove to help prevent it and I have the Caresia when I need more compression. The incisions healed so I have been fitted and have prosthetics. It will take some time to get used to.

I needed to go see the nurse practitioner at the oncologist's office last week because I had to have someone else look at my chest with me and tell me if the changes are normal or not. I don't know what normal is anymore and I am at the point of not trusting my judgment when it comes to self-evaluation.

People talk about denial when you see symptoms of cancer or hear the diagnosis but not often do people realize there is a denial component to being well again. It takes time to trust that my body will not betray me, that I will be able to recognize signs of a recurrence before it is too advanced to cure. It takes time to believe that there is "no evidence of disease."

I decided to move forward on the job change. I have healed enough and I can't live my life in fear that the cancer will come back. The home health position will be better professionally and financially and I think I am doing well. I start my new job with Health at Home on February 11. It is very difficult to leave the high school where everyone has been so supportive, but even in this change they all seem to understand why I am making this career move.

It is important to me that as I reenter my busy lifestyle that I don't forget the lessons learned. I am still making an effort to keep up with people (maybe not through the online journal as much though) and getting together with people on a more regular basis. People have always been the most important thing in my life and I don't want to get too busy for them. I have had a few breakfast, lunch, and dinner dates recently. Met some new friends at a scrapbooking retreat and I am trying to balance my life...a struggle for most of us.

So as I am moving forward you may not see as many updates but take it as "no news is good news" for now. I will update when I have a follow-up appointment, if anything changes or if there is something really on my mind.

TTFN (Ta Ta For Now) Marcy

Lucy: Sounds like a plan Marcy! Congrats on your new job and best of luck with it. You will be awesome and change is good sometimes. Love you!

Alan: Good luck with the home care nursing. It should be a blast. Personally, I enjoy meeting people and finding out their life stories. There's a lot of interesting people out there. Stay well my friend.

GG: Best wishes to you in your new job. I am sure you will love it. Love you.

LM: We will miss you at HHS Marcy! Thank you for all that you have done!!!

JY: Hi Marcy, you will be missed at D601. It was a pleasure to get to know you and walk some of your journey with you. I look forward to your fewer and more far between updates, meaning no news is good news! Please stay in touch and I hope that the home care position works out beautifully. Good luck! I'm sure you will be very good at it!

TH: Hi Marcy! We are going to miss you at HHS! You are so awesome! I always enjoyed our conversations when I was in your office! So happy that your new job is going to be a better position for you. SH is going to miss you very much also! We send you our love and big hugs!

FB: January 29, 2013

The first thing I do when I get home is take my shoes off, the second thing...take my breasts off. Getting my clothes and things ready for the next day, my breasts are laid out next to my scrubs. Weird.

Kitt: That could take some getting used to!

Marcy: A few women I know have said, "I wish I could take mine off when I got home."

Kitt: I'm not sure I'd even want to replace them but it's one of those things I really wouldn't know that answer to unless I had to deal with it...

Marcy: Honestly, it is more comfortable being flat, I mostly wear them to look "normal" for other people. I don't have any issues with needing them to feel like a woman.

As I moved through adjusting to prosthetics there were many times I would not bother putting them on. In the summer they became hot and heavy. I had some waterproof prosthetics that I could insert into the mastectomy bathing suit that I bought online. I wore it a couple of times and then switched to wearing the bottoms and a tank top when I went swimming. The prosthetics were heavy and when I leaned forward in a pool they would pull away from my chest. Ultimately, I knew my life was about my experience, not what others thought of them, and decided to live that way. And sometimes people surprise you. When I talked about cancer to people I just met, they would ask me what type of cancer I had. I would motion to my chest and say, breast cancer. It made me realize that people don't look at other people's chests as much as I perceived they did.

FB: January 29, 2013

Two students I haven't met before were in my office waiting for their mom when the brother says, "Are you the nurse that was here last year?" I said yes, the sister says, "So you're the one who beat cancer?!" We then talked a bit about cancer and treatment and being healthy again. Glad I could answer their questions.

EM: February 16, 2013

From: Marcy

To: Alan

Hi, I hope you are sound asleep.

Nothing good can come from sleep deprivation. I don't know what has gotten into me. I tried to offset my "research" by watching hours of Ellen YouTube videos to make me laugh. Dani joined me for some of it but I feel like someone needs to know what I honestly think and I believe you are the only one that can "handle the truth."

The truth is I don't believe I will be alive to see my five-year mark. If by some chance I do, I will die of shock if I reach the age of fifty-four (ten years). Considering Riley is fourteen now, that doesn't seem long enough. Why do I think this? Because I read too much. This last article, I know it was written in 2007, which makes me wonder how up-to-date it is, but it really got to me tonight. I think the medical community likes to think they are doing better with IBC but I am not convinced. Find me the research articles that show better outcomes. I am not trained to read some of these papers so I may be misinterpreting them or taking it out of context (kind of like when I read the Bible, ha ha). But I have always felt that most physicians don't really get it. They treat it the same as other breast cancers (almost), and then after treatment protocol they say, "No evidence of disease." Well of course there is no evidence, we didn't look for any. It is like a crime scene where the techs never go beyond the police tape. I feel like there is some evidence in there but no one is looking because they want to say it was gone. Then I think that I need to have a psych check. It is like what I was trying to explain in one of the online journal entries. I'm in denial that I am healthy again. I think the best thing I have going for me now is my hormone receptor status and being on Tamoxifen.

I don't think I will live long enough to retire, so I really didn't care about cashing in some of my retirement and I don't think I will add much more to it, other than what is automatically taken out from work. The good news is, because I feel this way, I think I am telling and showing the people in my life that I care and think about them, even with small gestures. Over all, I am happy, I drive around smiling, thinking I have a pretty good life. I do things with the kids, spontaneous get-togethers with friends or family. I mail cards to friends, call people and tell them when I am thinking about them. I stop by to hug people when I am in their area. I want people to remember that I did those things because I don't think I will be able to do them for more than three to eight years. I know it is crazy to think that way but I do. It does make me sad sometimes. Especially when I am sleep deprived. Overall I think it makes me appreciate the moments I have. I am grateful for what I have. I am just worried that the thing I won't have is a long life. Maybe this is God's way of making me be grateful for the time I have, the nagging feeling that I won't have a lot of it. Maybe you will be sending this to me on my five-year mark, ten-year mark, and beyond to say, "See, you were wrong, you are still here." Or maybe you will read this after I am gone and think, "I guess deep down she knew and she was right about the time she had left."

Am I reading these things wrong? Would you be willing to read this and tell me honestly what you think, is it a reputable paper? It sounds like a lot of data from early decades was missing but at least they say that. A lot of the jargon I don't understand. If you have any other resources can you can send my way. Especially any that actually paint a more positive picture of my long-term survival? I would appreciate it. I am thinking there aren't many. (Theoncologist.alphamedpress.org/content/12/8/904.full)

Some of the things that stood out in this one are:

• "Some studies have shown that a multidisciplinary approach can improve both local control and survival, with about 30% of patients living >5 years. Neoadjuvant chemotherapy is considered to be the main component of treatment. The presence of pathological residual disease in the breast and lymph nodes following neoadjuvant chemotherapy is considered an important adverse prognostic factor." ("Residual disease"; I am assuming that I had that due to the cancer still being in the breast tissue and six of twelve lymph nodes after the neoadjuvant chemotherapy?)

• "Other studies of patients with breast cancer have shown that pCR is associated with superior survival outcomes, but not necessarily for IBC."[2] (Yet this makes me think that even if I had pathologic complete response, it wouldn't matter.)

Overall, it is quite worrisome that the survival of these patients has not improved much over these decades, and not only the development of clinical trials to treat this group of patients, but a better understanding of the first principles for IBC, acquired through molecular biology, etiologic epidemiology, and animal models, is needed to improve patient survival. IBC patients have been and still are excluded from the majority of clinical trials, probably because of the rareness of the disease, the lack of knowledge on how to treat these patients, and also the poor advances made against this type of breast cancer. (Maybe this has changed in the five years since this was written... I would welcome any articles/studies, more recent that shows improved survival rates, because really, although people say not to look at numbers and statistics...from what I can tell, only 25 to 40 percent of women with IBC make it to five years, that means 60 to 75 percent of us die in that time. That is a lot. Those aren't really good odds.

Good night, Marcy

2.   Ana M. Gonzalez-Angulo, Bryan T. Hennessy, Kristine Broglio, Funda Meric-Bernstam, Massimo Cristofanilli, Sharon H. Giordano, Thomas A. Buchholz, et al., "Trends for Inflammatory Breast Cancer: Is Survival Improving?," *Oncologist* 12, no. 8 (2007): 904–12, http://theoncologist.alphamedpress.org/content/12/8/904.full.

From: Alan

To: Marcy

Good morning, I hope you had some decent sleep.

I couldn't figure out the best way to structure my reply so it might be a little jumbled. I subscribe to *Up To Date, Prescriber's Letter, 5 Minute Clinical Consult,* and others. They review a lot of these papers. This paper is a good one and considered "recent." The average quote in these sources regarding five-year survival rates is around 40 percent. They site all types of journal papers but none are "apples to apples."

Your interpretation of your situation, from scientific standpoint, is accurate. And I wouldn't lie to you or minimize your conclusions.

But, what does 40 percent mean to Marcy Browning? You're not spinning a roulette wheel one hundred times. One way I look at it is like this: In the next five years the cancer will reappear or it won't. *Your* odds of recurrence are really 0 percent or 100 percent because there's only one of you.

So live the way you feel your life should be conducted, but assume *your* odds of survival are 100 percent. They say it's better to believe in God and be wrong than not believe in God and be wrong.

I'd like to share a story I've only shared with Sophie. I had a best friend from kindergarten until we moved in fifth grade—Robert. We lived on the same block. We played baseball and floor hockey and traded baseball cards. Life in third grade was perfect. One fall day his dad was killed in a car accident. I couldn't process it. It's not right. How could he not have a dad?

I spent the next two years at 6 p.m. riding my bike as far as I was allowed waiting to see my dad's car come around the corner. It always did but the anxiety took its toll.

Every day since that I'm able to enjoy with family and friends is like an extra day and a day I'm grateful for.

Every day when I say goodbye to Sophie I wonder if this will be the last day one of us is here.

So I live like you live. Hug someone and tell them how much they mean to you. Have fun. Make good memories.

You're right about the stats and the data, but forget about it—it's not meant for you. It's meant for journal editors and conferences. I once asked an advisor at Merrill Lynch, "How much money will I need when I retire?" She answered, "When are you going to die?" So there you have it.

Alan

From: Marcy

To: Alan

Thank you. I like knowing my interpretation isn't way off but I also like the different options at looking at numbers and especially the confirmation regarding living life with gratitude and appreciation for people. Overall, I feel good today as I sit in the local community college parking lot and wait for Riley. He is learning to scuba dive.

Thanks for the feedback. Marcy

EM: February 19, 2013

From: Marcy

To: Alan

Subject : Home Care

Hi, I think I am going to like my job but there definitely will be higher stress times depending on the acuity and number of patients I have.

Today in training, I saw *two* women with breast cancer. They both had reconstruction... It really reinforced my decision to not do it. The incisions they have are ridiculous. One has it all the way across her lower abdomen and the other has it half way down the left side of her back...and those are just the donor sites, not even dealing with the expanders and breast incisions... *No thank you*, not for me. The other patient we saw today had the choice of going to the hospital today or trying the diuretic and possibly going to the hospital tomorrow. I really think she should have been in the hospital but maybe it will be okay. The next patient was discharged from home care and hospice is starting tomorrow. There were a couple others today also. I will go out again with another nurse tomorrow, then on to five days of OASIS [Outcome and Assessment Information Set, a medicare guideline for home health care] and computer training.

Tomorrow I have a follow up with the radiation oncologist, that shouldn't be a big deal.

Not doing very well with diet and exercise. If I can beat cancer, why can't I beat obesity? It is so hard! I was considering checking into Eight Weeks to Wellness and the chiropractic center nearby. It seems comprehensive and may give me the focused jump start I need to get back on the right track. I don't know how expensive it is though.

Things going okay with the chiropractor?

Take care.

From: Alan

To: Marcy

Hi, I totally agree with the reconstruction. The prosthetics are very natural. You still got it goin' on girlfriend.

As far as weight loss goes, set achievable goals. Make small gradual changes in diet. Do a treadmill or bike every day for a few minutes, cut out one bad food at a time.

I'm liking this chiropractor. He's cracking my back once a week. It doesn't hurt anyway. By the time he's done with me I'll be six feet five inches tall.

As with most things I have thoughts on breast reconstruction and what I've learned about women. It may be weird or off base but if you're interested in my thoughts I will share them with you.

My guess is your new position will be quite rewarding and enjoyable. I think it will take effort and time to get there. Sometimes that thought is daunting, but something like this is worth the effort. The satisfaction of hard work and time spent is far more sweet than the instant gratifications of our current times. Enjoy the ride.

Sleep tight.

EM: February 20, 2013

From: Marcy

To: Alan

Yes, I would like to know, what are your thoughts on reconstruction? I want to know if married women my age are more likely to have reconstruction because of their spouses and if single women my age opt not to have it.

TTYL

From: Alan

To: Marcy

I have many thoughts not in any particular order.

I think most married women do not have reconstruction if they're in a good relationship. I know I'd rather have my wife be healthy than worry about saline or silicone breasts.

From: Marcy

To: Alan

Without bashing on Jack (okay, never mind, I will be bashing him a little but it is the truth as I see it), we talked about this when I did the Avon Walk but seeing his behavior, how important sex and image are for him, I think he would have made things much worse and I am glad I am single.

From: Alan

To: Marcy

I think if I were dating a woman who had undergone mastectomies I'd care only about our relationship. Any decent man would too. A relationship is what matters, not breasts. As far as sex and intimacy, there's endless possibilities for erotic adventures and stimulation without boobs. Cosmo would lead us to believe that we all should be gold medalists in intimacy. It's not realistic. A good relationship is truly what matters. I base this not on my own experience but on the countless conversations I've had with men and women who somehow feel deficient in their sexual prowess based on some ridiculous standards from TV, movies, and magazines.

From: Marcy

To: Alan

Totally not worried about this. I don't think I will ever really want that kind of intimate relationship again but if I do, if they can't handle the chest flat they aren't the person for me.

From: Alan

To: Marcy

The main thing I've learned over the years is that women want to look nice. A very common encounter: A 78-year-old women comes in on a

Wednesday with a cold. She has a wedding this weekend and she wants to know if it's OK to get her hair done tomorrow. She bought a new dress and doesn't want to miss the wedding. She wants to look nice. I'd say 96 percent of women I've seen as patients—all ages, shapes and sizes—want to look nice. It might be a piece of jewelry, a dress, makeup, whatever, but it's a very common theme.

Another thing I've noticed is women look at other women as much or more than men do. Women worry more about the relative prettiness of other women a lot. Women make a ton of comments about other women's boobs or clothes, etc.

From: Marcy

To: Alan

That is true, women can be real malicious too.

From: Alan

To: Marcy

And quite honestly, I've never met a woman who was happy with her breasts. I've heard so many self-deprecating comments during exams about size, shape, etc. It's kinda sad to be held to a self-inflicted standard of an imagined perfection.

There's a ridiculous standard set for women—supermodel, movie actress. It's crazy.

From: Marcy

To: Alan

That's sad.

From: Alan

To: Marcy

Here's what I think, and this may get a little awkward. The prosthetics are very natural looking. You're an attractive woman. You're still young. My guess is you want to look nice, attractive, and feminine and you can, you absolutely can. I get that you want to lose a few pounds but don't ever feel unattractive if you don't get to your weight goal.

From: Marcy

To: Alan

I am really thinking I have handled the no-breasts situation well. Even with being called sir a lot for a while, I know I don't need breasts to be feminine. I don't care about that very much. The weight is an issue, partly for looks and feeling sexy but also because I have been at a good weight (probably last time was in 2008) and I liked how I felt then. The energy I have, the mood. The benefits of losing weight are much greater now than ever before. Not sure why I struggle with it so much.

From: Alan

To: Marcy

And if you find yourself in a relationship and he's a good guy then everything will be ok. There's adult fun to be had without boobs.

From: Marcy

To: Alan

True, very true.

From: Alan

To: Marcy

In sum, you made the right choice. And it's still OK to try to look nice. And you do.

Be good,

Alan

From: Marcy

To: Alan

Thank you! You are such a good person; I am proud to be able to call you my friend.

Marcy

CB: February 20, 2013

Follow-Up Appointment

Hi all,

I went to the radiation oncologist today for routine follow-up, he says there is "no evidence of disease." I will see him in another three months. Sometimes there are side effects from radiation that become evident later, just like there can be damage from chemotherapy that shows up later. No worries though, things are going pretty well.

I am not going to OT/PT anymore. I think now that the bad pain in the hand, arm, and shoulder is gone, the rest will just take time. I will just manage symptoms as they occur.

I started my new job and will be in training for a little while; a lot has changed in home care since I did it full time. I think I will like it though and it will be rewarding and well paying.

Yesterday I saw two women who just had mastectomies and reconstruction. It is such an individual decision. It did reinforce my decision not to have it. I can't see ever changing my mind on that. I am used to the prosthetics, for the most part.

My next appointments aren't until the end of March. I will see the medical oncologist and will be due for my yearly physical. That will be full circle from when this all started last March. I guess if I am looking at the bright side, I can say, "At least I don't ever have to have a mammogram again." As for the rest of you women out there, get them done!

I want to remember what it means to "live like you're dying" and continue to prioritize my life that way. People are most important, no one knows how much time they have left, let's make it count.

Take care, love ya, Marcy

P.S. Still having low blood pressure readings. I stopped taking it myself. Figured I felt okay, why obsess about it. Today at the doctor appointment the blood pressure was 88/63. If I take my beta blocker my BP is lower; if I don't my heart rate is too fast. I guess I will go back to taking half a tab and seeing if that works for the heart rate.

GG: Marcy you are so special.

CP: That's great news Marcy. Glad to hear you're doing well. Good luck in your new job.

DA: Hi Marcy, You were in my prayers last night and was thinking that I wanted to send you a note. I'm so glad to hear your report. Things are so much better. What a long year it has been for you but I think you have learned what we all need to learn—to live life intentionally. You have taught us all so much. Thanks for sharing your ups and downs and now your victory. You are an inspiration! Many continued blessings

Alan: You're doing great! Give yourself a pat on the back today. And take good care of those patients.

JH: I am so happy for you; you made it through so much!! Your spikey hair is *awesome*!! I bet it is nice to have hair to spike. Good luck in your home health job.

PH: Hi Marcy, Glad for the update and happy for you that things are going well! You look absolutely awesome and love your "do," as in hair do!!!! Love you.

CB: February 26, 2013

Relay for Life as a Survivor

Last year, weeks after signing up for Relay for Life, I was diagnosed with cancer. I didn't participate in the event as it was days after my first chemo. This year I *will* be there, maybe even speaking. Definitely taking a survivor lap. Please come to opening ceremony, donate, participate, and celebrate with me! Being there would not be possible without all of you.

Love, Marcy

Late winter and early spring of 2013 I spent less time posting on the CaringBridge medical journal site but cancer continued to be a daily topic. In between parenting, continued appointments to follow up with doctors, and OT/PT, I was starting a new job.

The home health position required training on the computer, refreshing some of the knowledge and skills that I had not used in some time and getting to know many new coworkers and members of the medical community. It proved to be a time of both getting out of my self to help others but at the same time it involved looking back on what had happened over the last year.

The Difference a Year Makes

CB: March 12, 2013

Checking In

Hi all,

Just wanted to check in with you all and see how things are going and update you on what I have been doing.

I started my new job at health at home one month ago. Lots of training, lots to learn but it is going well.

Other than that keeping me busy, I am working on a speech for Relay for Life. It is a challenge to really think about the events of last year and how it has changed the person I am today. I would love if you could come hear it or donate to the event.

Okay, about the prosthetics. It seems like I view them more as an accessory than a body part. I am more used to them now but have been frustrated that a lot of the shirts I wore before the surgery I can't wear anymore. The shirts don't fit right, even with the prosthetics on. I may have to avoid V- necks. I am very comfortable without breasts. It's almost like, when getting ready for the day, I decide if I want to put them on, like: Should I wear a watch, should I wear my breasts? On the weekends, why bother.

I am still frustrated with my physical weight. It isn't about appearance; it is about being uncomfortable. Just moving around my body when it is heavier is more of a task. I am going to get some help with that. I love Weight Watchers and think it is a healthy program but I think I need a little more accountability and guidance, so I am going to look into some other programs and see if one can give me the jump start I need.

Overall things are normalizing a little bit more every day. I am so happy spring is on the way.

Please keep in touch and come to Relay for Life if you can.

Love,

Marcy

Alan: I'll be there. I just might need a GPS to find it is all. But I'll be there!

JY: Hi Marcy, So glad to hear your update. I was just thinking about you yesterday! I'll look forward to seeing you at the relay!

CB: March 29, 2013

One Year Later

I can hardly believe that last year at this time I was trying to figure out how to tell my family I had cancer, worried about what it would mean, wondering if I had a future. Today, I got the tattoo I had been talking about, similar to Dani's but still my own. You'll probably think I am crazy. Well, that doesn't matter, most people know I am crazy BUT I almost didn't get "Survivor" written on the tattoo because I was afraid of "jinxing" myself. Isn't that silly?

My follow-up with the medical oncologist was uneventful. No tests, no labs. He asked if I wanted an MRI for the headaches or a CT scan because of the cough. I told him I could wait for a few more weeks, and see if it goes away.

I'm still stressing a bit about the Relay for Life speech, haven't thought about it in a week or so. Instead I have been focusing on the new job and learning all I can. It feels awesome to be caring for patients in their home again.

I hope to see you at Relay and thank you for donating. I have been trying to remember the lessons learned over the last year. As I am now back to work full time and trying to live a "normal" life. I don't want to forget that people are the most important thing to me and time has more value than money. I have been trying to call or write to people when I think about them and see and hug people when I can. I am grateful for you!

Love,

Marcy

Delivering a well written, meaningful speech was important to me. I worked for hours on it. I wrote a long speech that needed to be cut into the time frame allowed. I then called Miriam and Hannah and read the speech to them for practice. I clearly remember, sitting in my car in a parking lot where I could read my speech to Miriam without anyone at home hearing it yet. Edits were made, tears were shed, and I practiced again later by calling Hannah. More edits made, more tears shed. I was so excited but also anxious as this would be done at the high school where I worked during the time I had cancer. It would be in front of those students, families, faculty, and staff. I knew it would be emotional and I hoped it would be helpful.

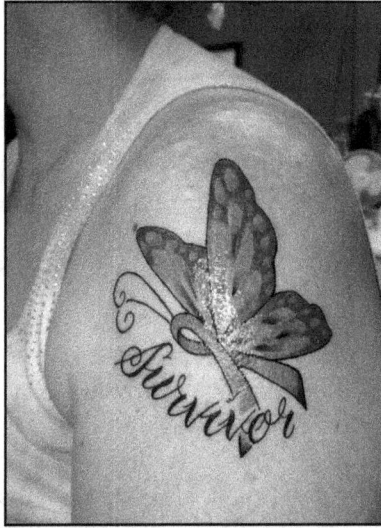

Figure 7-2. My breast cancer survivor tattoo

Miriam remembers my call and practice speech. It was hard for me to read the speech to her; it was hard for her to hear it. We didn't pretend objectivity to this nearly life-destroying event. She had been so afraid of my death, and when a close friend lives so far away it is even worse. She says now, "What I remember most was your strength. I was in awe of everything you handled while you were going through the treatment. How you continued to care for your family and work and love others." She continues, "I will always wish I had been closer and able to do more. But I'm so thankful for the people you had around you who were able to provide that support, the assistance getting to your appointments and caring for you on your bad days. I'm just grateful that you had what you needed to get through it, and that includes a whole lot of hard work and determination on your part too." I think hearing or reading the speech was the first time many heard the story all at once and the impact of hearing all the events at once made an impression.

CB: April 18, 2013

More Nervous

Hi all,

It's been a while and I guess that's a good thing. I have been busy with work and getting into the swing of things. A lot to learn, but it is rewarding being on the caregiving side of healthcare instead of being the patient. I feel like I have an even better perspective than I did before and I think my patients really can feel that I care and understand.

Soooo, tomorrow is the Relay for Life at Hamilton High School. I will be one of three speakers so I don't know exact time or order of things but the opening ceremony starts at 6 p.m.

Hope to see you there, please ignore my shaky voice.

My mom and I went to the survivor and caregiver dinner at Hamilton High School prior to opening ceremonies of Relay for Life. I thought she was given some well-deserved and long overdue acknowledgment for her support of me and my family. Walking around the high school less than two months after resigning from my nursing position was bizarre. Combining my roles of school nurse, survivor, former employee, friend, loved one, and now speaker was peculiar. I felt like all eyes were on me walking through the hallways and at the same time felt unrecognizable.

This was my first Relay for Life experience since I wasn't able to go the year before. Roger, Patti, Dani, and Riley met my mom and me there. As it was expected to be poor weather for the weekend, tents were set up inside. We walked around the cafeteria and gym looking at the set-ups people had selling food, crafts, and cancer awareness items. This was not just a breast cancer event and all types of cancer were represented. As we made our rounds many hugs and introductions were made.

Other friends and family started to arrive and meet us at our spot on the bleachers. Ron and Laurie, Liza, Jade, Alan, my dad, and his wife came as well. I knew with Alan's pain it was a great undertaking for him to drive out there, stand for that long, and sit on bleachers. He reminded me that after the speech he might duck out and not be able to find me to say good-bye. I understood and thanked him.

I was the second speaker and along with my speech I brought a basket up to the microphone with me. Dani and Riley sat on the floor among the other high school students and younger kids. There was a numerous rows of adults in a half circle of around where the kids were seated. I know they were taking bets on how far into the speech I could get before crying. Whoever said less than two paragraphs won. As the first tears came, I was able to make a joke about such a bet, laugh, and regain my composure. I frequently looked up to make eye contact with my family and friends, partly to trick myself into thinking they were the only ones there, partly so they knew when I was talking about the support I received they knew I was referring to them, but mostly because I really wanted them to understand how much it meant to me to have them with me.

During the speech I held up my basket and acknowledged the stack of cards and letters that I read over and over while lying in bed. I shared the examples of the gifts, talked about the luminaries lit, and all the power they have on reducing cancer's impact on the people in their lives and society as a whole.

After the speeches were done, the kids, my mom and I walked hand in hand the first lap of the relay, the survivor's lap. We all were fairly physically and emotionally spent and sat and talked for awhile, visited with some friends and went home that night. As I reviewed the events of the day in my head before going to sleep I relished the overall sense of peace, I hoped it would last.

CB: April 29, 2013

Relay for Life Speech, Uncut

My story is about breast cancer, but there are about 200 types of cancer and we are here in support of all people affected by all cancers. We are here to do something about it so that future generations don't have to. When I think about my personal story of cancer I think it's best to start it from when I signed up for Relay for Life in 2012.

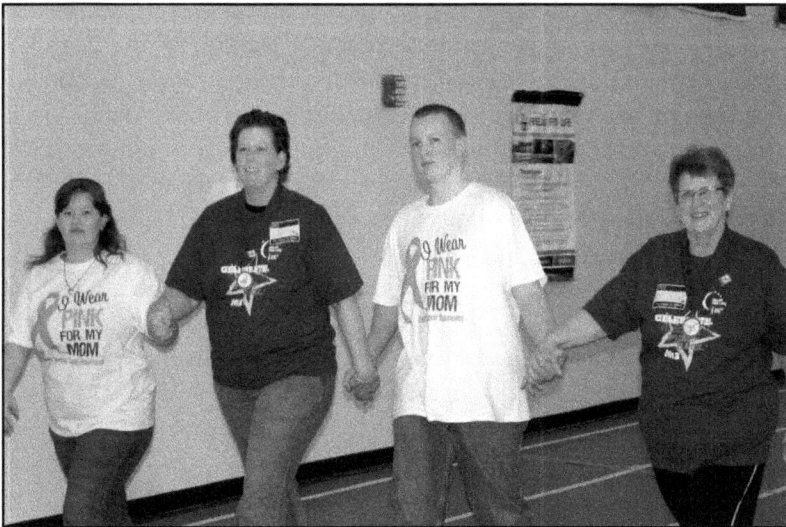

Figure 7-3. Dani, me, Riley, and Mom walking the Survivor's Lap at Relay for Life

I was working here as the Hamilton High School nurse and I wanted to be more involved. Little did I know when I signed up for the Relay on February 18 that just six weeks later my doctor would be calling me to say I had an invasive and aggressive form of breast cancer. Over spring break I had gone for my routine physical and yearly mammogram and I honestly believe if I had not done that I would not be standing here today. Inflammatory breast cancer makes up only 1 percent to 5 percent of all breast cancers and is automatically staged as at least a 3B. They saw from the scans that it was in a lymph node but not in any other organs. That was the good news I was trying to hold onto. I needed chemotherapy before surgery to keep it from spreading so a few days before the Relay for Life event at Jackson High School I started chemotherapy and was unable to participate in the event. Thank you for participating, for thinking of me and for the luminaries. You made a difference! Because of your support I was able to get a wig from the American Cancer Society to wear to my son's eighth grade graduation. Every one of you are making a difference.

I am going to tell you briefly about what it took to treat my cancer. I had a chemotherapy treatment every two weeks for four months and switched chemicals half way through. I had side effects making the last two months of chemo very difficult for me to get through. After chemo I had bilateral mastectomies with twelve lymph nodes removed on the side of the cancer. I was discouraged to find out that after four months of chemo there was cancer in six of the lymph nodes. I had side effects from that surgery, mainly related to fluid buildup at the surgical site and lymphedema from the lymph node removal. I had thirty-five radiation treatments with side effects and complications, mostly involving burned, peeling skin and infection. Before I could finish radiation I got sick with an abscess and cellulitis. Those infections caused me to be in the hospital for a week. I had IV antibiotics for seventeen days and another surgery in which some of the chest muscle was also removed. I had side effects from the second surgery as well, causing limited range of motion in my arm, pain, numbness, tingling, and weakness in my right arm. All of this caused me to lose a lot of time from my job here. Eventually I did physical therapy to help with some of those complications. The radiation that I expected to be done in October was finally finished on December 20. I received my last radiation treatment and at that point, in my mind, went from a cancer fighter to a cancer survivor! The day after radiation was complete I went on Tamoxifen, an oral hormone therapy treatment to prevent the return of the cancer.

Among all the feelings associated with a cancer diagnosis a major one is powerlessness. We are here today to prove that we are not powerless. There are things you can do as an individual, a loved one and as a cancer fighter to prove that we are definitely not powerless!

To prevent cancer for yourself... Live a healthy lifestyle. If you smoke—quit, get help if you need it. Eat healthier, move more. Get routine physicals and suggested cancer screenings such as mammograms, colonoscopies, and blood tests; whatever is appropriate for your age and gender. Learn your risks factors and your genetic history, then change the things you can.

If you have a friend or family member who has cancer, here are some suggestions of things you can do to help them with their journey. These are just some of the things done for me. Be creative. Being supportive doesn't have to cost money. A lot of these ideas don't take much time either but I knew I was loved and cared for, which gave me hope and strength when I felt discouraged and weak. I'm going to present these things in the form of a thank you for what my friends and family did for me. I may not even get to all of it but I want you to know that what you have done has made a difference. So... Thank you for:

- Sending me cards—I look at them frequently, even now.

- Sending me emails and calling, texting, or sending me messages on social media.

- Thank you for reading my online journal. Thanks for making encouraging comments.

- Thank you for the gifts in the mail, the flowers, fruit arrangement, balloons, and Lou Malnati's pizza, jewelry, music boxes, movies, and even a good luck penny from Vegas.

- Thank you for cleaning my house.

- Thank you for putting up plastic on my windows to keep out the winter draft after I had surgery and couldn't lift my arms.

- Thank you for going with me to chemo. For going to the doctor appointments with me and for helping me process and remember what was said.

- Thank you for waiting with my family, while I was in surgery.

- Thank you for visiting me in the hospital and after I got home.

- Thank you for buying a movie for me and watching it with me at my house.

- Thank you for hanging out at the amusement park with my son, Riley, and me so I wouldn't have to do it alone.

- Thank you for organizing my kids' birthday parties and graduation parties, so we could celebrate together.

- Thank you for caring about my comfort, for the handmade knitted prayer shawl and the comfy body pillow. For the candy to get the awful taste out of my mouth that I had from chemo.

- Thank you for going to pick up my medicines for me when I couldn't get off the couch and the burn cream when I couldn't leave work to do it.

- Thank you for the encouraging words, especially to the nurse who told me to "keep fighting" when I was coming out of surgery. I couldn't even open my eyes or speak yet, but I heard you.

- Thank you for letting me cry... I did a lot of that.

- Thank you for making me laugh, I did a lot of that too.

- Thank you for giving me time alone but for not letting me be alone for a long time.

- Thank you for the money you collected and donated to me directly and the money you donated to the Relay for Life and even the donation in my name to Hurricane Sandy Relief.

- Thank you for taking Riley to do things so he could get out of the house when I didn't feel well.

- Thank you for praying for me and putting my family and me on your prayer lists. Thanks for thinking about me and sending me good vibes.

- Thank you for buying the pink ribbon items, for the pink streaks in your hair, and pink t-shirts and hats. For making pink pumpkins and jewelry. For signing the pink fire truck for me, for participating in runs and events to fight cancer.

- Thank you for letting me sit around your campfire or hang out at your house and do nothing but watch Bears football. Thanks for cooking for me.

- Thank you especially to my mom and kids, who live with me. You saw me at my worst and held it all together.

Dani and Riley, I am so incredibly proud of you. My children are the reason I fought for my life. I love you.

If you are a minor and your parent has cancer you are not powerless. The best way you can help them is by taking care of yourself in whatever way you can. Most likely they don't want you to have to take care of them. They will be better able to take care of themselves knowing you are going to be responsible for yourself, your schoolwork, and your health. Hang out and spend time with them but still get out and enjoy your life. They don't want their struggle with cancer to hold you back. Talk to people if you are struggling, it is normal to need help during tough times and you deserve to get what you need.

If you are faculty or staff at a school and you are aware of a student with cancer or a student with a family member who is fighting cancer, spend some extra time keeping track of those students. Don't wait until you see signs that they are struggling. If it's a student with cancer, they need to know you have their back when they don't feel well and that you will help them get caught up. If the cancer fighter is a parent, they will feel more at peace and better able to do what they need to for themselves if they know someone is watching out for their children. The children will do better knowing you understand their struggle at home. They may be hesitant to ask their struggling parent for the help they need or ask you. Don't wait to be asked to support a student who is struggling.

If you are now in the fight against cancer, talk to your family and friends, tell them your feelings, because you will experience every feeling imaginable, and sometimes several at the same time. If you need to talk to a counselor do it. I did. Sometimes you just need to talk to someone about doubts and fears, someone who isn't a family member or friend. Let people help you. This has always been a tough thing for me, but I learned that sometimes you give help and sometimes you need it. It feels good to help others and others get that same feeling from helping you. Enjoy the moments you have with your family and friends. Explore the things that relax you. During chemo I listened to songs suggested by my family and friends. It made it feel as though they were with me. I strongly recommend creating an online journal web page. It's a wonderful outlet to keep people informed and get support from your family and friends as well as a place to vent your troubles when you need to.

Become a part of your healthcare team. Learn what you can about your treatment and don't be afraid to ask questions. Get a second opinion. It doesn't mean you don't trust your doctor; it's just to help you get on board with the plan and put your mind at ease. Take pain medicine if you need it. A doctor told me, "You don't get any points for suffering." You are stronger than you realize.

If you are a cancer survivor, what can you do now? I don't think many realize how hard it is to feel like a normal and healthy person again after going through so much in the battle against cancer. There is denial and there is doubt. "Is it really gone? Will it come back?" This is my current struggle and I am making a concerted effort to trust that my health is good and I can move on now. I will never forget the life lessons that I've learned. I want to look forward and plan for my future without taking today for granted.

As a survivor, I will fight cancer by sharing my story. I will look for ways to be involved. I am currently enrolled in a study being done by the American Cancer Society that will evaluate an online workshop for cancer survivors. I want a quality life. The treatments we have now have kept me alive but we need to save more cancer fighters with more effective treatments that have fewer side effects and fewer complications. Too many cancer patients die of complications from therapy; we need more research to prevent and cure all types of cancers and prevent recurrences. We need to continue to support cancer patients and their families. Your participation today will help move us forward on that.

You guys are awesome! As a good friend of mine, Alan, always says, "Now go make some memories."

Alan: Awesome! You did great last night. It was your night to shine. I saw your smile on the survivors' lap. It brought tears to my eyes.

Reflections

The immediate months following the end of cancer treatments proved to be what I think now was a honeymoon phase of recovery. There were holidays, a vacation, a new job, and celebrations of the end of cancer treatments. I still had many doctor appointments to go to plus physical and occupational therapy but I was trying to move forward with my life. As the confetti settled on the ground the dust was kicked up and choked me. I would continue to seek help from friends and family and the medical field to come to terms with the changes in me and the overall feeling that cancer could rear its ugly head and try to take me away from what I held most dear: the people in my life.

— *8* —

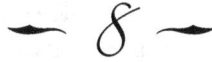

Survivorship

New Battles

CB: April 25, 2013

The Truth of the Matter—My Fight Continues

Hi all,

So I am back on the roller coaster. I know I should look to the future but feel sometimes I think I should have gone to a cancer treatment center. I don't think I got the most aggressive treatment and I worry still about the fact that I didn't achieve pCR (pathological complete response). I think it is a vicious cycle. I don't feel great so I worry, lose sleep, and then feel worse. I believe my mental health would be better if they would just do the damn PET scan. Depression? Food addiction? Obesity? Cancer? These diseases add to the fatigue, sleep deprivation and overall feeling of malaise. Society is much less supportive of things they believe are just a plain and simple choice and see the fight with weight and depression as a matter of will power. I wonder if we supported those with food addiction and depression as much as those with cancer, how quickly we would reduce all the problems associated with depression and food addiction. It doesn't do much for my self-esteem to think... Yeah I beat cancer but I can't beat obesity or depression.

Love and Hugs, Marcy

P.S. I still feel like I am fighting all of this but in a different way. I did join an IBC support group online and am meeting some IBC survivors of ten to eleven years (so far that is the best I can find).

One other thing: To my out-of-state friends who think they haven't been able to help because of the distance: I love you all. Thank you for listening to me, and keeping in touch, really you have done so much for me!

CB: April 27, 2013

On to the Lazy River

Hi, my friend sent me an email saying time to get off the roller coaster and into the lazy river. I loved that. Today I went to the amusement park with Riley and rode some coasters. Yeah, I know better but really wanted to do that with him. We walked around the park several times and now I am really sore and down for the count.

The online IBC support group has been very informative and interesting. When people are aware you have breast cancer all the breast cancer survivors rally to support you and it helped a lot, because there are many. Yet the whole time not many knew much about IBC. It scared me not to know any IBC survivors. My lymphedema therapist knew one before me, recently treated. My oncologist said they treated one woman who is an eight-year survivor. I found a few here and there, mostly five to eight year survivors but the further out in years the fewer I could find. I have found a few more in the ten- to eleven-year range through this private Facebook group and have heard rumors of a twenty-four-year survivor. Maybe they are out there but just don't participate in groups anymore. Many in the group are getting treatment now or in their first one to two years after treatment. Startling how many are dealing with recurrences.

I see the radiation oncologist May 20 and the medical oncologist's nurse practitioner in late June. If I am not feeling better physically and mentally by the June appointment, I am going to ask for a PET scan. If that doesn't go over well I may even consider going down to that cancer specialist's hospital. The more IBC patients they have on record the more data they can get for future changes. They are doing a lot of research and trials.

For now, I am going to put my feet up and relax. I hope you are enjoying the beautiful weather!

Marcy

Jade: It was so great to see you last week and you were amazing. After I read what you wrote, you reminded me of how I felt when I was done with treatment. It's hard to trust your body again after all you have been through. Plus, how unfair is it that we get cancer, lose our boobs, gain weight from the poison we have them infuse through our veins, and then we are supposed to go back to our life and wait anxiously for tests to be done on their schedule while we anxiously wait. If I interpreted you wrongly I am sorry but if not, I totally understand. That's why I said ten to fifteen years. Always praying for you.

PO: Thinking of you Marcy—be gentle with yourself... You have been through so much!

CB: May 16, 2013

Emotional Recovery

No one really told me about emotional recovery from cancer treatment. I feel like the expectation was that when the treatment was over, celebration happens and I move on. It's not happening like that for me.

I am sure there are a lot of factors contributing to my fatigue and headaches. Stress of a new job, being overweight, medication adjustments, thyroid being off, heart rate being off, all adding up to not sleeping well. I am exhausted and overemotional. I love my patients but I am crushed when I have to transfer them to hospice. I have many cancer patients right now and they are not ready for hospice but will be soon. It is so hard. I see families struggling to care for their loved ones and I feel powerless in many ways. With some patients I have "survivor's guilt" because I know they are terminal.

It has been a tough week. Sometimes I don't want to be a nurse anymore. I had to pull over twice today in between patients and cry. I went into my clinical manager's office and cried. She is a survivor too and thankfully knew exactly why I was crying. We discussed antidepressants but she also said the only one our oncology group says is okay while taking Tamoxifen is Lexapro and I can't take that (I did in the '90s and almost fell asleep behind the wheel—I don't need more fatigue).

Thank goodness the weekend is almost here. On a good note, my supervisor did my ninety-day review and I got all "exceeds expectations." I also got a MVP recognition based on a nice card one of my patients sent in. Now I just have to decide is it worth the emotional upheaval and the exhaustion. Big sigh.

GG: Marcy, you are amazing. Always remember God is walking with you. Look to him and he will guide you. Love you

JH: Hi Marcy. I know so much of what you are going through, and you have been through so much more than I have! I take Effexor (venlafaxine), an antidepressant, and it helps a lot. It also is safe with Tamoxifen and seems to help hot flashes too. Ask about it.

I know it's tough, posttreatment is so hard to get used to. I don't know why. If your job is not right for you, especially right now, you can change again. You need energy too, you give it out at your job and at home. Keep thinking about what YOU want to do. It does not matter what anyone else thinks—really, I mean it, not even kids. This is about you. And don't feel guilty or feel like everyone comes before you, IBC didn't feel that way, it picked you. Now is your time.

Alan: Your job is hard but vitally important. Would you want anyone else doing it for you? No, of course not. Is there anyone who could do it better? No, definitely not. You do good work for people and it matters. It takes its toll but it's as rewarding as it gets to comfort someone in a time of need. It's especially hard to be called upon to help others when you yourself are suffering. Hang in there!

Betty: I cannot even begin to imagine what you are going through. What I do know is that you *are* a strong woman with people who love you and care for you. You are always in my thoughts and prayers. Even though we are separated by many miles, you are always near in my heart. God will see you through all of this. Hang in there sweet lady. Love you.

Lucy: I'm sure there are so many reasons why you are so emotional—many of them due to the nature of your job and yes, what you have just been through. I'll email you, but give your body time to adjust and settle in. As you know, hormones can cause a multitude of issues. Love you dear friend!

SS: Marcy, I know exactly how you feel. The thing is, you would not be you if you didn't care. We have tremendous empathy for our patients, and it wouldn't matter if they were cancer patients or not...you just care and want to help your patients, no matter their age or their diagnosis. So often, we home health people, bring our patients home with us. You know that. I have to think, this is God's child, I am just a helper, He is in control...I can help, I cannot change things. Love you... Stay happy and healthy. Miss you at school.

DA: Hi Marcy, I know you have a really hard job. It takes a very special person to handle everything you are doing. I know that you have a great heart of compassion for your patients. They are blessed to have you for their nurse. I will pray for God's guidance for you.

Peace of Mind, Hard to Find

EM: May 19, 2013

From: Marcy

To: Brooke

Hi Brooke:

I am trying to work out a consult appointment. If I do, I will need time off to get to Texas, get the consult and testing, and get back. I am considering the last week in June or the first week in July while Riley is at camp, so I won't have to worry about him. Do you think I can work it out at Health at Home? I really think this will give me the peace of mind I need to move on with my life.

Thanks,

Marcy

From: Brooke

To: Marcy

We will work it out. You need this testing.

CB: June 6, 2013

A Long Way to Go for Peace of Mind

I have an appointment on June 13th at the cancer center. My specialist is the clinical director at the Inflammatory Breast Cancer Clinic. I think if he tells me that I am okay with the treatment I had and the cancer didn't get through my lymph nodes to any other place in my body I will believe it. All I am asking of him is to actually make sure there is "no evidence of disease." It is a long way to go and costly but my peace of mind is worth it, isn't it?

Alan: It's worth every cent and then some. Safe travels!

Lucy: I think that is a great step if it will give you peace of mind. It is your health and your life, so pray hard and do what you have to do! Love you!

JY: Marcy, I think it's a great idea no matter how far or expensive it is for your peace of mind. Good luck with everything and I'll look forward to seeing how the visit goes... Hang in there!!!

GG: You are worth it!!

JH: Your peace of mind is more important than anything, for you and for your family. You are so doing the right thing.

DA: Peace of mind is a priceless gift. I would do it too! You continue in my prayers.

CB: June 18, 2013

Texas

Hi, I have spoken to some of you and many have asked about my trip to Texas and if I am going to update the online journal site.

Yes, eventually. I left Texas very confused, concerned, and a little angry. I am still trying to process what was done and not done while I was down there. I will explain later...maybe this weekend.

Thanks for checking up on me, more info to come,

Marcy

CB: June 23, 2013

Whom Do I Believe? Where Do I Go from Here?

Hi, sorry about the silence. I really hate when people know how confused and distraught I am. I have been working on making sense of and accepting what happened, or didn't happen at the specialist and trying to figure out where to go from here. Even after all this time, I apologize if this is confusing. I am going to try to explain things and then tell you what is going on now but please be patient.

I have recently read this by Ann Landers: "Nobody gets to live life backward. Look ahead, that is where your future lies."

I don't want to live backward but I think sometimes I have to look back to make sense of today so I can look ahead to the future. Here are some confusing details.

I went to that cancer center because that is where one of the first clinics for inflammatory breast cancer is. They are one of the most active in care and research on IBC and have a phenomenal reputation. They are the experts. Before I say anything else I want to first give the physician credit for making sure he asked if I had questions and waiting for an answer, but of course I was just flabbergasted at what he told me and could not come up with anything until later when I was in my hotel room. Ten days later and I am still unsettled about what he told me.

My expectations: I had thought that he would

- Review my records, which he did.

- Ask me questions about my history, which he did (although partially, he only asked about my symptoms prior to treatment, not anything about treatment).

- Ask me about my current complaints, which he didn't, although they were on the questionnaire.

- Examine me, which he did, although his exam would have been more thorough if he knew or cared about what my complaints were.

- Make recommendations, which he did (I'll get to that later).

- And I was hoping based on that he would order tests to look for cancer, which he didn't.

So, what I was told by the Illinois doctors who assessed and treated me was that I have an aggressive type of cancer, based off the ultrasound and mammogram and biopsies. I had skin thickening observed by my primary care physician, and the orange peel appearance of the skin. I had itchiness and nipple discharge before that but ignored it (that's another story) and just went to my physical where the first concern was brought up. I never had a rash or redness, which is what most IBC patients have as a presenting symptom. Because I presented with skin thickening and the timing of the diagnosis was due to a routine physical and not breast symptoms, the IBC specialist totally blew my diagnosis out of the water and said I didn't have IBC (good news right?). If I had noticed it myself and gone to the doctor, *then* he may have thought it was IBC, but only if I had a rash. The surgeon did a skin biopsy after the physical exam and the reports from the mammo, ultrasound, and needle biopsies, but that is not what counts in diagnosing IBC. He then went on to tell me that most women with IBC have estrogen-negative and progesterone-negative cancer and are HER (Herceptin) positive and that I don't so I don't have IBC unless I am one of the 5 percent who are estrogen positive, progesterone positive, and HER negative. He also said the *grade* of my cancer isn't consistent with IBC—I thought it was just found early. Yet if he is using that as a reason to discount the IBC, he is contradicting that it is diagnosed by clinical exam not biopsy. He said he thinks from the reports that I had a slow-growing cancer and he believes because I had dense breast tissue that the mammogram in 2011 missed it. He also said if I had metastasis (spreading) it would have shown in the first PET scan. Although I don't understand because only one lymph node was shown positive on PET and there were six shown on surgical pathology. He said it wasn't that the one spread to the other during treatment, I had six lymph nodes involved from the beginning. If that was the case and what he said was true about the PET picking up if I had mets [metastasis], wouldn't it have also found the six lymph nodes? He said I didn't respond to chemo because all those lymph nodes had cancer before and that they would have showed scar tissue, not cancer, if I had responded. All this time I thought it had grown and moved into the other lymph nodes while I was getting treatment, even he said the chemo was ineffective. Also I thought the reason the doctor or I never felt a lump was because it grew fast and in sheets, like IBC does but he said it was slow-growing. So why didn't the doctor or I ever feel a lump...ever, even though it was 4.3 cm × 3.8 cm × 2.4 cm, the skin involvement was 7-9 cm. It just blows my mind that I have been thinking I had IBC all this time and that ALL of the doctors here are wrong. All the Illinois doctors said I had an aggressive, fast-growing, and invasive cancer. It was staged as 3B because of the IBC diagnosis. If Dr. Colby, the Spirit University specialist, disagreed with the diagnosis she didn't say so. The Texas doctor did say I had a high chance of recurrence because of the number of lymph nodes that were affected, yet he made it sound like Tamoxifen was the wonder drug. If Tamoxifen is so effective against this type of cancer (whatever type it is because the doctor only told me that it wasn't IBC, not what it actually was) then why would he say I have a high chance of recurrence? If chemo wasn't effective then couldn't it have spread from my lymph nodes from April to August and grown from August to December when I did start Tamoxifen? Is it really that effective that it would kill any metastasis that was growing, and how do we know if there was any spreading if I was never tested after treatment? Is it possible to not have severe symptoms and still have mets? Isn't that why so many people die, because it is found late only after they get really sick? Not having IBC is a good thing because the survival rate is much worse, but do I believe him? Were all my doctors wrong? I felt so alone with the type of cancer I had all this time and then found an IBC support group and now I am told I don't have it and now I don't belong there either. I do still have a high chance of recurrence though?

In my angry, judgmental opinion, he was too specialized with his own agenda and since I didn't fall into his criteria to help with his research, and I had already been treated, I was a waste of time. I think he would only be interested in me if I did have mets but I am not sick enough or have enough serious complaints to look to see if I have mets or if I lived there and was going to transfer my treatment there he may have thought I was worth the time.

I didn't send him records from Dr. Colby but the other doctors must have because he kept asking what she told me. He also states that he believes that Tamoxifen is more effective in my case than chemo was and that if there was cancer in other places the Tamoxifen would take care of it. By the time this came up I was already in shock that he said the mammogram missed it in 2011, my doctors got the IBC diagnosis wrong, and that no tests were going to be done. His recommendation: stay on the Tamoxifen and lose weight...hire a personal trainer, do yoga and meditation. Exercise an hour a day and eat healthy. He told me that part of it is getting mentally healthy and I said that was why I was there. For peace of mind that there was no more cancer in the body, and he said there isn't. But *how* does he know that if they don't look?

Maybe I need to complain more? I don't want PET scans every three months. I just thought I deserved one check after treatment, either a PET or bone scan and brain MRI. (I don't have lung or liver symptoms and am not worried that it spread there.) Also a follow-up echo or cardiac test due to my heart history and cardiac symptoms. I don't care if insurance will pay for it, they shouldn't be calling the shots, I will pay out of pocket. I asked when a person has chronic headache history and chronic arthritis how would they know if the pain they had was part of the old or if it was from something new. He said if it isn't in the joints to check it out. Okay, well, I have had pain in the shoulder blade and ribs where my breast used to be and he ignored that. My headaches are increasingly worse and I fall—sometimes when I bend down or squat to take care of a patient I almost fall over. I fell twice in front of other nurses and once in front of Riley. I lost my balance and fell on my stairs twice. I fell in the shower Wednesday morning (slipped) and hit my head. I have had double vision and blurry vision. A little better recently though, maybe the vision blur was from crying and stress after the appointment with the doctor. I didn't tell him about that fall either, although I put those concerns on the symptoms sheet where it asked. I lose my balance a lot but I am sure it is because of all the weight gain. The problem is doctors tell you to lose weight and do nothing to help. That is when he said I need an action plan and all the stuff about hiring a personal trainer, seeing a dietician, etc.

So after all that, he handed me a "survivorship" folder and said bye.

I am serious that I need a break from doctors. I don't know whom to believe. Do I give my treating doctors who evaluated me at the time more weight or the IBC specialist who reviewed my records? Sounds like it doesn't matter what my diagnosis is ;they all read what each other wrote and agree with the treatments and agree that testing isn't needed until I am really sick. So be it. They tell me to get mentally and physically healthy but they don't do what I need to get there, tests and support in weight loss. I don't feel like anyone in the medical community understands, I don't even want to be part of the medical community anymore sometimes. I don't want to talk about cancer anymore and I want to quit my job sometimes. I really love my patients though and want to help them; some of them feel as alone and hopeless as I do and yet I sometimes wonder if I can afford changing jobs and going into retail or working at Starbucks or something. I think if I didn't have to work I would do volunteer work and help single moms take care of their kids when they were sick so they didn't have to take a sick day. Or take the elderly shopping or to their doctor's appointments, help people organize or help sick people clean their house, anything to help people. If someone needed help losing weight I would walk with them, etc. Just help people and not charge them money for it....but I am not rich so I go to work.

I shared my concerns with some people. Most of what you read above was in an email to some of my medical friends. Since the time of the Texas visit I have lost six pounds. I have walked twenty to thirty minutes *every* day for the past seven days. Because another breast cancer survivor said, "I totally get it and I need to get healthier too, let's walk together." I have eaten healthy food 90 percent of the time. I am trying to be a better "survivor." I have to tell you though, the honeymoon of finishing cancer treatment ended a couple months ago and life has been a huge struggle. I am doing what I can to get stronger and healthier and move on. Yes, the cancer could come back. No, I don't want to live in fear of that anymore. Yes, I am disappointed that the medical community doesn't value the benefits a few tests can have on my mental health.

So there it is the whole truth... I hope I didn't confuse you too much.

Lesson learned. Cancer patients deal with this long after the active treatment stage is over, yet the support often drops off when the active treatment stage is done. I still feel more like a "fighter" than a "survivor."

Thanks for staying interested. I know this was a long entry.

Take care, Marcy

EM: June 15, 2013

From: Brooke

To: Marcy

Subject: I will keep working at it.

Okay... I read this last night and had to kind of sleep on it and reread it this morning. After I researched IBC a little. I am not sure if there is anything I can say to make you feel better. But I am going to give you my two cents and then give you a proposition...

First, let's see if I understand what this guy told you... He said he does not think you have IBC. It does sound like he had his own agenda and the fact that he did not believe you were an IBC patient, he was gonna move on. That sucks! *But* I do not believe this was a waste of your time.

After researching IBC and reading everything you typed to me this is what I understand:

- To be diagnosed with IBC there is 1) a rapid onset of symptoms, 2) signs and symptoms for less than six months, 3) erythema (red, pink, reddish purple, bruised looking—the *rash* he was talking about?) and a rapid increase in breast size with significant swelling, heaviness, or burning, 4) the erythema covers at least one-third of the breast, and 5) initial biopsy sample shows invasive carcinoma.

- Usually all IBCs are hormone-receptor negative, that is why Tamoxifen is usually not a treatment for IBC.

Tamoxifen is used in hormone-receptor-positive situations; the way that Tamoxifen works is it blocks the body's ability to make estrogen. This can cause estrogen-dependent cancer cells to stop growing and die. Tamoxifen is specific to breast cancer cells and can have this effect on breast cancer cells no matter where they are growing in the body.

Okay having said all that. I am not going to judge you. Don't ever think I would. I believe I was your friend prior to becoming coworkers, so don't worry about the fact that we work together.

Also I have felt the same way you do. Would it be easier for me and everyone else if I was not here? Believe me I know. But you are so important in so many lives—especially your kids! And your patients are so lucky to have you as well as your coworkers adore you!

I know you are angry. I get that. So be angry for a while. But I think this gives you the opportunity to bring the information you received in Texas back to your physicians. Ask if this doctor's claims are valid? It sounds like to me they may be. Tell them about your headaches and your balance and fall issues. Okay make them worse than they are... They need to check that out! These are valid concerns. Based on the fact that the cancer was possibly not IBC, was the treatment you received appropriate? Was it the same treatment someone would receive with invasive breast cancer? Don't stop pursuing it!

The Tamoxifen is also a discussion with your physician. If you are hormone-receptor positive, then Tamoxifen is an appropriate drug for you. It has been proven in many studies of its effectiveness. Believe me I know. I have researched it extensively through projects in school. And know that research shows premenopausal women should be on it for ten years, instead of five years. This is just information for you. You have the right to decide if you want to take it or not.

So try not to give up on the medical field. Be frustrated and mad. But hopefully you can take this information and use it here to find out more. To me it sounds like you had some form of invasive breast cancer. Which is what I had. I did not feel my lump because I had cysts in my breast and lumpy breast tissue to begin with. So the cancer was only seen with mammography, then ultrasound and confirmed with the biopsy.

So now that you are thinking... "I wish she would stop typing..." Here is my proposition. You and me become workout, eating healthy buddies! Interested? I have a few diet tips and we live close enough to meet and walk together. To at least get things started. You need the support and I need the support, so together we can do this. I used to work out all the time and was so much more mentally healthy than I feel right now. So let's see if we can help each other out. Give me a call when you get home.

You are going to get through this. And I want to help you and myself in the meantime.

Brooke

From: Marcy

To: Brooke

Your interpretation is spot on. Of the five criteria I had one, two, and five. But I think you are right on all counts. That is the way I understand Tamoxifen too. I guess the depression has made me want to let myself go—in fact the place I have been the most functional and valuable probably has been work. I think there may be confusion on the actual diagnosis but it sounds like they all agree the treatment was appropriate.

No, still not ready to see doctors.

Yes, I can be a health buddy with you, do you have a plan? Maybe after I get started and can see some progress and feel in control again, things will get better in many ways. Hopefully we can work something out. Tomorrow is Father's Day and so I will have to go to my family thing but can call you late afternoon, early evening.

Thanks Brooke, thanks for understanding.

From: Marcy

To: Brooke

I came across this documentary called *Hungry for Change* on Netflix [2012]. Have you seen it? If not, you should watch it…all the way through. It really sums up what I have been dealing with, especially at the end, the guy who talks about not being at the point of taking his life but welcoming death and how he got through that really hit home. Instead of telling myself to take away certain foods, it talks about adding the healthy ones. Heaven knows I have had enough taken away from me. I think that is part of my brain problem.

Bottom line, I will start taking the Tamoxifen again and keep working at getting healthy (not ready to go to doctors yet though). I can be healthy again. Okay, boob-less but healthy. I am putting pictures of a smaller and healthier me up on my desktop, maybe I'll print them and put them in my car during work to remind myself I did this before and I can do it now. Thanks for the email and I hope we can work together on this. I am motivated now but when the negative and fearful thoughts come back, it is hard to dig out of the hole.

Thank you for being a friend to me, for helping me make sense of my visit to the specialist and for not giving up on me.

Marcy

From: Brooke

To: Marcy

Brooke: Call me tomorrow later. When you can! We will start Monday! It will be fun!

CB: August 15, 2013

Fall

Hi all,

This won't be long because it is hard to type with a broken elbow. I fell at work and broke my elbow *and* ankle. Wasn't even that bad of a fall, usually "rolling" an ankle is mostly soft tissue injury. I do take calcium and Vitamin D and have for a long time. Called the oncologist for a DEXA scan to check bone density. Here is some interesting info.

"Women who have had breast cancer treatment may be at increased risk for osteoporosis and fracture for several reasons. First, estrogen has a protective effect on bone, and reduced levels of the hormone trigger bone loss. Because of chemotherapy or surgery, many breast cancer survivors experience a loss of ovarian function, and consequently, a drop in estrogen levels. Women who were premenopausal before their cancer treatment tend to go through menopause earlier than those who have not had the disease. Studies suggest that chemotherapy also may have a direct negative effect on bone. In addition, the breast cancer itself may stimulate the production of osteoclasts, the cells that break down bone."[3]

On a brighter note, I started the hospital's weight management program and am finally starting to lose some of this weight! Before my fall I was

3. "Breast Cancer and Osteoporosis," *WebMD*, accessed June 2017, http://www. webmd.com/breast-cancer/breast-cancer-and-osteoporosis#1.

walking one to two miles on most days. Seven out of the previous eight. GRRRRR.

I'll keep you posted, Marcy

Alan: I'll bet you were secretly doing mixed martial arts and that's how you really broke your elbow and ankle. So what did the other guy look like? Oh man, Marcy, sorry to hear about this. Keep your chin up.

JY: Thanks for update. What a bummer!!! will pray for a quick and speedy recovery!!! Just a little bump in the road...you have definitely survived bigger bumps!!! Hang in there.

CB: August 30, 2013

Radiation Recall Dermatitis?

Hello,

I noticed a rash on my right chest area where the cancer was and the mastectomy and radiation was. It extends from the front to the back and got more red from the time I noticed it until I saw the doctors today. They think it might be a radiation recall dermatitis, although the radiation oncologist who would be the expert on that is out of town. The medical oncologist put me on steroids and told me it should be getting better by Tuesday; if it is not improving or getting worse, may need to go for a biopsy or try different medications.

I do get to go back to work on light duty, three days a week starting Tuesday. I am out of the big boot and now using an ankle brace. Will start physical therapy next week. The elbow is doing well but still no lifting more than five pounds with it. I did get the DEXA scan and my bone density is fine!

Doing well on the hospital weight management program, lost fourteen pounds in three weeks. Now that I can walk, it will help the weight loss. He also said I could swim with my ankle and elbow but not sure I want to do that with this rash.

Overall, I'm moving along. Hope you all are well and have a great, safe, healthy Labor Day weekend.

Marcy

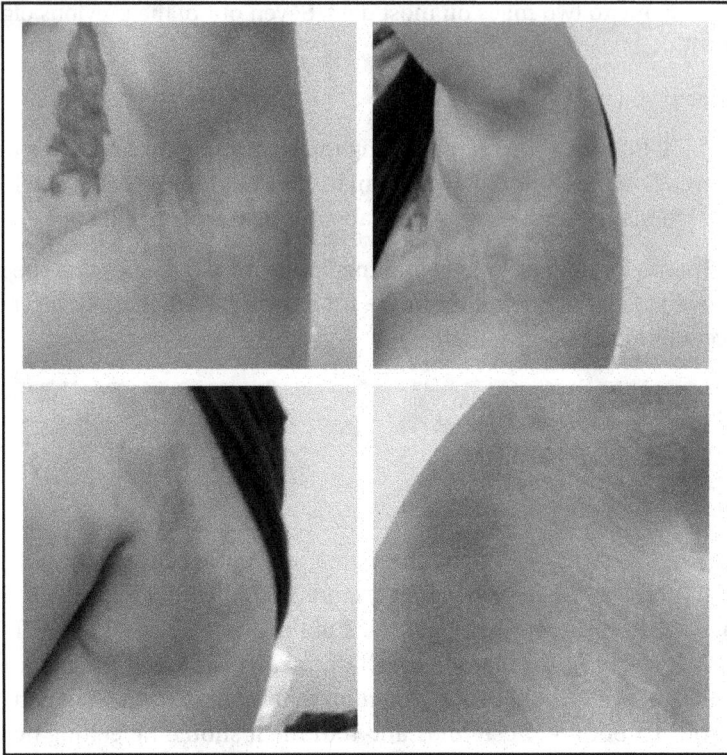

Figure 8-1. My rash that was called radiation recall dermatitis

CB: September 3, 2013

Round 2

Saw oncologist again today, he can't tell me what exactly this rash is but he put me on another round of steroids. The original rash improved but new rash developed on the arm. Still looks inflammatory... Unknown cause. If not better after this round I am supposed to call him but I am thinking if it isn't better after this round I should be seeing a dermatologist instead.

Was in the office on light duty today. For a field nurse being in the office is the equivalent of being sent to the principal's office or the library instead of going to recess. Will start physical therapy tomorrow. I have been trying to walk more with the ankle brace because the doctor said I could but may be overdoing it a little. I forget that it was only three weeks ago. Still swollen and sore but not terrible.

Hope you all had a nice weekend, Marcy

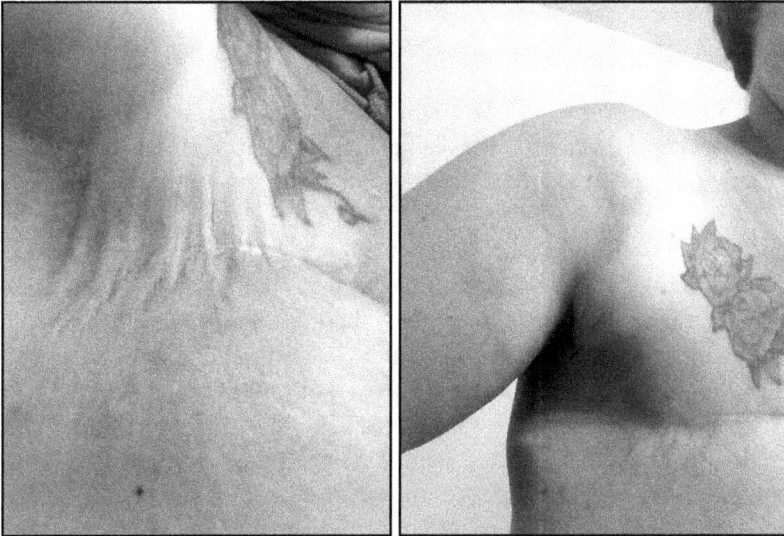

Figure 8-2. Axillary web syndrome (cording) [Left].
Rash and swollen area at end of scar [Right]

CB: October 10, 2013

Raising Awareness and Funds for Local Women

Hi all,

So on to the next phase of all of this. Who knew the posttreatment stage would be so difficult. I am getting better. I am healed from my broken bones and lost twenty-five pounds (still a long way to go). What good is all this experience if I don't share it with others? I share what I can in my professional life as a nurse, and I have shared with large organizations like Relay for Life, American Cancer Society, and Avon Walk.

Now is the time to take care of our local county folks. I have joined Joe and Tina from the Star 105.5 early morning show to do a fundraising walk. The money raised stays in our county. I am most likely going to be on the air with them next Wednesday sometime between 7 a.m. and 9 a.m. Please listen and if you can, support us and the walk. Joe lost his Mom to breast cancer and was very supportive while I was going through treatment. He even signed the pink truck and sent a picture of it to me. He always encouraged me to keep fighting! It is the things like that that keep us fighters going.

Thanks for all you have done to support me.

Love, Marcy

Alan: I'll be listening!

DA: You look so good! Hope all the healing is going well. The doors are always open. You have such a story of hope to share. You've been through a lot but have come out on the other side. Keep sharing your hope.

I invited Dani and Riley to come with me and sit in the studio while I talked with Joe, Tina, and Clinto. The kids were excited about going. It was important enough for me to have Riley there that I took him out of school for the morning. Being in a radio studio was something none of us had ever done and I think it made us all feel special. Riley even asked them to autograph his hat, which they happily did.

Joe talked to their listeners about the upcoming fundraising walk and how we had shared some private messages during my treatment. He had been through breast cancer by watching his mom go through it three times. It was personal to him and I wanted my kids to hear that. We talked about the diagnosis, the importance of talking to people, and once again it was reiterated that my reason is my kids, that they kept me going. We stressed how little shows of support make a huge difference and discussed the pink fire truck he signed to encourage me to "Keep Fighting." Years later, Dani and I saw that truck again in the parking lot of the grocery store. It was a reminder to always keep fighting.

CB: October 16, 2013

Thank You Joe and Tina at Star 105.5 Radio Station

What an awesome experience to be in the Star radio studio with Joe, Tina, Clinto, and my kids. I hope it will help educate people and inspire.

My kids had a great time and everyone was so welcoming. Looking forward to the walk on Sunday in Woodstock. If you are there look for me and my sister-in-law, Patti, who joined our team. Thanks again.

Patti and I participated in the Care 4 Breast Cancer Walk with Joe's team. The energy and number of participants at this event was incredible. Patti and I walked and talked and toward the end of the walk we all met together so we could cross the finish line as a team. It really does take a team of people to care for one person with cancer and I was reminded of this when I started reflecting back on my journey. Joe continues his community support and continues to walk in this event, increasing his team participant number goals and money collected goals, surpassing them year after year. I have routinely participated in another walk that is usually held on the same day. Although we are walking in separate events in nearby counties every year, I always remember his passion and energy as well as his diligent memorialization of his mother as he teaches his sons about her. I actually wondered if my children did lose me from cancer if they would help other women in this way. When I see a cardinal I not only think of my dear grandmother who died of stomach cancer but I think of Joe's mom and know they both must be proud of the fighting spirit they instilled in us.

The next months were spent trying to get back to as close to a normal lifestyle as I could. Medical appointments were slowing down. I did normal parenting things in the life of a mother of a high school student. I brought Riley to school activities, Sea Cadet activities, and went to football games. I wanted to shift my identity away from being a cancer patient, fighter, and survivor—I just wanted to be Mom, daughter, aunt, nurse. As much as I tried, my thoughts often consumed me. I continued to struggle with weight management and with a depression that I didn't speak much of.

At that time, the depression could have been situational, genetic, or from hormonal changes. I didn't think of harming myself directly, but there was a long period of time when I stopped taking my Tamoxifen. If the cancer came back and I died from that, my family would get the love and support they needed, and the life insurance they needed, because my death would have been cancer related. Society is empathetic to cancer suffering and is supportive of families that lost a family member from cancer. Society is not supportive of depression or families that lose a loved one from suicide; they would not have the support or the life insurance benefits. At the time, I focused on what wouldn't be lost with my death. I also knew being overweight would increase my risk of cancer recurrence because increase in body fat increases circulating estrogen, and my type of cancer flourished in estrogen. I couldn't seem to pull myself out of depression. I continued to work and struggle with my weight, losing weight then gaining it back and more. I had reached almost 210 pounds on my five-foot, eight-inch frame.

My focus started shifting again as my kids and I talked about a tattoo over my mastectomy scar. We saw many examples on Facebook: bouquets, lace bras, even a peacock ran over some women's scars. I knew as I began planning that I would be able to only cover the left side; if I can't have blood pressures, or needle sticks in the right arm I wasn't confident that tattoos on the side the lymph nodes were removed would be safe.

It was Dani who said, "Mom, you should get a phoenix." The more I thought about it, the more I thought I would like a tattoo over the scar on the left that was a symbol of coming out of the ashes brighter, stronger, and more beautiful. The mythical bird does this repeatedly, and I need to repeatedly remind myself that even when my depression wants me to feel like nothing, I can grow out of that and into something beautiful.

CB: January 30, 2014

Phoenix

Haven't updated in a while, don't worry, I'm still doing fine. Wanted to share two things with you.

(1) I am changing oncologists. Strange story. Was kind of upset for a while. Although I felt like my oncologist treated my cancer appropriately, I never really had that great of rapport with him. Loved the nurses and nurse practitioner but never really felt like my oncologist knew me from any other person walking in his door. To me, rapport with your medical team is important. I met his partner when I was in the hospital and asked to switch to him. The oncologist said (through his office staff, of course) if I didn't stay with him, I had to leave the practice, he would not allow me to see his partner. So I left, and he sent me a certified letter dismissing me from his practice. I am excited to say, I found a new oncologist who I think I will feel confident in. I take care of a lot of his patients in the home care environment and they really seem to like and trust him. That appointment is next Wednesday.

(2) I was going to wait to lose weight before I got my phoenix tattoo but I figured that would take too long soooooo...I started it today. It will take multiple sessions to complete. For those who think I am crazy... I find the mastectomy tattoo less risky, more beautiful, and less expensive than breast reconstruction. I have taken care of many women who are getting reconstruction and am so glad I didn't do it. It is a very personal choice without a right or wrong answer. I just know I am glad I went this direction.

Out of the ashes.

Love ya and miss ya,

Marcy

Alan: The tattoo is awesome. I will always have a fondness for the phoenix since it is the little-known mascot of my school. The phoenix rules!

LM: Marcy, you are such a strong woman! I will see you this summer! Enjoyed our last visit so much. XO

DA: Good for you—on both counts. I'm glad you found someone you are comfortable with. That's huge. Wow! What a tattoo. It will be beautiful when it is finished! Can't help but ask…did it really hurt? I'm too chicken to get one. It was great to see a post from you, was thinking of you this morning.

JY: Hey Marcy, so glad to hear you found a new doctor. I think you're right and the rapport is SO important!

JH: *Love the phoenix!! So* appropriate and meaningful!

CP: Glad to hear you found a new doctor. It is important to talk openly with your doctor. Way to go on your tattoo! Love you.

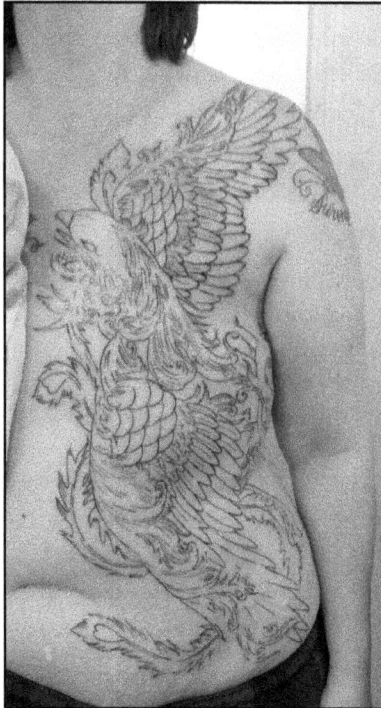

Figure 8-3. The outline of my phoenix tattoo

Both Dani's breast cancer pink ribbon butterfly tattoo and mine were done by Nikki Harris. We had been in to see her a few times about the size and style as well as colors. I knew this piece would be a time and financial commitment but what I didn't know was how therapeutic this process would be.

The design itself was a custom drawing from Nikki after discussing in detail what I wanted and sending her different examples of phoenix tattoos, which detailed things I liked and didn't. Her art was made into a stencil and she had it in three pieces. She resized them and placed the body and wings on, we discussed placement and made the adjustments that we wanted. The design extended from my left shoulder down to my hip. She removed and replaced it multiple times until we were satisfied. She then drew in the tail feathers to curl around the wings and body of the phoenix. I think that process took almost two hours and that was even before the ink was poured and that tattoo machine was touched.

The outline took almost four hours to tattoo. She explained that the outline had to be done in this sitting to complete the design, especially after placement of the transparencies and the hand-drawn feathers. As you can imagine, we talked a lot, we laughed a lot, and we sang a lot. Kam, the receptionist, would frequently come in to check on us or grab something that Nikki needed. I talked to her frequently as I was waiting for Nikki to get set up for my appointments.

CB: February 8, 2014

New Oncologist

I met with Dr. Richards and can see why his patients adore him. As a home care nurse I have cared for many of his patients, and he is one of the doctors I work with who will come to the phone and talk to me about the concerns and questions I have on our patients. This saves time and phone tag and allows for a collaborative discussion. Everyone at his office has always been great to work with as well, his partners and physicians covering for him have been receptive even when I have to page them on a weekend for a new patient or problem. If you are the type of person who gets offended if a physician has to leave the room during your appointment, he would not be the right physician for you. In my mind, knowing that he will politely excuse himself to address an important issue immediately makes me feel secure that if I needed him, he would be there for me as well. When I walked in, there were two of my patients in the treatment area; some may feel uncomfortable with that, but my patients and

I have a close relationship...they invite me into their home and I know them and their families. The one patient told the nurse, "You take good care of her." Makes me teary-eyed to feel how much they care about me, just as I care about them.

On to the visit. He was very mindful to understand where I was at in the cancer treatment and monitoring process. He listened, asked questions, and did his exam. We even had some nice conversation about tattoos. I warned him ahead of time. Dani thought I should have let him be surprised. He said he wondered how many more he would find as he did my exam, LOL. We seem to have similar philosophy on the surveillance of my health. This is one of the reasons I was unsettled before...I didn't like the "wait until you are sick or symptomatic and then we will check you" approach. My previous oncologist didn't even do labs; those where only done by my primary physician. Dr. Richards talked about the tumor markers CA15-3 and CEA: although not always specific, those blood tests could detect a recurrence eight months before symptoms even begin, are paid for by insurance, and are "simple" blood tests. The reason I write "simple" is because my veins aren't what they used to be and since we can't use my right arm, it decreases the choice of veins. Three nurses and four sticks later, I left without labs being done. I went back the next morning after pushing fluids and peeing all night and was able to have my blood drawn. Ugggh, I hate my veins.

So although I have a bit of anxiety about waiting for lab tests—all right, a lot of anxiety (wish I had some Xanax)—I am glad to know that he understands I need something more than a physical exam of looking and poking to believe I am cancer free. He said that many oncologists don't use tumor markers in this way. Some believe it doesn't matter because if there was a recurrence to stage 4, a cure would be unlikely for me. But we both agree that the value of eight months or more, in time and quality of life, is worth the surveillance. These are some of the reasons I liked him.

It is worth the few days of anxiety to have several months of peace of mind.

Physically, I can't say that I feel great but I am not going to bother you with my list of "minor" complaints. My problem has always been self-evaluation, as to what is minor and what needs to be addressed are often difficult for me to decide on. It is easier to be a nurse to my patients than to myself. So, I will wait and see on these issues. I am one of those patients who sometimes thinks, "I know what the doctor is going to say," so I don't bother calling.

When I first started home care full time last year, the oncology patients were very difficult emotionally and at times still are. I am coming to believe though that my experience gives me a little something extra to offer them. I like that something useful can come from the hard times I have had in life.

I will let you know how the labs turn out (I am sure they will be fine).

Take care my friends, Marcy

P.S. My next tattoo sitting is February 12, will touch up the outline and start the colors. Very excited.

CB: February 10, 2014

Peace of Mind

Hi all,

Tumor markers are good! Glad to know that and to know Dr. Richards will keep an eye on things.

TTFN, Marcy

CB: February 12, 2014

Tattoo Progress

Hi there,

So I sat for a couple more hours on my phoenix tattoo. More outline and started some shading. It will have color but *man*, this is a *huge* project. I am sure I will run out of funds and have to slow down on the appointments after a couple more sittings.

The thing about Nikki is this—not only is she a fantastic artist but she figured me out in no time and now there are rules when I see her. 1) No work phone calls or checking work voice mail during Marcy and Nikki time and 2) when I am in Nikki's space I am not allowed to make any self-deprecating remarks.

I think I handled most of the body changes well with the mastectomy. The biggest physical issue I have is the weight, especially messages given to me while I was growing up and during my marriage. There is societal pressure to be thin and the fact that I am not really is a deep-seated issue that I have to deal with. I have always known this was an issue for me, but I really didn't realize how negative toward myself I can be. I would not allow anyone to talk to me the way I talk to myself and that has to stop. It will definitely stop when I am with Nikki.

So thank you to Nikki for the beautiful art where my scars are; I don't mind looking at my chest anymore, in fact I can't stop right now. I love my Phoenix and she isn't even halfway done. Thank you for calling me out on the way I verbally abuse myself.

Another lesson learned. It takes time to change but I am aware it needs to happen.

I hope you are all well and being kind to yourself.

Love, Marcy

Alan: Looking good!

GG: You are amazing and beautiful.

CB: February 16, 2014

Gut Punch

I feel like I keep getting punched in the gut this weekend. Just opened a letter saying I was denied additional life insurance through work due to my "history of breast cancer and my build"—even they don't think I can lose weight and remain cancer-free. I'm going from tears to bawling today. My kids better be successful because I will not be leaving them much.

Grace: I know what it feels like to be punched and punched again, just as you do. BUT, I know that we get back up and keep on going, just as you have shown us time after time after time. Don't think about what you're leaving to the kids ($$$$$)! I know that you will leave the most important thing in the world—your love for them as one of the most incredible moms I've ever known! I love you! Grace xoxo

CB: February 18, 2014

This Made Me Cry

This just in: I sent a private message to someone I met through friends on Facebook who is also a breast cancer survivor. This is my message and her response to me.

Marcy: I really appreciate all your comments and sharing your experience with me. I am not sure many understand how hard "survivorship" can be. The support cancer patients get during the active treatment stage is great but many don't understand the aftereffects of fighting this disease and how it can continue to affect your life. Thanks for sharing your life with me.

Her: You are part of my social media support circle. We do need to be able to help each other through what we never expected—the neverending reminders that we are surviving something. Thanks for all of the courage you have shown facing survivorship while being a full-time single mom. The tattoo is such a sign of you reaching out and embracing. We can still feel young in spite of this disease trying to make us feel old, I so see that in you. Cheers!

I hope I can meet her in person someday!

There was a three-month gap in CaringBridge posts and I didn't have much to say about my health on Facebook either. Looking back, it is startling to me how short my memory can be. All the lessons learned about living life, making time for people, and doing what you enjoy began fading as I brought work home and slipped into other old habits. I went through the motions of life, without truly living it.

While I was sitting on the couch trying to catch up on the charting I had from home care patients during the day, Riley snapped me out of it. He was sitting across from me when he looked at me and said, "Mom, work has you all day and you come home and work more." That was a wake-up call I needed. He was right. When I looked back at my calendars to fill this gap between posts, there was nothing except work and appointments. No time scheduled with friends, no movies, and no outings with the kids, which I had always tried to do with them together and individually once a month. Nothing to bring enjoyment to the life I struggled so hard to save.

I talked to Ron and Laurie about this. Although they are some of the hardest working people I know, they plan a vacation every year during their slow time at the garage. They told me about the cruise that was planned in February 2015 with their friends, their eldest, and his family. A cruise? Now there was a fantastic idea. I had wanted to go on a cruise even when I was married and it never happened. What was I waiting for? Laurie gave me the name of her travel agent and I immediately requested the time off work and put my money down on it. Since I was not sure if I would ever get another opportunity to do a cruise I made sure to book a balcony room and start saving money to enjoy every last activity and excursion possible. I extended the idea to Miriam well in advance hoping she could be my shipmate.

A more everyday pursuit was in regard to fitness. I had been trying multiple things to get more active and lose weight. I had success in the past and was a lifetime member of Weight Watchers. I had tried to return to that, and then I tried a medically supervised very low calorie diet and weight loss program. There was nothing that I tried that helped me to make the long-term changes and lose the weight I needed to.

The heavier I got, the more difficult my home care nursing position got, the more tired I became, and the more depressed I got. The more depressed I got, the more tired I got and the less active I was. It was such a vicious cycle. I recall having to use the rail bars on the stairs in my house to pull myself up them. I recall being short of breath when I had to go upstairs at a patient's home carrying my nursing bag, and the embarrassment I felt if I had to kneel or bend down because I was not being able to get back up well. I was often in an awkward position while providing care to my patients and I felt I could have managed better at a more reasonable weight. I was a hypocrite talking about activity and healthy lifestyles and nutrition while I struggled with my weight myself. Whom could I help, if I couldn't help myself?

Between the physical stress of my job and Riley pointing out I was always working, I reduced my hours to four days a week. I was able to maintain medical coverage while reducing my hours. This helped tremendously yet I still felt very guilty for doing what I needed to do to take care of me, which was work less. Guilt was a predominant emotion from single parenting days, a poor marriage, and now since the cancer diagnosis.

I had a home care patient who had the lap-band weight loss surgery and had some success with it. I decided to make an appointment for a consultation and schedule to have the lap-band put in. I felt like I needed to do something right away, especially when I started looking at the weight limits for some of the excursions on the cruise: I was not going to pass up zip-lining in Belize, which, along with the crystal cave tubing, was the only excursion with the entire thirteen-person group. This seemed to be just the motivation I needed to do something about my weight, my health, and my life.

CB: June 19, 2014

If You Are Inclined to Help

So, I am not the type to ask for monetary help for myself. Yes, I have done fundraising for different causes but would never have thought of it to complete this very big tattoo project. My close friend, Lola, started this fundraising page online after she called my tattoo artist to get an estimate on what it would take to complete the phoenix tattoo. Understand that if I had gone with reconstruction—which is what I think most of society expects—insurance would have paid for it. I had thought about a tattoo, and Dani came up with the Phoenix, which seemed fitting. So far it has cost $1,500. I have a lot more to do. If you would like to be part of this project in a monetary way, you can donate on the website. I have my next sitting on June 26th.

All of my recent oncology follow-ups have been good. I am actually looking into a gastric sleeve surgery due to my weight. I've had the consult and am appealing the insurance denial. Apparently I am not quite fat enough.

Take care, do fun things with the people you love this summer. Life is short.

Love, Marcy

CB: July 1, 2014

THANK YOU

I want to say thank you for all the generous donations to offset the cost of my large phoenix project. I am putting it on hold short-term to get gastric sleeve surgery on July 16. The insurance finally approved and I am more than ready to kickstart my weight loss and get active again. I will then finish my tattoo and go on my cruise in February. I also wanted to tell you I started on online support group that was part of the study I am participating in for American Cancer Society. It is called Surviving and Thriving and it is six online lessons and discussion, one a week for six weeks. We are in week two. I am finding a lot of similar stories, struggles and support as well as getting some suggestions and hope that although my body will never ever be the same, I can get used to and even love my "new normal." That is what I am working toward. The aftereffects of cancer, as you know, have been very difficult for me. The depression and obesity have been so rough. I really am working on it, and appreciate all of your help in this and for not forgetting about me just because my "last treatment was done." Although I am currently not getting cancer treatment, I will always be a cancer patient, but that doesn't mean I can't thrive. So stay tuned, some fun changes are coming!

Love, Marcy

P.S. Thank you for the donations for the tattoo. *Thank you,* especially thank you to Sasha. I got the $500 check today and was absolutely flabbergasted. Thank you!

Alan: You deserve a cruise my friend. Enjoy!

The next six months I was focused on health. July 4 I took my family to Arlington Park Racetrack. Although I grew up in a neighboring town, I had never been there. We had reservations at the Million Room for dinner and racing, then we were going to stay for the fireworks. I was so uncomfortable in my body. I had no clothes that fit to wear to a nice dining experience and had to borrow some. I was 240 pounds by this time.

Two weeks later I had the vertical sleeve gastrectomy surgery. There was more pain than expected since the surgeon had to fix a severe hiatal hernia as well. Recovery was grueling. I was tremendously weak and my diet advancement was slow. I worked through it, did what the doctors told me, and gradually saw improvement in my energy level, my activity level, and even my sleep. Patti routinely walked the mile to my house to go on walks with me. We walked in my neighborhood at my speed and for the distance I could tolerate and then she would walk the mile back to her house.

As the pounds melted off, my confidence and self-esteem started improving again. I was happy more often. In October I took my fitness up a step and joined Snap Fitness health club. The owner and I talked frequently about life, cancer, health, kids. To me it was more than a health club. I felt empowered there. I had belonged to may health clubs in the past but none made me feel as capable of reaching my goals or as comfortable and proud of myself. I gave myself permission to spend money on a personal trainer as I knew strength training would get me to my health and fitness goals faster and more safely. The trainer took the time to listen to my history and my medical conditions and she developed a plan according to them.

Nikki and I resumed working on my phoenix tattoo. My goal was to have it done for the cruise in February with my friends. I could feel the active support of my network of friends dying off at this time, and sometimes it felt hard not to fade with it. But still donations came in for the tattoo and allowed me to finish a testament to strength and survival that would last the rest of my life.

I met the goal for the tattoo just as I had met my goal for weight. I was beginning to feel stronger physically, emotionally, and mentally. Stronger than I ever have in my entire life. My posture was better, I stood up when I walked and held my shoulders back. I spoke with confidence. I was taking the time to do what I needed to do for me. Life was improving.

In December I changed the direction of my career. I felt I could make a great impact for hospice patients and their families. With the encouragement of Patrice and Brooke, my nursing mentors, I moved forward with this change. I had much to learn about end-of-life care, but it was in line with a newfound purpose in life.

Alive and Living

Blog (B): *Flight of a Phoenix*, January 20, 2015

New Purpose

During my cancer treatment I used a medical website to post updates for my family and friends. I have found that there have been many things I have wanted to write about over the last year but didn't feel that I could put it all on a medical support page. I will be transferring the content from that site to this one, where I can write about many topics such as health and fitness, cancer, family, spirituality, healthcare field and nursing, adoption, and whatever else crosses my mind. There will be a poetry section as well. There will also be a link to my daughter Jo's blogs (more on this in a minute— I am saving the best news for last).

So the cancer and health update: Still hanging out with NED (no evidence of disease). I have been to my radiation and medical oncologists as they have requested and they say things are looking good. The purpose of going to the radiation oncologist is to monitor for after effects of radiation that could effect the skin, lungs, and heart. The medical oncologist I switched to is great; I feel like he knows and is interested in me, not just my disease. I have been having chronic headaches and had a MRI and saw the neurologist. No signs of cancer in the brain, and the headaches, although they are frequent, are mild and localized in a certain area. As you all know from previous CaringBridge posts, the two years posttreatment I struggled with depression and weight gain. I finally did something about this.

In July I reached my all-time highest weight of 240. It was affecting my work, mobility and worsening my depression. Spring of 2014 I had signed up for my first cruise ever. So excited to do this with friends, I was looking at the choices of excursions and saw that I would be excluded from things that I want to do, such as zip lining due to my weight. That was the last straw. I began the process of getting approved for weight loss surgery. On July 16, 2014, I had a vertical sleeve gastrectomy. I often say that my oncology team saved my life but the surgeon gave it back to me. As of this morning I am 157.8, down 82.2; BMI from 37.6 to a normal 24.7. The goal I had with my surgeon is 155 by my personal goal is 150. I work out with a trainer lifting weights and walk. I haven't felt this good physically in a long time. I see muscle definition and consider myself a strong woman again. The depression is going away and I am considering going off the medication for it soon. I will be talking to my primary care physician about this next month.

Career Update: Although I loved working in home care with my patients and the staff there, I still felt something was missing and I wasn't quite where I needed to be. This was before I lost all the weight and my back was hurting being out in the field too. A mentor of mine called me to ask me to work with her at a privately owned home health company; she just took a director of nursing position and wanted me to work for them as clinical supervisor. I loved working with Patrice, and again the staff there was great but both Patrice and I decided this wasn't the place for us. She asked me if I considered home hospice. At one time in my life, not too long ago, I think I was too emotionally fragile with the recent cancer. I had been losing weight and working with a personal trainer and feeling strong. Patrice went back to a company she worked for previously, closer to her home, and I got hired at JourneyCare. JourneyCare is a fantastic company. Everyone there has been incredible. I have a lot to learn but really feel like this is a calling for me. I was meant to do this. Maybe this was the reason I have been through what I have. This is part of my purpose in life. I am also planning on doing the online RN to BSN completion program at Purdue-Calumet University and then getting my certification in palliative and hospice care.

My phoenix tattoo is basically complete, we will take one more pass to fine tune the color and shading after I get back from my first cruise ever!

That's all great news, right? So what could be better than a new direction, career goals, healthy kids, feeling healthy and strong, and having no evidence of cancer? Drum roll please... Being reunited with the child I placed for adoption more than twenty-eight years ago. Here is the rebirth announcement I posted on Facebook:

"On 11/17/1985, I gave birth to Steven Douglas. He was then placed for adoption on April 28, 1986, and became Joseph Mason. We have been reconnected this week. I couldn't be happier or more proud of her. Please welcome my daughter Josephine Stephanie back to our family."

So again, I want to thank all of you who followed me during my cancer journey and helped me through the struggles as well as celebrated with me when I was soaring. My life really is better now than it has ever been. Stay well.

After receiving a letter in the mail from my first-born child, all of the conversations with the friends who were somehow connected to the adoption process were validated. The infant who was assigned male at birth and whom I had raised for over five months had contacted me. Immediately, I reached back and was able to be with her during a pivotal time in her life as she transitioned from male to female and became the woman she is today. The work I was doing to survive and thrive in my life I was able to pass on to her.

As we got to know each other, we did a side-by-side timeline and we realized that if I had tried to contact her during my cancer treatment, it would have been more than she could bear, as she lost her stepsister to breast cancer just prior to my diagnosis. It proved to me that continuing to seek advice and keep my child's best interest a priority was the right thing to do.

B: *Flight of a Phoenix*, January 23, 2015

Don't Rob Me of a Good Death

So before I try to explain what this statement of "Don't rob me of a good death" means, you may need a little bit of background on me. I have been a nurse for almost twenty years in a variety of settings including home care. Last month I felt called to go into hospice care and believe this is where I will spend the second half of my nursing career, specializing in end-of-life care. I am a cancer survivor. In 2012 I spent more time thinking about death and dying than most people who are in their forties with teenagers at home should have to.

The reason I am writing about this now is because it has become clear to me that end-of-life care is misunderstood. How clearly the word hospice is misinterpreted (seen as giving up) and how people suffer and their families suffer when it isn't necessary. Although I am new to hospice I have identified what I believe are some of the reasons we don't allow the people we love to have the "good death" that they deserve

No one wants to lose the people they love. I think we need to be taught better coping skills and life skills. Death is just as much a part of life as birth is. Whether we are afraid of not being able to live without the person who is dying or we are afraid of what dying may look or sound like, it is unfair to push someone "to be a fighter." It is unfair to make them feel guilty or weak for not going to one more chemotherapy session or not wanting to go back to the hospital to control their pain or breathlessness because we don't want to face the facts and allow them to die on their own terms.

Society has put so much focus on "fight the good fight," "losing the battle to cancer," "staying positive," and "not giving up" that we are afraid to be honest. We are afraid to say, "I know this treatment isn't going to cure me, in fact it may put me in the hospital and cause me to have painful procedures and may even shorten my life from complications. I am ready to stay at home and manage my symptoms and disease process so that I can make every moment I have left count." We want a miracle cure, instead of acknowledging that the miracle may be that we are allowed to die at home in comfort with the people we love close by. We don't want to hear this from our loved ones. We don't want to hear our physician say, "You are dying." Physicians are trained to heal the sick and injured. Maybe some are afraid if they are honest in the prognosis they have failed as a physician. Maybe they are not trained well enough as prognosticators. In fact, some physicians and healthcare people are uncomfortable with having those conversations at all. We can't say the words death and dying. I know I was never taught to have the end-of-life conversations in nursing school. More and more often I am reading and hearing stories from people who say, "If I knew they were that sick, if the doctor told me he was dying, we would have gone home and just been together, we would have done things differently. We only had hospice a few days before he died." A day or two of hospice isn't enough. It is not enough time to provide the teaching and support for the patient and loved ones that they need to be comfortable and have a good death.

I know someone who is going through this now. Eight years ago he was diagnosed with prostate cancer. I met him four years ago. I watched him tend to his beautiful yard and flowers. When he wasn't out in the yard for a while I knew that the cancer that had spread to his spine was being treated with radiation to alleviate the pain. This would not cure it but would shrink it enough so that he could have a quality to his life and do what he enjoyed. Recently he had a large lump on his neck; the prostate cancer had spread. He has gone through some extremely exciting new cancer trials but the cancer has spread even further. He has said to me he is grateful for the extra time he had and he is just worried about his wife. The day after Christmas he started chemo again. We know it isn't going to cure cancer. We are unsure if it will extend life but we do know now that the life it is giving him is one of pain, and illness. What if instead of having chemotherapy to extend his life only to end up sicker, we focused on what we could do to prepare his wife for his death and after? What if we set up support services while he was alive so that he knew her needs would be met? This didn't happen and he got his second round of this chemotherapy treatment this week and was taken to the hospital with fever, dehydration, and confusion.

My question is: Why is this happening? Does he really want to extend life to spend it confused, in pain and in the hospital? Does his family really want to see him suffer like this to have him on earth for an extra couple days or maybe weeks? Why not have that conversation and get him into hospice earlier? His symptoms could be managed. His concerns for his spouse could be addressed and we could prepare both of them for what to expect during the dying process. We could help them make every one of life's moments matter. Studies have shown that when hospice is started early people often live longer than expected. I would add that they live better.

So I had that conversation with his wife last night. I gave the information to her so that they can make an informed decision on when to start hospice and what benefits hospice can provide. I gave her my support and a hug. Then I went to my room and prayed that no matter what decision is made that he has a "good death." That he dies comfortable, at peace with the people he loves prepared and around him, if that is what he wants.

When it is time for me to go, I hope I know in time to have hospice so that I can prepare myself and prepare my family for the dying process. I want my family around me, having fun, laughing, listening to music, singing, and saying goodbye. I want hospice to keep me comfortable and keep me out of the hospital. I want to be at home. That to me would be a "good death" and I hope no one tries to rob me of that by calling 911.

My company often says, "Your loved one's last moments becomes your lasting memory." My job is to make those things meaningful.

It was already the end of January and the cruise was two weeks away. Shopping for a bathing suit and clothing for the cruise was a daunting task. I was never a person who loved shopping to begin with and after having a bad experience with the mastectomy swim suit I was not looking forward to shopping at all. I had shared my concerns about shopping with a former coworker, Iris. She excitedly offered to go shopping with me. She was previously a Victoria's Secret employee. She was confident she could help me find something. I never in my wildest dreams imagined I could wear anything from that store again after the mastectomies and weight issues.

I grabbed my foam breast forms and shoved them in my purse. I was hoping that by using them instead of the waterproof ones that they could be folded and put into the small hole in the top part of the bathing suits. Having lighter ones may also prevent them from pulling away from my chest. After meeting Iris at the mall, the very first place we went was Victoria's Secret. Iris walked in confidently and immediately went to the bathing suit section. Pulling down a bikini top, she asked to see the foob. I dug it out of my purse as she removed the thin insert from the bikini top. She folded the foam and put it inside. I couldn't believe what my eyes were seeing. I thought, that's cool but I will never find something I look good in and feel comfortable in.

While I just stared at bathing suits and decided I couldn't wear them, she pulled out bathing suits and told me, "You are going to try all these things on. You can't tell if they are going to work if they stay on the hangers." As I was in the dressing room Iris coached me. The very first suit was snug around the top so the forms wouldn't pull away from my chest. The bottoms were a beautiful blue and there were thin shorts to wear over them when I wanted. I tried every suit on she gave me and surprisingly had many choices. She taught me that there was also special tape that I could use to secure the top to my chest. With a new poise I brought my selection up to the counter. It was the first one I tried on. We walked out with smiles and maybe even a bit of swagger.

We went to another bathing suit store and I bought a one-piece. Shopping with Iris was fruitful and fun. By the time we were ready for lunch at the Cheesecake Factory I had bought three dresses, two bathing suits, a few tops, and some shorts. I don't think I had ever in my life allowed myself a self-indulgent shopping spree. It felt extraordinary. A whole new joy came into my life, and I've shopped differently ever since.

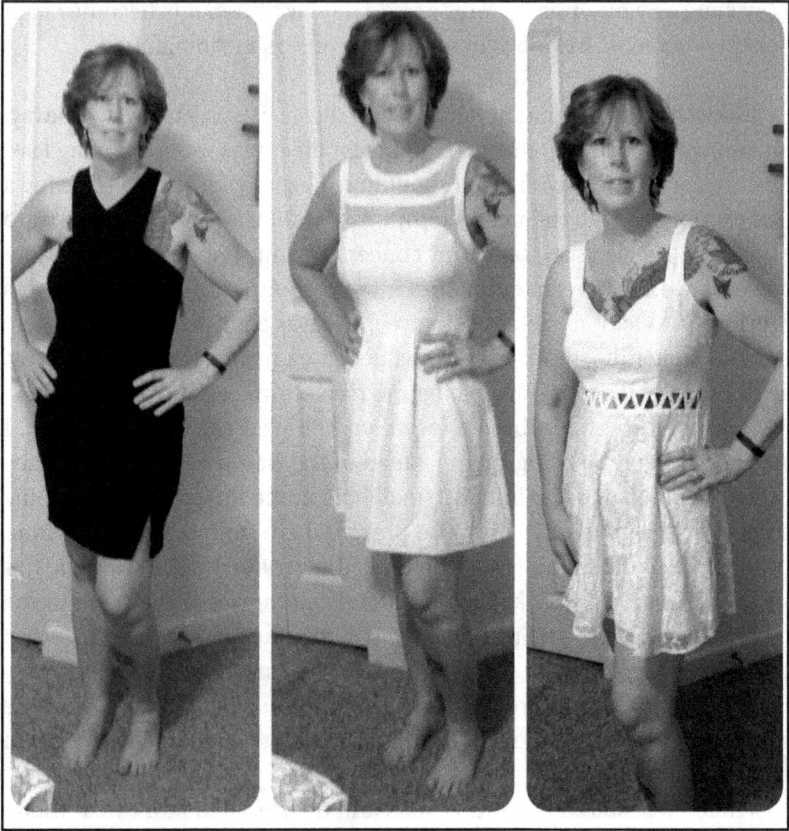

Figure 8-4. The picture I emailed to Grace to show her my new dresses for the cruise

EM: February 4, 2015

From: Grace

To: Marcy

Wow!!!!! Beautiful. Inside and now outside too! Love your hair too! Guess I just plain love you! Xoxo

To: Grace

From: Marcy

Thank you. I love you! I get teary when I think about how long I have known you, how you have always been there for me and my kiddos and how grateful I am for you. Even if we haven't seen each other in a while I know you are just a short drive or a phone call or email away and I hope you know that about me too.

I love you, Marcy

From: Grace

To: Marcy

Always and forever. xoxoxoxo

B: *Flight of a Phoenix*, February 14, 2015

Caring for Body, Soul, and the Whole

Too often assumptions are made when someone is unable to speak or express themselves. We assume that there is nothing going on in their brain, that they are unalive.

I imagine in their mind they are saying, "I'm not dead yet."

They are looking for a connection. Their eyes are closed but maybe they can hear.

When I was in my early twenties I was depressed and suicidal. I attempted suicide twice in two weeks. Although I was getting better at it with practice, I still failed in killing myself. What I remember though is being in the emergency department, my eyes closed, semiconscious, and getting my stomach pumped. One nurse said to a coworker, "If she does this again we should just let her die." In that moment I was thinking, why can't you just let me die now? Did they think I couldn't hear them, or did they know I could hear and they were just being cruel?

That was in the early '90s. Fast-forward to August 2012. I was being wheeled out of the operating room after just having bilateral mastectomies for stage 3B breast cancer. Either a nurse, or tech, I really have no idea who, leaned down next to my baldhead and commanded me in a gentle voice, "Keep fighting." I couldn't open my eyes or speak but I heard her. The chemo was done, the surgery (at least that one) was done but I had no idea how much fighting was left to do. I remembered her and when times got so rough I wasn't convinced I'd live, I could hear her commanding me to "keep fighting" and so I did. I spent multiple times trying to kill myself in the past but now I wanted to live and had an illness that could kill me. She knew I might be able to hear her and she was not being cruel, she was being compassionate and encouraging. Someone thought I had value and acknowledged my fight so far, empowering me to go on with the fight. What a difference from the voices that I heard saying, "We should let her die" that were harshly spoken about me in the early '90s. I was alive but not living back then. I needed help, and I wonder looking back, wasn't it obvious? Instead of the help from the medical field, what I got was more feedback that told me I wasn't worthy. They proved to me that I wasn't worth the effort to find out what the problem was. They were satisfied to treat the illness (in this case overdose), not the whole person. They didn't treat the pain, the emotional pain. I think that is still too common of a theme in the medical field. I have spent a lot of time on both sides of the medical field, as the patient and a nurse. My oncologist and my medical team treated the cancer, but the aftereffects of the cancer treatment caused me to be unalive again instead of living. (More on that next time.)

After the corrective jaw surgery that I had for developmental defects, my jaw was wired shut. I carried paper and pen to write what I wanted to say and often the person I was communicating with gestured for the paper and pen to write back to me, assuming I couldn't hear them because I couldn't speak. Why are we as people or as medical professionals assuming that the people we love or our patients that we care for are unalive when they are quiet or locked in their mind?

Being a "well-seasoned" nurse but new in hospice, I have a lot of experience both professional and personal that I use to benefit the people I care for and their families. Being new to palliative and hospice nursing I still have much to learn. I have many patients with advanced Alzheimer's or dementia from various causes like brain cancer. Many of them are noncommunicative and don't open their eyes. If they say more than one or two words at a time it is nonsensical speech. Should I assume that they don't hear me and not talk to them? Should I assume that since they don't recognize me, my time isn't well spent? Should I also assume that they don't have anything they need me to know or want to express to me? Absolutely *not*. That would be a great disservice to them and their loved ones. I still need to do what I can to reach them and to encourage their family and friends to do the same.

We meet as a team to discuss the best plan of care for our hospice patients. The disciplinary team includes our medical director, nurse case managers, CNAs (certified nursing assistants), LPNs (licensed practical nurses), chaplain, and medical social workers. Our goals for our patients are different from most medical professionals. First we don't make the goals for the patient and family, we assist them in making their own. The goals usually are things like this:

- I don't want to go back to the hospital again.

- I want my pain and symptoms of my disease to be managed at home.

- I want to get kidney dialysis a couple more times so that I can attend my child's high school graduation.

- I want to leave the hospital and be extubated (have the breathing tube removed) at home, so I can die in my own bed, with my family around me.

- I want to go to teach piano lessons again.

- I want to go on one more date.

- I want to make a video for each of my children.

Our job is to make those things happen. We may have volunteers go for a piano lesson, or a volunteer go on a date with a ninety-year-old woman, bring her flowers and dance, or sing with her. We may bring in a therapy dog, assign an art, music, or massage therapist to treat the entire person's wellbeing. The chaplain may go to their home with communion or arrange for someone to receive several sacraments in one day. For us in hospice it is about making those moments matter and we are taught that the patients' end-of-life experiences are their loved ones' lasting memories. We want it to be calm and meaningful. As I have said before there is such a thing as a "good death." But what about "making moments matter" as I mentioned? How do you "make moments matter" in someone who seems unalive?

B: *Flight of a Phoenix*, February 22, 2015

Alive vs. Living

Bon voyage family and friends! As posted on Facebook by my shipmate and high school friend Miriam, "Marcy and I are going off the grid for the next week. No work, no union appointments, meetings, stress! Unless you have the emergency number (if you are not one of our kids, you likely do not), you will not be able to reach us. And kids, unless it's a completely severed body part (toes and fingers don't count) and you are bleeding out, don't call. Really—don't call. Love you."

The first cruise ever in my life and we have excursions planned at every port. This morning though we are taking some down time on our "Day at Sea" to write and relax. Today I am Alive *and* Living. When I asked Miriam what those two words meant to her, her response was, "Alive is with breath and living is with soul."

Why am I writing about this? In 2012 I didn't think I would be alive let alone living. Now I am on a cruise ship with my computer propped up on my lap, listening to and watching the waves from our balcony room. Preparing for shows, meeting people and an excursion at every port. I am very grateful to my medical and oncology team for saving my life. They kept me alive through the months of chemo, radiation, and two surgeries. They saved my life when I had complications that landed me in the hospital. I thought surely I would never make it out alive from that complication. After the treatment was over there was a honeymoon period, a time to just to be grateful no more treatments needed. That honeymoon period didn't last long and I will tell you why.

Although I have been known to say that I have gained more from cancer than it took from me, I had to take stock of what damage was done financially, physically, emotionally, mentally and spiritually. I didn't care much for this inventory.

Financially, I cashed in some of my retirement money and used what little I had in savings due to all the time off and needing to continue to support my two children and my mother, who thankfully lives with me and helped me through the rough spots.

Mentally, I was still going through chemo brain, having a difficult time remembering, and using wrong words. At the same time I was starting a new job in home health nursing to help recover some of the money I needed to use from savings.

Emotionally, I felt weak. I was not sleeping well and being fearful that the cancer wasn't completely gone or would come back. It was almost crippling.

Physically, with being chemically induced into menopause to reduce the estrogen that feeds the cancer cells, also mucked up my emotions. The steroids and the medications made it difficult to lose the weight. I could always lose with Weight Watchers. I was back down to 180 pounds from 215 pounds after gaining weight dealing with my bad marriage and divorce. The oncology team told me that during treatment it is not the time to worry about losing weight. It came on little by little until I was 240, which is 90 over my goal weight. I was too tired after work and too heavy to get any significant work outs in. So I just continued to eat to try to manage my depression. Depression caused by the situations in my life and the aftereffects of the cancer treatment itself.

At that point I was alive but not living. When my fifteen-year-old son one night asked me to put my work computer down and said, "Mom, they [my work] get you all day, do you have to work at night too?" those words caused my heart to ache. My teenage son, asking me in such a way to join him in the land of the living. I realized that I fought cancer to stay alive, especially for my children, and what am I doing now? Taking all of that ,life I was given and spending too much time with work and taking care of everyone other than myself and the family I fought to be here for.

So what did 2013 and half of 2014 look like for me? Those of you who followed me on the medical journal website know that I was gaining weight and having issues with depression. In July 2013, I had gone to the specialists at MD Anderson in Texas. They didn't want to hear about how fearful I was about the cancer coming back. All the physicians were telling me that body fat would increase the estrogen levels and my risk of the cancer returning. One specialist spent a good deal of time reviewing my records to tell me I didn't have the type of cancer the medical team in Illinois thought I had. I needed to take the Tamoxifen to prevent cancer's return, eat healthy and exercise one hour a day... He handed me a folder on "survivorship" and dismissed me. In other words, I was alive and not living. I resented this physician. I resented his implications that it was "just that easy" to get my life back and get control and confidence in my body and myself again. I flew back home with my tail between my legs and even more depressed than I was when I flew to Texas. Time for antidepressants, again. Just another oncologist to tell me I wasn't doing a good enough job surviving. They were right, I was alive but not living, yet no one in the medical field was giving me concrete help to get my life back on track.

My friends signed up for a cruise, this cruise that I am on now. I always wanted to go cruising so I used my income tax return and paid for it over a year in advance. More depression about my weight came into play when I discovered that the excursions that I wanted to do would exclude me because of my weight. I tried Weight Watchers again. I tried a medically supervised very low-calorie diet. I couldn't maintain that type of diet to have the weight loss stick.

That is when I saw the bariatric surgeon, thinking I could get a lap-band. He explained to me that they are moving away from the lap-band and that I would be a good candidate for vertical gastric sleeve. I would be meeting with the surgeon and nutritionist.

July 16, 2014, I had the vertical sleeve gastrectomy. He also said that I had a hiatal hernia that was worse than they expected and he fixed it. The hernia repair made the recovery from the surgery go slower. That was step one in taking control over my life again. After some of the weight started coming off I started working with a personal trainer for weight lifting. I was eating better, exercising, and changed jobs. The pounds decreased and the confidence increased. The more I moved, the more weight I lost. The more weight I lost, the more in control I felt. The more control I felt over my life, the more life I started living. I changed jobs to a new position in hospice care and I applied to go back to school into an online RN to BSN program.

On February 9, less than a week to go before the cruise began, I hit my weight loss goal. I called the surgeon and spoke with his assistant, Mary. I told her that I feel like the oncologists and medical team saved my life but that she and the surgeon and their team gave it back to me. I was in tears, thanking her for helping me to live my life again. The change physically, emotionally and mentally has been astounding.

I have a newfound confidence in myself, feeling of worth and looking forward enough to my future to go back to school. As a side note to my dietary changes and gym membership, my mom has also joined the gym, is eating better and losing weight as well.

Today on the cruise we saw a show called the *Motor City*. Miriam and I sang and danced with the cruise ship entertainers after the show and she looked at me and said…"This is living." Yes, tonight I knew I was alive and living well. "Celebration" by Kool and the Gang was heard many times. Seems to be a theme lately. Miriam and I danced to this on the cruise with the performers on the cruise ship. Yes, a celebration! Let's live and celebrate life.

My dear grandma Bollman used to say, "The worm has turned" when something that previously wasn't going her way began to improve. I believe in my life the worm had turned. Most of the year my time was spent balancing my hospice nurse job, time with my family, and time for myself to continue working out and writing. There were periods of time when I

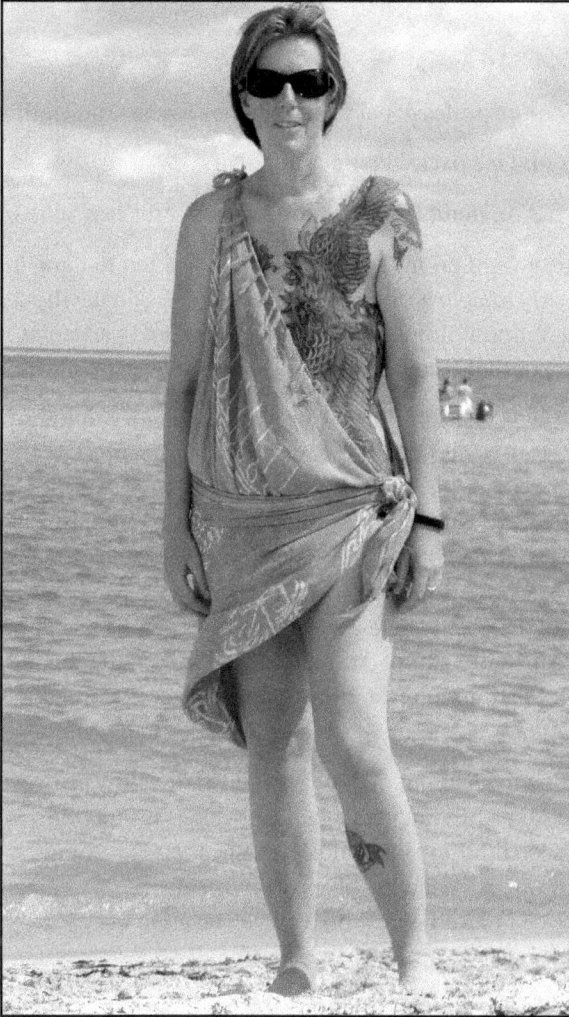

Figure 8-5. On the beach in Cozumel

felt normal and even joyful. Times when I could forget that I had cancer. I
didn't talk about it every day. It was a period of time when I was learning
new things and looking forward to new opportunities. I felt I had value. I
was healing. I was living

I continued to participate in the Making Strides for Breast Cancer walks
with my former coworkers, led by Brooke. Each year I check in at the
Survivor table, I proudly don my survivor sash and update the number of
years on my survivor sticker.

B: *Flight of a Phoenix*, March 21, 2015

On the Road Bike Again

Bicycle tune-up, professional bike fitting, new gear, and clothing: $900

Band-Aids and ice packs: Pennies to dollars

First time out on Road Bike in over five years: Priceless

I knew after I went on my bike ride today I wanted to hang out at home and write. My topic has changed from what I originally thought I would be writing about. I did not realize the impact this particular ride would have on me or that I would have such a desire to share it with you.

I'll share a little background on my cycling history to help you understand why this is significant for me. I started cycling regularly around 2002, when I was married. We rode together mostly and with the kids. I did my first 100-mile group ride in June 2007, without my husband. I felt so accomplished. I was at my Weight Watcher lifetime member goal weight of 155 pounds on my 68-inch frame. Our weekend rides varied from twenty-five to fifty miles. Toward the end of my marriage and during my divorce in 2010, I stopped riding. Having gained weight and becoming depressed, I had no interest in my bike. My heaviest weight at that time was 216.

I was starting to snap out of that funk and get healthy again in 2011–2012 and joining Weight Watchers again was down to 180 pounds. In March of 2012, I dusted off my bike, took it to the shop for a tune up, new tires, chain...the works. While my bike was in the shop, I was diagnosed with breast cancer. I picked up my bike and it stayed in the garage for the next three years.

When I was getting chemotherapy, my oncologist told me not to worry about Weight Watchers, not to worry about my weight at all. So I didn't. During my treatment I was drop kicked into menopause from the chemotherapy, put on steroids, tired and didn't move much, depressed, gained weight. The "survivorship" was just as hard as the treatment. The doctors now started telling me that I was too heavy and the excess fat would increase the chances of the cancer coming back. I was about 220 pounds then. I tried many things for weight loss, including going back to Weight Watchers. I tried a medically supervised very low calorie diet. I would lose a little, gain a lot. I was tired, depressed, not moving much and gaining weight at a rapid pace. My heaviest weight was 240 pounds in July of 2014.

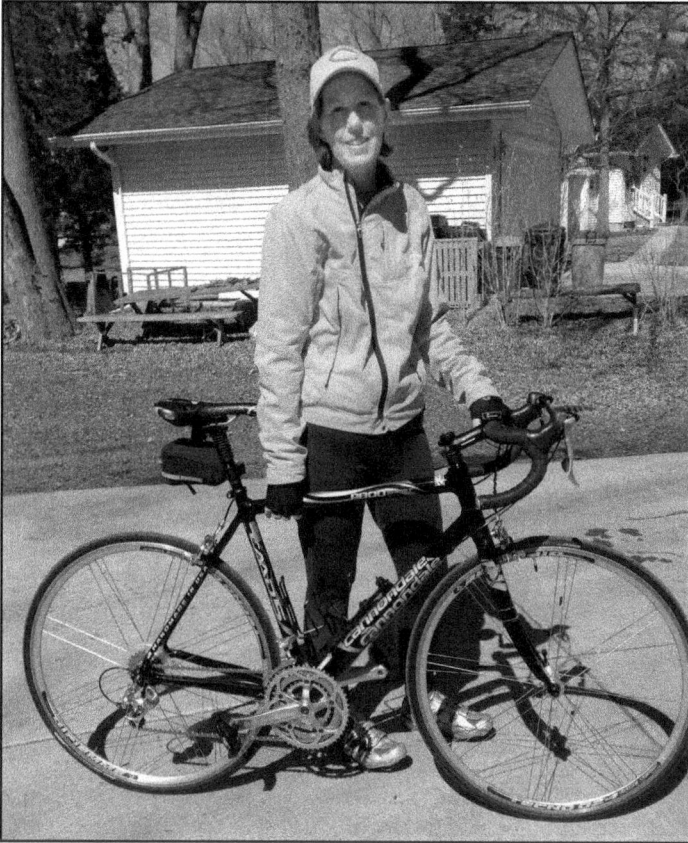

Figure 8-6. I'm geared up and ready to ride again

I hit bottom and decided on weight loss surgery. July 16, 2014, I had a vertical sleeve gastrectomy. Some think surgery is the "easy option." Wake up! It is not an easy option; it is not an easy decision. The risks and pain are not easy. Society's judgments are not easy. The lifestyle changes are not easy. It is worth it! At least it has been for me. I am now working out with a personal trainer, eating healthy and wanting to get on my bike again. I have surpassed my Weight Watchers goal of 155 pounds and weigh 144 pounds! My high school weight fluctuated between 140 and 145.

So once again, having not used my bike in about five to six years I took it to the bike shop. Invested in everything it needed and everything I needed to hit the road again, including a professional bike fitting. I found it made a world of difference in my ability to stay on my bike and in my efficiency when I did this just before my century ride in 2007.

The nutritionist has been asking me to come to the bariatric support group, so today was my first time. I thought it would be a great day to start riding again and rode my bike to the group. It was a nine-mile ride out, nine-mile ride back. Surely, I could do that ride for my first time out in over five years.

The ride *to* the bariatric support group: My neighborhood is a little hilly with narrow streets. The first few miles of my ride were spent getting used to the gears. I didn't realize until three to four miles in that I was in the high gears used for cycling downhill. No wonder I was struggling. I had to relearn gear shifting, which levers do what on the right side and left side. Refreshing my memory on clipping in and out of the pedals was also a challenge. I managed to be able to do this on the way there without falling. Adjusting to the position on the saddle, shifting my weight back when I was going uphill, and heels down for a more efficient pedal stroke were things I had to remind myself to do. It used to come naturally after I learned it the first time. After about four to five miles in, I was comfortable with the gears. The new issue was the numbness starting in my right hand third and fourth finger. I worry about this. The cancer treatments caused neuropathy for which I needed occupational therapy. I am concerned this may be an issue. Yet, I think...if this is the worst of it, I will be okay. It is a bit cold and I wish I had cycling gloves with the full fingers. Still, cold fingers and ears are not going to keep me from getting back on my bike. I pulled into the hospital for the meeting with an overall sense of well-being and confidence. I was slow but got there... Nine miles in forty-one minutes.

The bariatric support group was great. I loved meeting those who are on a similar journey but have their unique story. Many of us exchange information so that we can support and encourage each other in between the monthly meetings. I felt proud to be a part of this strong group of people.

The ride *back* home: The sun was shining more than it was at 8:30 this morning when I left my house. With the sun though came the wind. I set out knowing that if I just could not make it home, my mom was on standby to come and get me. The problem with this route was the roads. I often drive these roads and wonder why cyclists are on them. There isn't a lot of shoulder area, curving and two lanes, no passing zones. Not the safest roads. There was no other way if I wanted to ride my bike that I could go that would be any safer. I pressed on, learning to use my mirror again, positioning it, checking blind spots, using signals and praying that the cars and trucks would give me just a bit of wiggle room. Thank you to all of the motorists out there who pay attention to those of us on bikes. A few miles into the ride home, the wind was getting to me a bit. I could feel my legs burning at times but that wasn't a concern; in fact, it was desired. I continued to try different handle bar positions. I had never been one to use the drop bars but my goal this year is to become competent and comfortable with that. I was starting to feel tension in my shoulders and neck. Posture is so important and I have a hard time remembering to relax and drop my shoulders. Even when I am lifting weights, my trainer has to remind me at times to watch my shoulders. I pulled over. I didn't need to pull over on the way there but on the way back, it was a different story. I realized I was struggling partly from the wind but mostly from not eating. I took out my protein bar and took a few bites. Having the gastrectomy puts me in the position of deciding am I going to eat or drink. I can't eat and drink at the same time. I hydrated on the way there and during the meeting but what I should have done was to eat the protein bar when I got there. Lesson learned.

I decided I was not going to call my mom to bail me out. I told myself, "You are going to ride the rest of the way home, even if it is at two miles an hour and you have to stop five times. No matter how long it takes you are finishing this." I stopped one other time for a few bites of protein bar. I got home in forty-seven minutes.

I thought as I was pulling into my driveway that I was happy with this, first time out in a long time. I slowed down, clipped out of my left pedal, but before I could get out of my right, started falling over. I caught myself with my right hand and while I was lying in my driveway unclipped my right pedal.

So overall, I am pleased with my first ride. I have a lot of refreshing to do before my weekend bicycling trip that I signed up for in June. I think I may need to go get an x-ray on my hand but am going to try RICE first. Rest, ice, compression, and elevation.

Overall, I am happy. I am happy with my health, my activity level, and my new life. No, it is *not* easy. It is easy to sit on the couch. The effort *is* worth it!

I did not go through cancer treatment, obesity, and depression to fix those things and not live my life.

On the Road Bike Again—Part Two

It has been over a month since I wrote part one of my challenge to get on my road bike again. Partly due to weather, partly time and mostly due to excuses. This post is going to be a look into how my mind works. It is partly self-talk during my second ride of the season, partly things I want you to know about me, and maybe some things that might help you, if you need to borrow some self-talk. I was also writing some parts of this post in my head, knowing I might forget what I want to say. This kept my mind occupied as I rode by myself on this ride.

Yesterday I invited my local friends to join me on a bike ride. No takers. It is always so much harder to motivate myself to get out there and to do a long ride when there is no one with me. Still, I need to get some miles in before some weekend biking events I have scheduled. I got my biking gear out and my bike in the car and told myself, "Just go first thing in the morning, shoot for twenty miles and see what happens."

I decided the Prairie Trail would be a good place to go. This is what I am most familiar with. I rode this trail a lot when I was married and with my children. Off I went with my coffee and protein drink to park my car and head out on my lone ride. I had everything I needed including a music playlist on Spotify, which I figured would come in handy. I was amazed at the appropriateness at some of the songs at key times. I will name them and honestly, the timing of them during my ride I am not making up. The playlist was created by someone from the walking challenge I am in and was on Spotify. I had "1,000-mile challenge ultimate playlist" on shuffle and had no idea which songs were on the list.

I had a few goals for this ride:

- Use drop-down handlebars as much as possible

- Get in twenty miles

- 12–14 MPH

- No falls

I was comfortable the first few miles in the drop-down position. I was thinking about the two weekend bike trips I plan on taking this summer and hoping that if I have any issues with soreness with saddle position I would get that worked out before the first weekend ride. The only thing I didn't really like about the drop-down position was I felt like it was harder to look ahead at the terrain. I was reminded on a couple of the sections of bike path that when riding through standing water, the water hugs the tires and then spits on the back of you. Yep, wet butt. I continued to think about my position, pedal stroke, relaxing my shoulders, and keeping my heels down: All the things that I had gotten used to before I took a five to six year hiatus from my bike.

My thoughts shifted to being somewhat proud of myself for just being out there on the path. I thought about all the trips that were taken on this path with my family, with my former husband. We had some belly busting laughs, some scary injuries, and some explosive arguments. It was starting to get a little lonely. I looked at my odometer and I had only gone four to five miles. I was starting to feel tingling in my fingers of my right hand and my thoughts took me to some of the rides I did in 2005. One in particular was the Springfield Century. I didn't do a hundred miles as intended. By the time I rode sixty-two, my left hand was so weak I could not hold silverware tight enough to cut pancakes. Turned out I had cubital tunnel syndrome and would need an ulnar nerve transposition surgery to keep my hand muscles from continuing to atrophy. The issue I am having this time I believe is related to the surgeries for breast cancer I had on the right side and the nerve damage associated with it and possibly some neuropathy from the chemotherapy as well. I debated with myself for a while on if I would seek any doctor's opinions on this or just, "shake it off." Back to the 5 miles I had ridden, that's it. I switched to look at how long I was riding.. Twenty-eight minutes, that's it? I am tired already.

This is where the first self-talk, mental gymnastics, mind game came into play. I told myself, it doesn't matter if you get in twenty miles, just ride out for forty-five minutes, you are almost at thirty, you can do fifteen more minutes, and then you can turn back. I got to the area that was changed from the last time I was on the trail. A large bypass was built and I was curious about how they diverted the bike path as it was built directly through where the bike path used to go. It was a nice downhill and a bit curvy, I was thinking, "This is a welcome break, I think I will coast here, too bad it will be uphill on my way back."

I could feel my pace slowing down when "Feel This Moment" by Pitbull, featuring Christine Aguilara, came on and made me start thinking about how nice it was to be outside, being able to ride my bike, being healthy and the next few minutes went easier.

I was coming to the point of a bridge that was significant to our family rides. When the kids were little, or even just when it was my husband and me, we always stopped on this bridge to play "pooh-sticks." I told myself I would stop on the way back but I had to keep going until the turn around point. For the next few miles I had to think about what I remembered was further up. There was the Otto engineering factory. I am just going to ride there, and then I will turn around. When I got to the factory, I thought, I can't be too far from the Dairy Queen, I'll just go there and sit on the tables for a break and then turn around. Just as I decided to continue on, the next song on the playlist was "We Are the Champions." On the way out, it was still early enough there weren't many people on the trail. Only one cyclist passed me.

I do not consider myself a cyclist; when people ask, I usually just say, "I ride a bike." I was never as avid as my ex: if given a choice, I avoid days that are too cold or windy. I will ride in the rain if I get caught in an unexpected rain, but will not start a ride if it is raining.

I was keeping a decent pace at that point when I got to a section where I almost got myself killed. I saw the car coming but thought they had a stop. When I realized the stop sign was on the bike trail and for me, I clutched my brakes while simultaneously clipping out of my pedals. I could feel my back tire lifting off the pavement as I screeched to a halt. I am sure that car had some choice words for me. He waved me through but at that point, I had already stopped and really needed to get my wits about me before pushing off again. A few short blocks later, I was at my turning point.

Shortly after I started on my way back, a cyclist was behind me. I could see him in my mirror and hear his bike but he made no effort to pass. I thought, "Really, I am just starting and am very slow, just pass me, you aren't going to get much from drafting off me." He finally passed and went barreling down the trail. I could not believe how inadequate it made me feel. I started to let the negative thoughts drift in, how slow I was riding, how I struggled to get in ten miles so far when there was a time when ten miles was practically nothing. Just then, the Andy Grammer song "Keep Your Head Up" came on.

The "pooh-sticks" bridge was coming up, the perfect opportunity to get off the saddle for a minute or two. Again, my thought shifted to all the family rides, and games. When riding with younger kids, it is all about occupying the mind, not as much about limitations in ability. I starting thinking about my son and his cycling accomplishments, then got back on my bike to press on.

The tingling in my fingers was turning to numbness and I was starting to feel the ischium bones again. I am going to need to get this worked out before the longer rides. I was getting a little antsy in my saddle.

I was back to the point of the bypass bridge and it saddened me a bit when I saw the diversion the trail took. The Prairie Trail Bike Shop that was in Algonquin was gone. I am riding the bike that Sam sold me all those years ago.

As I am going under the bypass, I have a bit of momentum to go back up the incline but not a lot. I started thinking as someone went whizzing by me on my left about momentum. Momentum is so helpful at times but when I really thought about it, there is not a lot of growth when I am riding the wave of momentum. As I sat back on my saddle, pushed down, and pulled up my pedals I thought, this is when I get stronger. I was thinking about working with my trainer: when I am struggling and pushing, she keeps saying, "slow, slow, slow." My muscle fibers are burning. They will grow from that. Don't we sometimes want to ride the momentum? It is easier. I am stronger now from having to slow down and push through. Pushing through my divorce, the cancer, the depression, and obesity made me a stronger person. My speed kept falling below 10 miles an hour on the inclines. I pushed a little harder trying to stay in the double digits. I had to battle my self-talk that was saying, "You are not fast enough, and you are weak." I decided I would scrap the goal of 12–14 MPH. The speed is not important, the important thing today was that I was out there and I just need to keep the pedals going around in circles.

As I was finishing up my ride, "Right Now" by Van Halen came on.

That strong, single woman made it back to her car.

Now back to the goals of this ride:

- Use drop-down handlebars as much as possible: I used them for half the ride

- Twenty miles: Yep, made it

- 12–14 miles per hour: Decided this goal was not worth pursuing at this time

- No falls: I didn't fall, or get hit by a car. No bandages or ice packs needed.

I got back in my car and started to head home. In just a few minutes, my Garmin activity tracker buzzed at me and said, "Move." This cracked me up, after all those miles, since I only had in 945 steps.

It was a good ride. Although I would much rather have had company, I did it! I kept myself company by writing this in my mind and reminiscing about past rides, enjoying the moments and looking forward to future rides.

B: *Flight of a Phoenix*, October 23, 2015

Breast Cancer Awareness

Since I was diagnosed with stage 3B breast cancer, this is my third Breast Cancer Awareness Month. Honestly, I felt like if I kept seeing pink I would vomit. It is bad enough to be "aware" I had cancer every time I look in the mirror, get dressed, shower, or hug someone. When I do those simple daily things I am reminded that I almost died and could have a recurrence of a deadly disease. I was plenty "aware" of breast cancer without having a sea of pink everywhere in front of me. In fact, I never even liked the color pink, but once you have breast cancer it is assumed that pink is your color. While undergoing cancer treatments and immediately afterward all the pink is comforting to tell you people are helping through breast cancer awareness events and in particular with the pink awareness ribbons. I even have one tattooed on my arm. It surprised me how different I felt about it this year. My awareness is going back and forth between fear and paranoia to feeling as if I am stronger and more confident than I have ever been in my life.

At the end of September, I put in an offer on a house: the first house I was buying on my own. I am a single mom and daughter of my seventy-seven-year-old mother who lives with me. Three years ago when I was being treated for cancer, I never thought I would live long enough to buy a house, or be able to retire. Having my offer accepted was exciting and yet terrifying.

I discussed my fears with my children, Jo (29), Dani (22), and Riley (17). My daughters understood, but my son didn't really want to hear about it. I think, having to be the "man of the house," he couldn't even think about the "what-ifs." He saw me at my sickest and I think he doesn't want to visit those thoughts again. I told my daughters how paranoid I was. The overwhelming fear that if I bought a house and have a huge loan, the cancer would come back. I would be leaving my mom and the two kids, who still live at home, with a house to pay off with my life insurance and the uncertainty of where to live.

You are probably thinking it is nuts to even entertain thoughts like that. I imagine anyone who has been told they have a high risk of cancer recurrence would be paranoid. Since I did not achieve pCR (pathologic complete response) to chemotherapy, I am at a higher risk of breast cancer recurrence. When my cancer was discovered it was already stage 3B. The fact is after four months of chemotherapy, I had cancer in six out of twelve lymph nodes. When I started chemotherapy the scans only showed cancer in one lymph node. I do not trust my body. There is an unsettling feeling that something in my body could destroy me. The little rashes I have, the prickly pains where I shouldn't have them, and the fact that my body doesn't look or feel normal due to the surgeries makes it hard to evaluate. I go for my checkups and am always told there is "no evidence of disease."

My daughter Jo said, "You are fine but if it does come back, we will deal with it together." Dani said, "Shut up, Mom, you are fine." I love those girls! So I pressed on with the house buying process.

Toward the end of September, I had planned on doing a photography shoot to take portraits highlighting my phoenix tattoo done by Nikki Harris but I cancelled. I was so overwhelmed, panicky, and worried. I just couldn't calm my nerves and I knew it would be difficult to capture the photos I envisioned in that state of mind.

I managed to reschedule for October 18. The last weekend to pack before my move but the day I knew I had to do it. With all the pink I was being forced to look at it during Breast Cancer Awareness Month it was harder and harder to deny to myself that I still felt fragile.

October 18 I was also scheduled to do a breast cancer walk with my former coworkers and friends. Of the thirteen of us walking, four have had breast cancer. The walk was at a beautiful nature preserve. This was the place I went in April of 2012 to do a photo shoot before I lost my long hair. The plan was to do the walk in the morning and then in the evening do the photo shoot with Kamila Angelika. The day was more than I could have hoped for. It was so empowering to be at the walk with other women who have known the same despair and hope that I have known. Walking and chatting with those who are further ahead on this road gave me comfort in knowing I am not alone in my thoughts. They nodded in understanding and told me what I was feeling was normal. It also felt gratifying to be able to support those who are coming after me by remembering where I came from and reminding them "better days are coming." A strong group of survivors and their supporters. So maybe pink is okay today, maybe I can embrace Breast Cancer Awareness...today.

I had been thinking for a while what I wanted my photos to portray. The story I wanted to tell. People need to realize that it doesn't matter how someone looks on the outside, they still may have scars underneath. You could learn from them unless you judge them. You see, with my prosthetics on and my "normal clothing" I don't look like I have had a disease such as cancer, and you wouldn't know I have tattoos. You may just see a woman. A woman with kids who has a career as a hospice nurse. But under the wrapping there is more, so much more. The photo shoot, in my mind, should be a progression from the "wrapped woman" to the one that emerged after the cancer experience. The Phoenix.

In the past I saw myself as not really "photo-worthy." I was a bit nervous, not about the photographer or taking my top and prosthetics off but of spending all the time taking photos and having none turn out.

Kam chose a beautiful field to shoot some of the photos in. This was becoming fun, I felt a bit like a model. Off in the distance there was a woman and her horse. We watched them a little and she watched us as we took some of the first photos. We shot some photos to show me in the prosthetics, and then some showing what the actual prosthetics looked like.

Quite some time went by and she said nothing to us, until I took my top off. It was then that she yelled over to us. "Do you have permission to be on the property?" There was a for-sale sign on the property and we weren't going to be there long or do any damage. Kam yelled back a simple answer: "No." The woman with the horse continued, "Well if the owners drive by, you may be in trouble." Instantly, I felt wrong, dirty, like I was doing some sort of nudity photo shoot. Being very uncomfortable and ashamed of my body now I asked Kam if we could go somewhere else. Kam and I discussed why the woman with the horse chose that timing after watching us for so long and not saying a thing. We suspected she thought this was some type of pornography shoot as she wasn't close enough to see my tattoos or mastectomy scars and probably only saw bare skin. After taking a step forward in my confidence in the appearance of my body, two sentences from a stranger set me back two steps.

Kam knew of another place that would be good and we still had enough time before it got dark. We went to a barn near her house. The experience of those photos was phenomenal. As Kam and I walked, shot photos, and talked and I told my story, I felt more confidence and pride.

The process of getting the phoenix tattoo was a healing process and photographing the tattoo, photographing *me*, helped document the process. I feel stronger, proud, healthy, and liberated.

I have learned that once a cancer patient, always a cancer patient. It doesn't end on the day of the last treatment. Cancer may be cured but its physical, mental and emotional effects don't go away. I know my fears and paranoia will always be there in the back of my mind, waiting for a moment when I feel weak. Those thoughts may shake me but they will not cause me to fall. I will look at myself, my tattoo, and my photos and be reminded I am stronger than I was before.

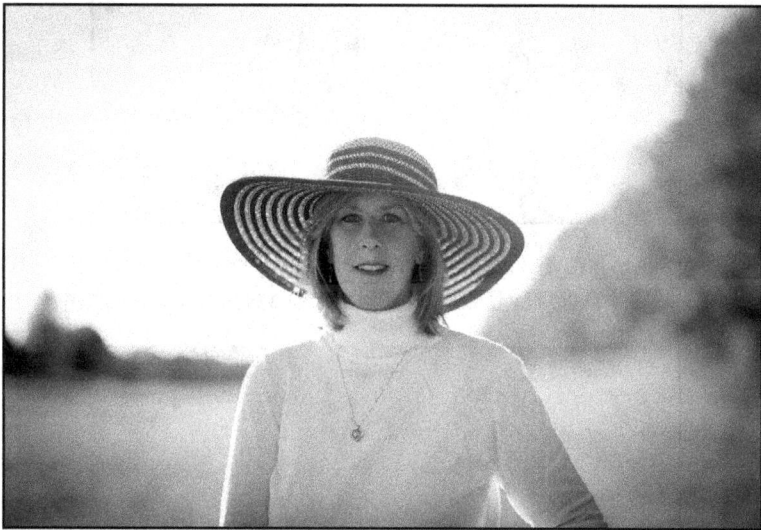

Figure 8-7. One of the first photographs I felt beautiful in (photo by Kamila Angelika Photography)

The daunting burden of discovering my "new normal" and learning to trust my health and body was a task that would take years, and, as I am beginning to accept now, one that may never fully come to an end.

Denial at time of diagnosis is expected and understood. It serves a function in allowing a cancer patient and their loved ones time to process the news that will surely be life-changing. I found there is a denial after treatment is done, denial that I was cancer free and could be healthy again. In my case, I had missed a sign of breast cancer months before diagnosis, which is something I have not even to this day discussed with my family:

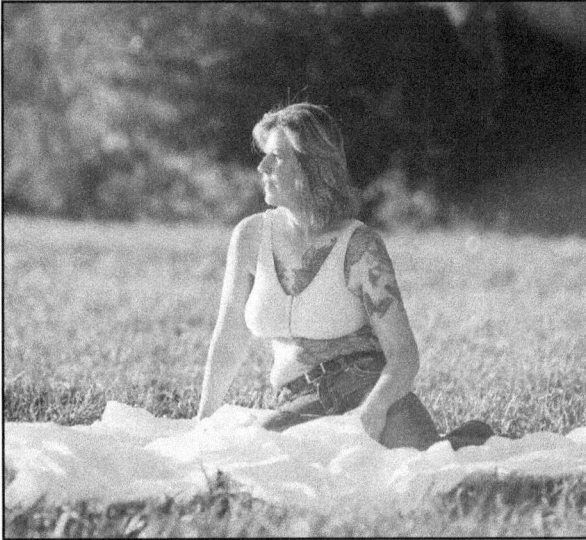

Figure 8-8. With my prosthetics on (photo by Kamila Angelika Photography,tattoo by Nikki Harris at The Living Gallery Tattoo Parlour)

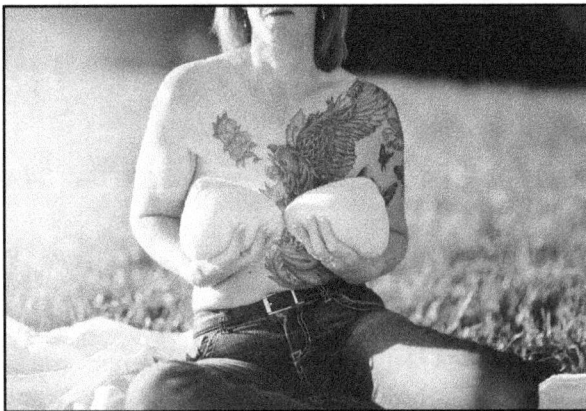

Figure 8-9. Holding my prosthetics (photo by Kamila Angelika Photography, tattoo by Nikki Harris at The Living Gallery Tattoo Parlour)

I had gray nipple discharge. After looking it up on medical sites, I convinced myself that it was not a significant finding unless it kept happening sowhen it didn't continue, I forgot about it. I had not mentioned it to my physician during my annual exam because I really didn't pay much attention to it. I had been paranoid about lumps and bumps being breast cancer in the past and it had never been anything to be concerned over... How could I, a seasoned nurse, ignore the significance of nipple discharge in

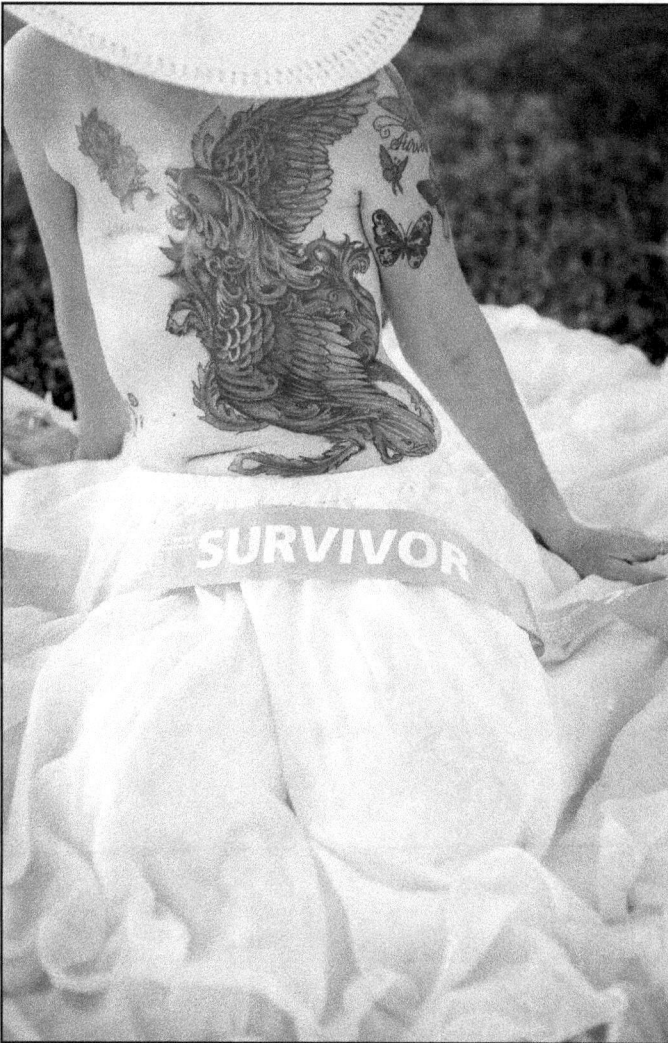

Figure 8-10. With my survivor ribbon (photo by Kamila Angelika Photography, tattoo by Nikki Harris at The Living Gallery Tattoo Parlour)

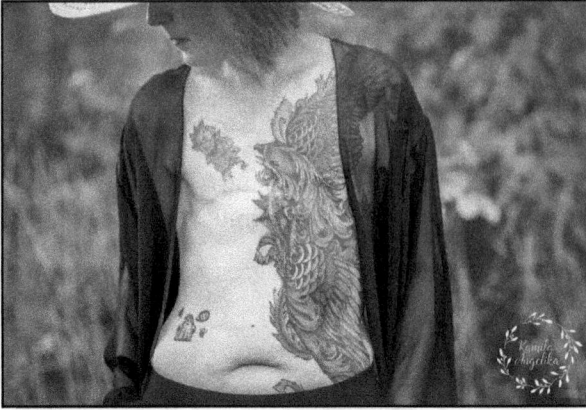

Figure 8-11. Showing my phoenix tattoo (photo by Kamila Angelika Photography, tattoo by Nikki Harris at The Living Gallery Tattoo Parlour)

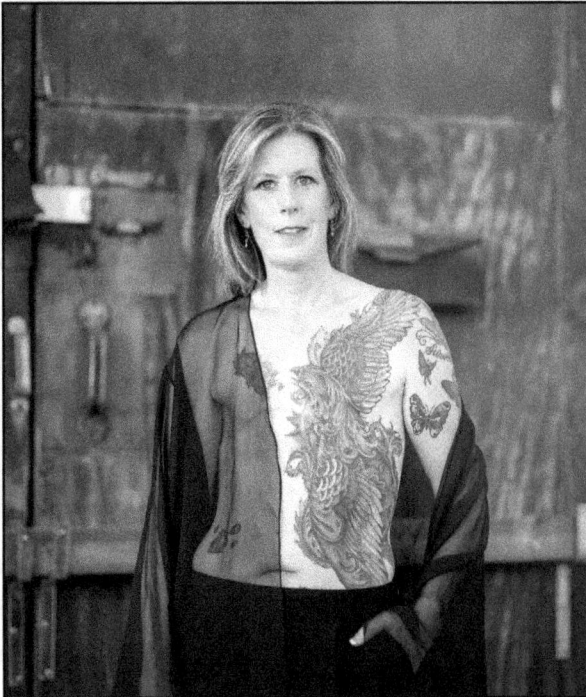

Figure 8-12. Showing my phoenix tattoo (photo by Kamila Angelika Photography, tattoo by Nikki Harris at The Living Gallery Tattoo Parlour)

a woman who was in their forties? As I type this and reflect on this, I still tear up. I still feel responsible for the advanced stage of the breast cancer. Assumptions could have killed me. I still feel guilt for what I put my family and friends through. This has been why trusting not only my body's ability to alert me that something is wrong is arduous but also trusting my ability to identify which signs and symptoms are significant.

Epilogue

Better Days Are Here

Putting this book together was more challenging than I had anticipated. The editor suggested certain areas of the book have more reflection and detail, filling in some information and gaps between the blogs, emails, and journals. I had a hard time with this for a few reasons. First, the stress of the early diagnosis affected my memory because emotionally, humans have a self-protection mechanism for such traumas. I was aware of my survival mode but until writing this I had not fully grasped how deep that went. I also had "chemo brain" and my memory during that time frame is poor. If I hadn't written most of the book via journals and blogs at the time it was happening I don't think this type of book could be possible. Reflection about what actually happened is also more painful than I expected. I thought all my thoughts and feelings were an open book, but in actuality there were times in the cancer experience when I felt incredibly alone even with over a hundred people checking in on me, leaving supportive comments, sending flowers, and so on. Sometimes I didn't even feel understood by other cancer survivors and that was just as painful as the physical effects of treatment. There were times I wanted to die and only fought for my children; the time to spend with the young ones, and the chance just to meet the oldest.

There was a realization that has come from working on the edits and adding new content to this book. As I asked my friends and family to help me with remembering certain aspects of my cancer diagnosis and treatment, I have come to understand that as hard as moving into survivorship was for me, it was hard for them too. They were neglected by society after the treatment phase was over. They still had to process what it did to them to watch and help someone they love go through something so difficult. Asking those questions have given my mom, kids, and other family and friends the opportunity to say, "I was so scared when_____" and, "I really thought you were going to die when_____." These are the things they never expressed to me previously. These are the things that family and friends don't often express because they are told, as the patient is told, to have hope and stay positive. I now understand that I never considered how difficult "survivorship" is for my loved ones.

My friendship with Alan, who shared a fellowship in healthcare as a physician and in suffering from his chronic pain, became an invaluable source of understanding and support. These interactions and the "behind the scenes" emails back and forth made it clear to me that chronic disease and acute disease often have the same effects on a person's ability to live a fulfilling life. The outpouring of support for someone who has cancer is unyielding but a chronic pain sufferer often has their concerns minimized, or worse, is treated like a drug seeker or attention seeker. It is my belief that not only does society need to recognize the long-term adjustments that are required of a cancer patient, it needs to recognize the complex and serious nature of chronic pain. We both found humor to be particularly helpful in easing some of the heartache we had that was difficult to share with others.

I received a letter from my firstborn child, Josie, in December 2014 inviting me back into her life. We have learned we have an abundance of commonalities, from physical appearance, mannerisms, and sense of humor to the love of writing and the desire to share our stories. We are in the process of writing a trilogy. The first two books will be individually written by each of us. Josie's will cover her life up to the day she wrote the letter to me and with anticipation and hope put it in the mailbox. Mine will be from the time I found out I was pregnant with her at age sixteen until I received that letter. The final book we will write together and share how she was able to transition into our family and her birth family, and the impact that having her birth-mom in her life had on her transition from male to female.

Things I have done and often continue to do since being diagnosed with cancer: air-boat ride in Florida; take ballet, tap, and hip-hop dance classes; learning to ride a motorcycle and saving to buy a Harley-Davidson; joined a women's hiking group; and attended Chicago Open Air (three-day heavy metal festival) with Riley and crowd-surfed to some of my favorite bands. I have resigned from my position as a hospice nurse to pursue my dream of being an author and speaker.

I have plans for a high school alumni cruise, hiking in the Rocky Mountains, and a dog-sledding trip with the women's hiking group. There are so many more things on my life list—the term I prefer over bucket list.

Things I can no longer do since being diagnosed with cancer—Nothing! Having cancer did, in fact, give me more than it took, most importantly quality of life. Better days did in fact come and in a way I never thought possible.

Acknowledgments

To my family and friends: I wish I could list all of you individually. Please know that you all helped me in so many ways that it would be an impossible task to list them. You showered me with your love, hugs, and constant encouragement; you bathed me with your strength, and held me up when the world was collapsing. You met me wherever I was, even when I was in a dark place, and for those things I can never repay you. This book is my attempt to make you all realize the impact you have in making the world a better place. There is still good in this world and I know it because of you. I love you.

To Alan Kanter: You always knew the words that would bring me hope when I lost faith and laughter and when I felt such deep despair. You gave me strength when I felt too weak to lift my head. You met me wherever I was in my thoughts and emotions. By being the voice of reason, you kept me afloat when I was sinking. You believed in me when I didn't believe in myself. Without you I would never have believed "better days are coming" or that I deserved to have them. It wasn't until I really put this book together that I realized my story was also your story. I couldn't have done this without you, which is why a percentage of any proceeds will go to your charity of choice, the Animal Cancer Foundation.

To Dorothy Wagner, my patient and friend: You allowed me the privilege of reading the letters, stories, and history you wrote before dementia tried to steal your life. If someday my memories fade, others may read my words to me like I read your words to you. You inspired me to start writing again. My hope is that I may not forget the lessons learned in my life and my words will give others goose bumps, tears, and joy, the same as your words have given me. And that they will be a reminder of the meaningful lives we had.

To Nikki Harris: Thank you for making your tattoo chair a place where I spent hours learning not to be self-deprecating and learning instead to see my chest as a beautiful part of me.

To Kamila Angelika: Your photography made it possible for me to see the beauty in myself both with and without prosthetics.

To Chang2 Studios and Steve Tramte: Thank you for your photography.

To Carrot, Frankie, and Rogue for sitting by my side and on my lap while I worked on this book. Thanks for your company and drying my tears.

www.ingramcontent.com/pod-product-compliance
Lightning Source LLC
Chambersburg PA
CBHW062153270326
41930CB00009B/1524